DISORDERS OF
PERIPHERAL NERVES

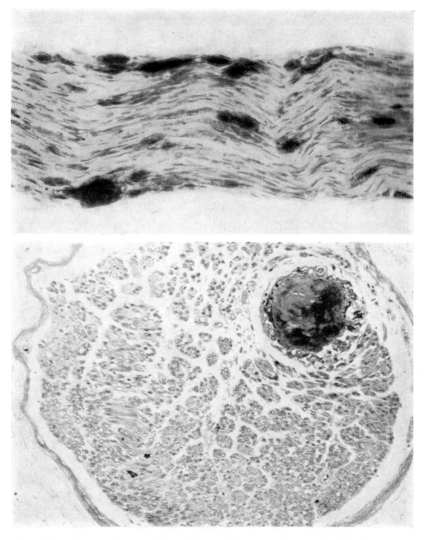

Top: Metachromatic material staining red-brown with cresyl violet in a sural nerve biopsy from a child with metachromatic leucodystrophy.

Bottom: A red-staining mass of amyloid within a transverse section of a sural nerve fascicle from a patient with the Andrade type of familial amyloidosis. Methyl violet stain. (Kindly provided by Dr P. J. Dyck.)

Disorders of Peripheral Nerves

W. G. BRADLEY
MA, BSc, DM, MRCP

Consultant Neurologist to the
Newcastle University Hospitals Group
and the Durham Hospitals Group,
and Professor of Experimental Neurology,
University of Newcastle upon Tyne

FOREWORD BY
JOHN N. WALTON
TD, MD, DSc, FRCP

Professor of Neurology and
Dean of Medicine,
University of Newcastle upon Tyne

BLACKWELL
SCIENTIFIC PUBLICATIONS
OXFORD LONDON EDINBURGH
MELBOURNE

© 1974 Blackwell Scientific Publications
Osney Mead, Oxford
85 Marylebone High Street, London W1
9 Forrest Road, Edinburgh
PO Box 9, North Balwyn, Victoria, Australia

First published 1974

ISBN 0 632 00081 3

Distributed in the United States of America
by J. B. Lippincott Company, Philadelphia
and in Canada by
J. B. Lippincott Company of
Canada Ltd, Toronto

Printed and bound in Great Britain by
William Clowes and Sons Limited
London, Beccles and Colchester

TO NINA AND
THE BOYS

Contents

vii

Foreword

The introduction of new neurophysiological and pathological methods of investigation of peripheral nerve function in health and disease has led to many important advances in knowledge within the last twenty years. Not only do we now know much more about Schwann cell function, axoplasmic flow, and mechanisms of neuromuscular transmission, but techniques of motor and sensory nerve conduction velocity measurement and the methods which have been developed for studying single teased nerve fibres histologically have indicated that whereas segmental demyelination and axonal degeneration frequently coexist in many disorders of the peripheral nervous system, some forms of neuropathy are predominantly demyelinating, while others are mainly axonal, sometimes resulting from disease of the parent anterior horn cell, sometimes from a 'dying-back' process of damage to the axon itself. The results of such investigations carried out during life have immeasurably increased our understanding of neuropathic processes so that a much more comprehensive and logical classification of the polyneuropathies, often upon an aetiological basis, is now possible than was the case only two decades ago.

Whereas a number of major works have been published on peripheral nerve disease and dysfunction, notably those by Sunderland and by Seddon, no short and succinct yet comprehensive monograph upon this topic is available. Dr Bradley has now repaired this omission. His book is logically constructed, clearly written, short but yet complete, and I believe that it will be deservedly successful. Successively he considers the progressive evolution of knowledge about the peripheral nerves throughout the ages, current knowledge of their structure and function, methods of investigation and the diseases and dysfunctions to which they are subject. Wisely for differential diagnostic purposes he considers briefly those disorders of the spinal cord and of the neuromuscular apparatus, not primarily due to

damage to the nerves themselves, with which the neuropathies may sometimes be confused and he has also included a commentary upon autonomic
dysfunction. The book is lavishly and effectively illustrated and many will
find useful the short concluding chapters on treatment, classification and
the aims of investigation.

I believe that this lively but readable monograph will be especially helpful to senior medical students, postgraduates and practitioners who wish to
know more about peripheral nerve disorders than standard textbooks provide. But the book is so well provided with references to the recent
literature that many neurologists, clinical neurophysiologists and neuropathologists will find it an invaluable addition to their libraries for the
valuable overview of the subject which it gives.

John N. Walton

Preface

The clinician confronted by a patient with peripheral nerve disease may have a number of daunting memories flash through his mind. He will remember that there are many hundreds of causes of peripheral nerve disease. He may recall some of the basic facts about the anatomy, physiology and biochemistry of the peripheral nervous system which he once learnt. He may strive desperately to recall how to amalgamate these memories with diagnostic intent.

The aim of this book is to cast light into this murky confusion, giving emphasis throughout to the clinical problems. The book is intended for physicians, including neurologists, with no specialized knowledge of peripheral nerve disease. It is hoped that it will be equally of value to those in training and to those intending to embark on a programme of research on the peripheral nervous system. An appendix of technical methods in pathological investigations is included.

The peripheral nervous system consists of three parts; first, the motor neurons, the perikarya and the first part of the axons which lie in the spinal cord; second, the primary sensory neuron, the central branch of which also lies in the spinal cord; and third, the autonomic nerves. A peripheral neuropathy may be defined as a disease affecting any of these parts though by convention diseases of the posterior columns of the spinal cord are usually excluded. The cranial nerves may be considered part of the peripheral nervous system, and as such are affected by many of the diseases described in this book. In addition, they are uniquely affected by a number of diseases. Conventionally the cranial nerves are therefore excluded from general considerations of peripheral nerve disease, a principle which has been followed in this book.

The clinical separation of diseases of the central and peripheral nervous system, of neuromuscular transmission and of the muscle, and the accurate localization of the site of the lesion in the peripheral nervous system are often difficult, requiring both knowledge and clinical skill. The book is therefore divided into chapters with a logical progression. The first chapter gives a historical outline of the development of knowledge of the peripheral nervous system through the ages. After that, the early chapters deal with the basic structure and function of the normal peripheral nervous system, the clinical features of peripheral nerve disease, and the methods of investigating the peripheral nervous system. These are followed by a chapter describing the basic disease processes, before a presentation of the details of many of the individual diseases of the peripheral nerves. The following chapters on diseases of the autonomic nerves, of the perikarya, of the roots, and of neuromuscular transmission and the skeletal muscles are designed briefly to cover the full range of conditions which must be considered in the diagnosis of peripheral nerve disease. The clinical presentation is then rounded off by a synopsis aimed at making it easier to come to a diagnosis in any patient with a peripheral neuropathy. The treatment of peripheral nerve disease is considered in the penultimate chapter, and the book is rounded off by a review of where we now stand in our understanding of the peripheral nerve, and what we may hope further to learn in the next decade.

Acknowledgments

It is a great pleasure to acknowledge the stimulation, encouragement and help given to me over the years by Professor John Walton. Many other colleagues have also indirectly contributed to this book as the result of many hours of lively discussion. In particular I want to thank Dr Arthur Asbury, Dr Peter Thomas, Dr Peter Dyck and Dr Albert Aguayo. I am grateful to Professor John Walton, Dr Peter Thomas, Professor Edwin Clarke, and Dr John Dickinson for critical reviews of the manuscript.

A number of the figures illustrating the text have been kindly provided by colleagues either from unpublished material or from their books and papers. The names of all these colleagues are acknowledged in the text, and I wish to express my thanks to them. In addition I am grateful to the following editors and publishers for permission to use previously published figures: Professor J.N.Walton and Messrs Churchill Livingstone for permission to use figs. 4.8 and 4.9, 5.4 and 5.5, 6.1, 6.2 and 6.6; Professor J.N.Walton and the Oxford University Press for permission to use fig. 2.15 and tables 2.1 and 2.2; Professor G.H.Bell and Messrs Churchill Livingstone for permission to use fig. 2.19; Professor I.A.Boyd and Messrs Churchill Livingstone for permission to use fig. 2.20; Dr F.O.Schmitt and the publishers of the *Neurosciences Research Program Bulletin* for permission to construct fig. 2.22; the editor and publishers of the *Journal of Neurology, Neurosurgery and Psychiatry* for permission to use figs. 4.5 and 5.6; the editor and publishers of the *Scottish Medical Journal* for permission to use fig. 4.6; the editor and publishers of the *Journal of Physiology* (*London*) for permission to use fig. 4.19; the editor and publishers of *Archives of Neurology* (*Chicago*), the American Medical Association, for permission to use fig. 4.22; the editor and publishers of the *Journal of Cell Science* for permission to use fig. 2.6; the editor and publishers of *Acta Neuropathologica*

(*Berlin*) for permission to use figs. 2.21 and 2.23; the editor and publishers of *Brain Research* for permission to use fig. 2.23; Professor S. Sunderland and Messrs Churchill Livingstone for permission to use fig. 2.11.

The encouragement and forbearance of Mr Per Saugman and Blackwell Scientific Publications is also acknowledged with gratitude.

I

History of the Peripheral Nervous System

The chronicle of the names of those responsible for advancing knowledge of the peripheral nervous system is a list of the most famous physicians and scientists through the ages. Peripheral nerves by their accessibility and relative simplicity provided a ready experimental tool through which knowledge of the whole nervous system developed. This chapter is only a brief outline of the highlights of this history. Opinions often differ about to whom each new idea or invention should be ascribed. Every such idea or invention is based on what went before. Accuracy is also difficult because of the scanty information available in many cases after the interval in time. It is hoped that by picking out a few of the more famous names and by showing the way that knowledge developed this chapter will provide some navigation lights through the dark mists of antiquity. It is also hoped that this chapter will whet the appetite of some to become interested in the history of scientific knowledge of the peripheral nervous system. In compiling the chapter, the author has drawn heavily upon a number of sources, particularly *The Human Brain and Spinal Cord: A Historical Study* by Clark and O'Malley (1968) and *Garrison's History of Neurology* by McHenry (1969).

Though man had observed nerves from his earliest carnivorous days, their significance was not appreciated. The Greeks did not distinctly separate nerves from tendons and ligaments, and the word 'neuron' was used indisciminately for all three structures. Hippocrates (460–370 BC), the Greek physician, described in his writings the brain and peripheral nervous system. Herophilus of Chalcedon (*circa* 300 BC) recognized the function of the nerves in carrying messages, and recognized separate sensory and motor functions. Together with Erasistratus of Chios (*circa* 310–250 BC), he believed that 'animal spirits' flowed from the ventricles of the brain down the hollow nerves to make the muscles swell, and thus to shorten. This concept occurred throughout the history of investigation of peripheral nerve function for the next 2000 years. It was still being advanced by Malcolm Fleming in his book *An Introduction to Physiology* (1759), and still continues today in the field of axoplasmic flow.

Galen of Pergamum (129–99 AD), the great physician of the second century, whose works held sway for the next millenium was also a great experimental physiologist and anatomist. His studies, which especially concerned the central nervous system, included observations of the effect of cutting the spinal cord and peripheral nerves in animals.

Little advance in knowledge occurred during the Dark Ages. William of Saliceto (*circa* 1210–77), the ablest Italian surgeon of his time and professor at Bologna, was the first to resuture divided nerves. The Renaissance saw the blossoming of anatomical studies. Leonardo da Vinci (1452–1519), the Italian artist, sculptor, inventor and scientist, produced many beautiful drawings of the human body including the cranial nerves, brachial and lumbar plexuses. His observations after section of his own digital nerve demonstrated to him the sensory function of nerves. Bartholommeo Eustachi (1520–74), the Roman anatomist and physician, produced beautiful drawings of his dissections of the autonomic nervous system, which were eventually published in 1728.

Jean François Fernel (1506–88), physician to Henry II of France, wrote one of the first works on physiology. He developed the concept of unwilled or automatic motor acts such as blinking of the eyelids and respiration during sleep. Thomas Willis (1621–75), the great English neuroanatomist whose illustrations were prepared by the equally great architect and artist, Sir Christopher Wren, introduced the term 'neurology' deriving it from the Greek word for sinew or bowstring.

The Dutchman, Antonj van Leeuwenhoek (1632–1723), was one of the earliest microscopists. He examined the peripheral and cranial nerves over many years, recognizing minute tubules which were the nerve fibres. He was uncertain whether his observations proved or disproved that the nerves were hollow. The concept of involuntary or reflex actions was further developed by René Descartes (1596–1650), the great French philosopher. The Mechanistic Theory was illustrated by the withdrawal of a limb from a fire, and it was believed that the motion was achieved by 'animal spirits' flowing down the nerves and into the muscles. The inherent excitability of nerve fibres was recognized in the Vitalistic doctrine advanced by Francis Glisson (1597–1677), who was at the same time Regius Professor of Physic and a busy physician in London.

Jan Swammerdam (1637–80), the Dutch embryologist and microscopist, introduced the nerve-muscle preparation which was later used to demonstrate the excitability of nerve and muscle. He showed that crushing a nerve induced contraction of the muscle, and that there was no change in its volume. This disproved the concept of the inflow of 'animal spirits' during contraction. Stephen Hales (1677–1761), a Teddington clergyman, showed the reflex activity of the spinal cord in decapitated frogs which hopped and contracted their limbs in response to a prick. More than a hundred years later Sherrington took up this method to investigate the function of the spinal cord. Felice Gaspar Ferdinand Fontana (1730–1805) the Italian naturalist, performed rather similar horrific experiments upon the heads and bodies of decapitated criminals. In addition he described the nerve axon and what later proved to be the myelin sheath.

Luigi Galvani (1737–98) though not the first to recognize the presence of electrical forces in animals ('animal electricity'), was the one who was mostly responsible for popularizing and investigating this property. In his day, he was a physician, obstetrician, anatomist and physiologist in the University of Bologna. His experiments began in the early 1780s, and were published in 1791. They stemmed from the observation that frogs hung by brass hooks through their spinal cord from an iron fence exhibited contractions. This observation lead eventually to the establishment of the physics of the electrolytic potentials of metals, and the voltaic battery. He also demonstrated that it was possible to stimulate a nerve by the injury current of another excitable tissue.

One of the earliest biochemical studies of the nervous system was that of Louis Nicholas Vauquelin (1763–1829), who in 1811 isolated phospholipid from brain. Also in 1811, Sir Charles Bell (1774–1842), the Scottish surgeon, physiologist and anatomist who did much of his research in London and in 1836 became Professor of Surgery in Edinburgh, described experiments which demonstrated that motor function lay in the anterior roots, and not the posterior roots. François Magendie (1783–1855), the French experimental physiologist, in a report published in 1822, enlarged upon this finding and showed that sensory function lay in the posterior roots.

With the invention of the achromatic microscope, the science of histology rapidly developed. Christian Gottfried Ehrenberg (1795–1876), the Professor of Medicine in Berlin, working with unstained water-mounted material, described the presence and structure of neurons in the posterior root and sympathetic ganglia in 1833. In 1836, Robert Remak (1815–65) clearly recorded in the embryo rabbit the presence of the axon remaining in the centre of myelinated nerve fibres after the myelin had been squeezed away, and also recognized unmyelinated nerve fibres (the 'fibre of Remak'). Remak was a Jew born in Poland who was Professor *extraordinarius* of Medicine in Berlin. The Czech patriot Jan Evangelista Purkyně (1787–1869) reported on the structure of cells and their processes in the central nervous system, including those in the cerebellum bearing his name. He was in turn Professor of Physiology and Pathology, first in Breslau and later in Prague. He recognized the connection between neurons and axons, and his work contributed to the basis of the Cell Theory.

In 1839, Theodore Schwann (1810–82) while working in the University of Berlin was led by his own and other studies to enunciate the Cell Theory that the body was composed of individual units or cells. He also identified a vague sheath with a nucleus outside the myelin sheath, which is now termed the cell of Schwann. Schwann was a German who later became Professor of Anatomy first in Louvain and later in Liège.

The earliest systematic description of diseases of the nervous system was by Moritz Heinrich Romberg (1795–1873), who was Professor of Pathology in Berlin. From 1840 to 1846 was published his *Lehrbuch der Nervenkrankheiten des Menschen*, which included descriptions of many diseases of peripheral nerves. Earlier, in 1821, Bell had described conditions causing facial palsy. In 1848, Robert James Graves (1795–1853), a widely-travelled Dublin physician better known for his description of thyrotoxicosis, recorded an epidemic of peripheral neuropathy he witnessed in Paris in 1828. The secondary degeneration of nerve following transection of the hypoglossal and glossopharyngeal nerves of the frog was fully investigated by Augustus Volney Waller (1816–70). His first reports appeared in 1850. He followed the progression of degeneration of the distal parts of the nerve fibres, finding that the proximal parts remained intact (fig. 1.1). The conclusion of his work was that the nerve cell was responsible for the nourishment of the peripheral parts of the fibres. Waller was born in Kent and practised medicine in London in the early years of his life before travelling to various centres in Europe to become an experimental physiologist.

Around this time physiology and particularly electrophysiology was blossoming. In 1850, Hermann Ludwig Ferdinand Von Helmholtz (1821–94) measured the speed of conduction of nerve impulses by means of a special galvanometer of his own construction. At the time he was Professor of Physiology in the University of Konigsberg, and he later held the chairs of Physiology at Heidelberg and of Physics at Berlin. From 1841 onwards

Emil du Bois-Reymond (1818–96) undertook a prolonged study of the electrophysiology of nerve and muscle, identifying the electrical polarization of the resting membrane, the action potential and recognizing the essentially identical nature of the process in the two tissues. He was born in Berlin of Swiss-French extraction, and was Professor of Physiology in Berlin.

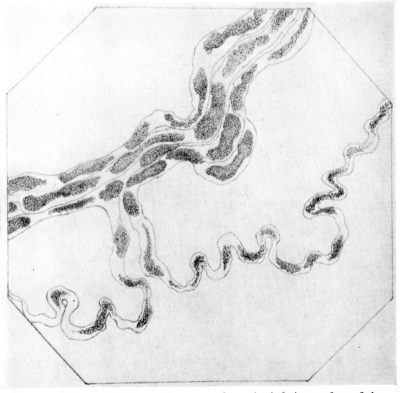

Fig. 1.1. Disorganized muscular nerve, from the inferior surface of the tongue, five days after section. (*From* Augustus Waller 1850. Experiments on the section of the glossopharyngeal and hypoglossal nerves of the frog, and observations of the alterations produced thereby in the structure of their primitive fibres. *Phil. Trans. Roy. Soc. Lond. B.* **140**, 423–429, fig. 3.)

Guillaume Benjamin Armand Duchenne of Boulogne (1806–75) developed clinical electrophysiology, applying the principle of the induction coil discovered by Michael Faraday in 1831 to the investigation of nervous system diseases. The major summary of his work *De l'Électrisation Localisée* was first published in 1855. Though Duchenne never held an appointment in any Paris hospital, he haunted the wards searching for clinical material. The publication of his clinical expertise and knowledge was largely due to the efforts of Charcot. He was however an argumentative and difficult man. His many contributions included descriptions of motor neuron disease, the muscular dystrophies, especially the pseudohypertrophic type, and various obstetrical palsies. He separated the diminished or absent response of denervated muscle to faradic stimulation from the normal response of myopathic muscle. He examined the pathology of the muscle and the spinal cord in motor neuron disease and acute anterior poliomyelitis, and noticed

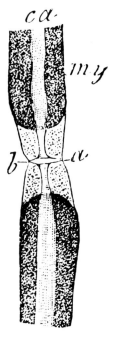

FIG. 1.2. Drawing of the node between two myelin sheaths. (*From* Louis-Antoine Ranvier 1875. *Traité Technique d'Histologie*, fig. 256. F. Savy, Paris.)

the pathological similarity of the condition. His work extended into electrotherapy and the production of mechanical aids for the disabled.

Paris also saw the work of the foremost physiologist of the nineteenth century, Claude Bernard (1813–78), who was Professor of Physiology from 1854. His studies were the clear exposition of the experimental approach, and were summarized in the classic texts *Leçons sur la Physiologie et la Pathologie du Système Nerveux* (1859), and *Introduction à l'Études de la Médicine Expérimentale* (1865). Among his many studies elucidating the function and mode of action of many parts of the nervous system, his discovery that curare impaired neuromuscular transmission opened the way

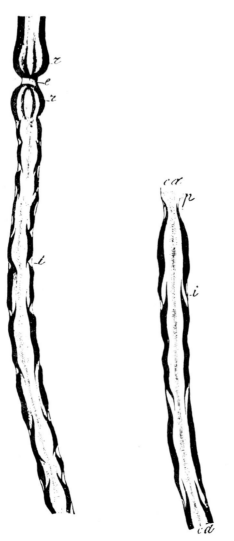

FIG. 1.3. Drawing of myelin sheath incisures. (*From* Ranvier 1875. *Loc. cit.*, fig. 258.)

for the investigation of synaptic transmission, neurotransmitters and the whole field of neuropharmacology.

In 1871, Louis-Antoine Ranvier (1835–1922), Professor of Histology in Paris, fully described the interruption in the myelin sheath, which now bears his name, and which had previously been recognized by others but thought to be an artefact (fig. 1.2). He also depicted oblique incisures (fig.

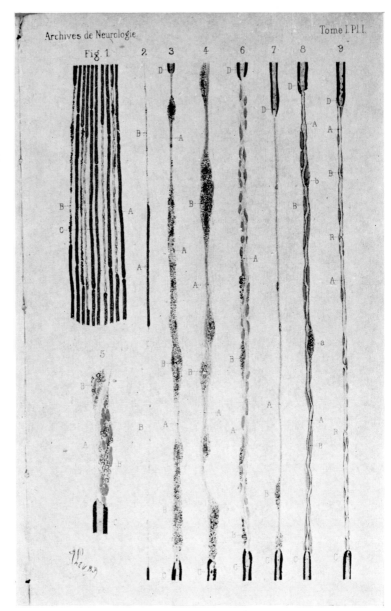

FIG. 1.4. Drawings of myelinated fibres showing segmental demyelination in lead neuropathy in the guinea pig. (*From* A. F. Gombault 1880–81. Contribution a l'étude anatomique de la névrite parenchymateuse subaiguë et chronique-névrite segmentaire péri-axile. *Arch. Neurol.* (*Paris*) **1**, 11–38, plate 1.)

1.3), which were later described by H. D. Schmidt in 1874 and A. J. Lantermann in 1877.

The understanding of peripheral nerve disease began to take shape around this time. In 1859 Jean Baptiste Octave Landry de Thezillab (1826–65), the distinguished French physician, described 10 cases of a disease associated with ascending paralysis and sensory loss. Whether such cases were due to peripheral nerve or spinal cord disease was debated both before and after this report. The findings of pathological changes in the peripheral nerves first in 1866 by Louis Dumenil, and later in 1903 by (Sir) Edward Farquhar Buzzard (1871–1945), who was later to become Regius Professor of Medicine in Oxford, confirmed that the disease was a peripheral neuropathy. The study of Guillain, Barré and Strohl (1916) was later clearly to delineate the syndrome of post-infectious polyneuritis.

From experience with gunshot wounds of the major peripheral nerves during the American Civil War Silas Weir Mitchell (1829–1914), the foremost American neurologist of his day, and his colleagues wrote the classic text *Injuries of Nerves* in 1872 in which was described causalgia. In 1880 A. F. Gombault first described what he termed 'névrite segmentaire périaxile', and which is now termed segmental demyelination. He identified this both in lead neuropathy in the guinea pig and in various lesions of the peripheral nerves in man (fig. 1.4). Loss of the myelin sheath without loss of the axons had previously been noted in 1868 in the central nervous system by Charcot. In 1883, Joseph Jules Dejerine (1849–1917), who later succeeded Charcot as Professor of Neurology at the Sâlpetrière, described arsenical neuropathy.

In 1886, Jean Martin Charcot (1825–93) and Pierre Marie (1853–1940) in France, and H. H. Tooth in England independently described peroneal muscular atrophy. Charcot was the greatest of French neurologists, for whom the Chair of Neurology at the Sâlpetrière in Paris was first created. Marie was perhaps Charcot's ablest pupil, though he did not succeed to the Chair of Neurology which had been Charcot's until the age of 65 years. Charcot was responsible for the elucidation of the clinical and pathological features of many neurological diseases including amyotrophic lateral sclerosis, bulbar palsy, tabes dorsalis, and the muscular atrophies. In 1893, J. J. Dejerine and J. Sottas described the condition of hereditary progressive interstitial hypertrophic neuropathy of childhood.

Meanwhile a long argument continued concerning the microscopic structure of the nervous system. Joseph von Gerlach (1820–96), Professor of Anatomy at Erlagen, found that carmine stained the central nervous tissue, and concluded that his preparations showed a network of innumerable interlacing fibrils. From this he advanced the theory in 1872 that the brain consisted of a syncytium or nerve net. Camillo Golgi (1843–1926), Professor of Histology at Pavia, supported this theory from his work using metal stains of the nervous system, which was first published in 1883. Santiago Ramón y Cajal (1852–1934), the famous Spanish histologist concluded that his studies of metal-stained preparations of the nervous system demonstrated the presence of separate cells. Heinrich Wilhelm Gottfried von Waldeyer (1836–1921), Professor of Anatomy at Strasburg and later Director of the Anatomical Institute in Berlin, was responsible for giving a name to the theory which eventually prevailed. In 1891 he summarized the great body of evidence starting from the Cell Theory of Schwann, and named the basic unit or cell of the central nervous system the *neuron*. The battle was, however, not finally resolved for a number of years. In 1906 when Golgi and Cajal were jointly awarded the Nobel Prize for Physiology and Medicine, Golgi insisted on continuing the argument.

Among Cajal's other discoveries was that of the *bouton terminaux* on nerve cells which offered the anatomical basis of synaptic physiology later to be developed by Sir Charles Scott Sherrington (1857–1952). Sherrington was in turn Professor of Physiology at Liverpool and Oxford, and was the foremost neurophysiologist of his era. In 1894, he investigated the composition of the peripheral nerves, showing that motor nerves had larger afferent fibres than cutaneous sensory nerves. In 1906 he published *The Integrative Action of the Nervous System*. This work laid the foundations for all modern concepts of central nervous function, including the interaction on a nerve cell of impulses arriving at different synapses, a term which he introduced.

The turn of the century also saw the active investigation of the physiology of sensation by Sir Henry Head (1861–1940). These studies with colleagues including W. H. R. Rivers were undertaken both at Cambridge and at the London Hospital where he became physician. Head was one of the major founders of modern British neurology.

The beginning of the twentieth century also saw the elucidation of the pharmacology of the autonomic nervous system, which had an important bearing upon the understanding of all synaptic events. In 1886, Walter Holbrook Gaskell (1847–1914) demonstrated the bulbar, thoracolumbar and sacral parts of the autonomic nervous system, and suggested the presence of two antagonistic parts, one excitatory and one inhibitory. John Newport Langley (1852–1925) applied nicotine and cocaine to individual autonomic ganglia in the elucidation of their separate functions. In 1905

Thomas Renton Elliott (1877–1961) discovered that adrenaline had an action similar to stimulation of the sympathetic nervous system, and suggested that adrenaline was released by sympathetic nerve activity. These studies were carried out in Cambridge, though he later became Professor of Clinical Medicine at University College Hospital in London. In 1907, W. E. Dixon similarly deduced that muscarine or a muscarine-like compound was stored in parasympathetic nerve endings. Sir Henry Hallett Dale, the greatest pharmacologist and chemical physiologist of the beginning of the twentieth century, who was Director of the National Institute for Medical Research for 14 years, was responsible for much of the further elucidation of synaptic chemistry. In 1914 he discovered acetylcholine in extracts of ergot, and distinguished its nicotinic from its muscarinic effects. In 1921 Otto Loewi (1873–1961), Professor of Pharmacology in Graz, identified a chemical 'Vagusstoff' which is released from the stimulated vagus. Dale and Dudley in 1929 showed this to be acetylcholine. Eventually in 1936 Dale and his colleagues, Brown and Feldberg, demonstrated that acetylcholine could activate striated muscle.

Sir Archibald Garrod first suggested in 1908 that diseases might be due to inborn errors of metabolism. This has formed the basis of the understanding of a large number of inherited diseases in man. An ever-increasing list of inherited and acquired diseases of the peripheral nervous system has developed during the twentieth century. Most of these still await the penetration of their dark secrets by the piercing light of biochemistry. However diabetic neuropathy, first described in 1917 by Albert Pitres (1848–1928), Professor of Medicine at Bordeaux, is now understood in part at least from the biochemical standpoint. As a result of a series of studies initiated by Sir Rudolf Peters in 1929, the neuropathy of beriberi is now known to be due to thiamine deficiency. The neuropathy of pernicious anaemia, which was one of the first to be investigated by quantitative histological methods by J. G. Greenfield and E. A. Carmichael in 1935, is now known to be due to cyanocobalamin deficiency.

Electrophysiology took a major step forward in 1922 with the studies of Joseph Erlanger and Herbert Spencer Gasser (1888–1963) in St Louis. They studied the compound nerve action potential, demonstrated the range of nerve fibre conduction, and many other features of the excitatory wave and refractory period of nerve. Their book *Electrical Signs of Nervous Activity* (1937) is a classic. Later the work of Edgar Douglas, Lord Adrian, Alan Lloyd Hodgkin and Andrew F. Huxley elucidated the mechanism of polarization of excitable resting membranes, and the induction of the action potential, as well as the function of the myelin sheath and nodes of Ranvier. It also led to the application of nerve conduction studies to clinical practice by Robert Hodes and colleagues in 1948.

The discoveries adding to our understanding of the peripheral nervous system and its dysfunction have come so thick and fast during the last fifty years that to chronicle them would take many volumes. A distillate of these discoveries makes up the remainder of this book. In the following chapters it has proved impossible to provide a historical review of each topic. All that has been attempted is to provide a skeleton of references, from the bare bones of which the interested reader may reconstruct the flesh of history.

HISTORICAL SOURCES

CAUSEY G. (1960) *The Cell of Schwann*. E. &. S. Livingstone, Edinburgh.

CLARKE E. and O'MALLEY C. D. (1968) *The Human Brain and Spinal Cord: a historical study*. University of California Press, Berkeley.

McHENRY L. C. Jr. (1969) *Garrison's History of Neurology*. C. C. Thomas, Springfield, Illinois.

MAJOR R. H. (1945) *Classic Descriptions of Disease*, 3rd edn. C. C. Thomas, Springfield, Illinois.

2

Structure and Function of the Nerve

STRUCTURE

Structure of nerve fibre

Two main types of nerve fibre are found in peripheral nerve, *unmyelinated* and *myelinated*. The unmyelinated nerve fibre consists of an axon of 0·2–3 μm in diameter invaginated within a *Schwann cell*, sometimes termed a Remak cell. From 1–10 such fibres lie within each Remak cell (fig. 2.1). Myelinated axons range in diameter from 1–15 μm in man and lie singly within a chain of Schwann cells, each of which forms a *myelin sheath* around the axon by a process of circular rotation of the mesaxon (fig. 2.2). The signal for the Schwann cell to form myelin, or to accept multiple axons without forming myelin comes from the axons rather than the Schwann cell. If a myelinated nerve such as the phrenic is implanted into an unmyelinated nerve such as the postganglionic sympathetic plexus, Schwann cells which had not previously formed myelin will now do so and myelinated axons will regenerate in the sympathetic plexus. Similarly un-myelinated axons may convert myelin-forming Schwann cells into typical Remak cells when regenerating into a nerve such as the recurrent laryngeal nerve which previously had only myelinated nerve fibres.

The boundary between one Schwann cell and the next on myelinated nerve fibres is clearly demarcated by a *node of Ranvier*. The boundary between each Remak cell is less clearly demarcated because of interdigita-tions of the cytoplasm. Each Remak or Schwann cell has the typical organ-elles of any other cell in the body, including mitochondria, Golgi apparatus, rough and smooth endoplasmic reticulum, ribosomes, microtubules and microfilaments, glycogen granules and lipid droplets (see fig. 2.2).

The axons contain smooth endoplasmic reticulum and mitochondria, and numerous microtubules and microfilaments. Microtubules here are termed neurotubules, and are about 24 nm diameter. They are composed of a wall of about 5 nm thickness, and a central core of about 14 nm. The microfilaments, here termed neurofilaments, are also tubular, but smaller with a diameter of about 10 nm, the wall being of about 3–4 nm thick with a central core of low electron density of about 3 nm. Both are unbranched

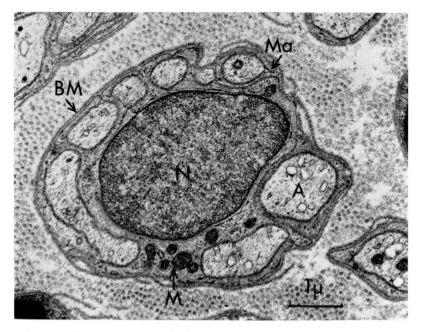

FIG. 2.1. Electron micrograph of a normal Remak cell containing eight unmyelinated axons (A), from the sural nerve of a child. Ma—mesaxon of unmyelinated nerve fibre, BM—basement membrane, N—nucleus, M—mitochondria.

and run linearly in the axon. The larger the axon diameter, the smaller the proportion of neurotubules. Neurotubules are particularly prominent in unmyelinated nerve fibres. The function of the neurofilaments and neurotubules are discussed under *Biochemistry* (page 50 *et seq.*). The myelin sheath is concentrically laminated with a periodicity between lamellae as indicated by x-ray diffraction studies of unfixed myelin of about 18 nm in peripheral nerve. The appearance under the electron microscope depends on the method of fixation. With primary fixation in glutaraldehyde followed by osmic acid, the periodicity is approximately 15–18 nm (150–180 Å) between the major dense lines, though other fixatives cause more shrinkage and a decreased periodicity. Between the major dense lines lies a less electron-dense intraperiod line. Both are double in appropriately fixed material viewed at ultrahigh resolution, and are believed to be formed by the fusion of the internal and external parts of the Schwann cell plasmalemma respectively (fig. 2.3). The clear zone lying on either side of the intraperiod

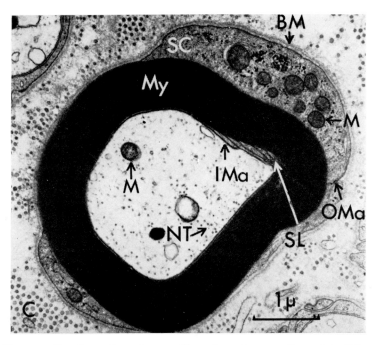

FIG. 2.2. Small myelinated nerve fibre of sural nerve of an adult. SC—Schwann cell cytoplasm, My—myelin sheath, OMa—outer mesaxon of myelin sheath, IMa—inner mesaxon of myelin sheath, SL—Schmidt-Lanterman cleft, NT—neurotubules.

line is thought to correspond to the hydrophobic lipids of the membrane, which are dissolved in the processing for electron microscopy. The chemical composition and structure of the myelin is further described on page 54 *et seq.* The structure outlined here, and the chemical composition described below explain the high electrical resistance which is a feature of the myelin sheath (see pages 42–43).

The number of myelin lamellae is linearly related to the axonal circum-
ference (Friede and Samorajski 1968). Thus the larger the axonal diameter,
the thicker the myelin sheath. The distance between the nodes of Ranvier
(the internodal length) is also related to the diameter of the myelinated nerve

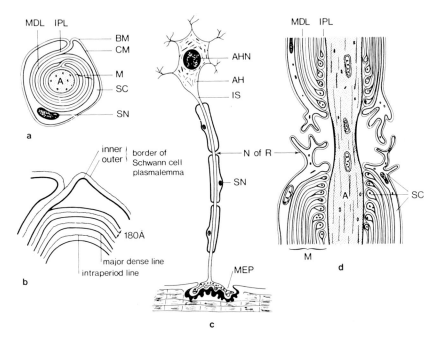

FIG. 2.3. Diagrams of the structure of a myelinated nerve fibre.
a Formation of the myelin sheath (M) by wrapping of the Schwann cell
(SC) membrane (CM) around the axon (A). SN—Schwann cell nucleus,
MDL—major dense line, IPL—intraperiod line, BM—basement membrane. *b* High power drawing of the inner mesaxon to show the formation
of the major dense line from the union of two inner borders of the Schwann
cell plasmalemma, and the intraperiod line by the union of two outer
borders of the Schwann cell plasmalemma.
c Diagram of an α-motor neuron. The anterior horn cell (AH), with its
nucleus (AHN) and initial segment (IS), lies in the spinal cord. The axon
is invested with Schwann cells separated by nodes of Ranvier (N of R), and
the terminal ramification lies in the motor end plate (MEP).
d Diagram of the structure of a node of Ranvier. The interdigitating processes from adjacent Schwann cells almost occlude the nodal gap.
Schwann cell cytoplasm (SC) lies superficial to the myelin sheath, and
also in pockets splitting the major dense lines where the myelin becomes
applied to the axon.

fibre. As can be seen in fig. 2.4, the internodal length of an adult limb nerve fibre with a diameter of about 12 μm is approximately 1·0 mm, while that of a fibre of similar diameter in the adult facial nerve is only 0·5 mm. The suggestion has therefore been made that the internodal length is proportional to the extent of growth of the nerve fibre from the time of myelination. The limb nerves grow in length during development to a greater extent than does the facial nerve. However this cannot be the whole story for the internodal length of the smaller diameter fibres is similar in both the facial and limb nerves.

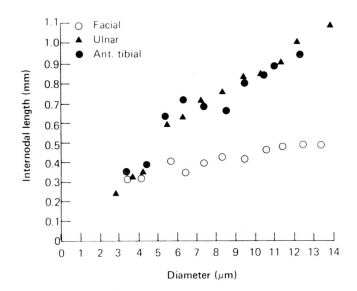

FIG. 2.4. Relationship between the mean internodal length and myelinated fibre diameter of the facial, ulnar and anterior tibial nerves of an 18 year old girl. (*After* Vizoso 1950.)

In some areas small pockets of Schwann cell cytoplasm remain within the myelin sheath, splitting the major dense line. These are seen where the myelin lamellae are attached to the axon at the node of Ranvier as shown in fig. 2.5. They are also seen as a series of such pockets of Schwann cell cytoplasm arranged as an echelon towards the axon which under the light microscope appears as a funnel-shaped cleft in the myelin sheath. These were first described by Schmidt (1847) and Lanterman (1877), and are usually called *Schmidt-Lanterman incisures* (Hall and Williams 1970) (fig. 2.6). The pockets of cytoplasm often contain one neurotubule which therefore

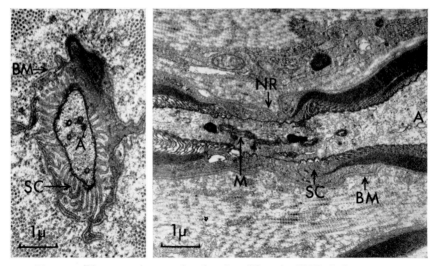

FIG. 2.5. Electron micrographs of nodes of Ranvier (NR). *Left*, transverse section. Interdigitating fingers of Schwann cell cytoplasm (SC) lie closely packed around the axon (A). *Right*, longitudinal section.

The pockets of Schwann cell cytoplasm lying between the lamellae of the myelin where it is applied to the axon are clearly seen.

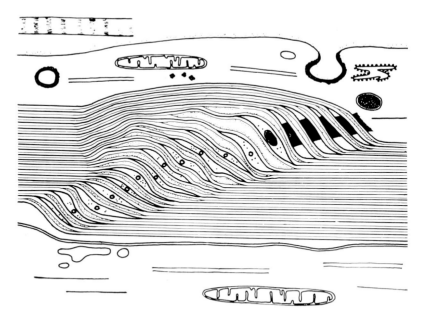

FIG. 2.6. Diagram of the structure of a Schmidt-Lanterman incisure. (*From* Hall and Williams 1970.)

presumably forms a complete helix from the superficial Schwann cell cytoplasm to the region of the axon. No other subcellular organelle is usually seen. Areas of dense thickening of the myelin lamellae (desmosomoid stacks) are often present. The frequency of incisures varies from nerve to nerve in the body, but in any one nerve, they are more frequent in younger and regenerating fibres, and are only present in fibres with more than 20 myelin lamellae. The funnel more commonly points away from the nearest node of Ranvier. The earlier arguments about whether Schmidt-Lanterman incisures were simply artefacts of fixation have been refuted, both by their stereotyped ultrastructure, and the observation of the behaviour of incisures *in vivo* under physiological and pathological conditions. Their function is discussed on page 64 *et seq.*

The node of Ranvier is more than a simple gap between two Schwann cells and their myelin sheaths. The normal distance between the myelin sheaths is less than 0·3 μm, and the distance is inversely related to fibre diameter. Adjacent Schwann cells have finger-like projections which interdigitate and to a large extent occlude the node (fig. 2.5). In addition the basement membrane of the Schwann cells is markedly thickened with large amounts of acid mucopolysaccharides, and there is an electron-dense subaxolemmal band within the axon. The function of this organization is discussed on pages 42–43.

The motor nerve fibres undergo considerable branching along the whole of their course from the spinal cord to the muscle. One anterior horn cell may innervate from a few to many hundred muscle fibres depending upon the individual muscle. The anterior horn cell, its peripheral branches and the nerve fibres which these innervate are termed a *motor unit*. The branching occurs both in the nerve trunk and within the muscle, arising at the nodes of Ranvier. Similar branching is also present in sensory nerve fibres.

Structure at ends of nerve fibres

Perikaryon

The axon of a myelinated nerve fibre arises from a cell body, the *perikaryon*, lying either in the posterior root ganglion or the anterior grey horn of the spinal cord. The perikaryon of an unmyelinated nerve fibre lies either in the posterior root ganglia or autonomic ganglia. A number of differences exist between the neurons of the anterior horns and posterior root ganglia. The posterior root ganglion neuron is a unipolar cell, whose single axon divides

into a central branch running in the posterior root to the spinal cord, and a
distal branch running to the peripheral sensory endings. On the other hand
the anterior horn cell is a multipolar cell with many minor processes,
termed dendrites, and one main process, the axon running to the peripheral

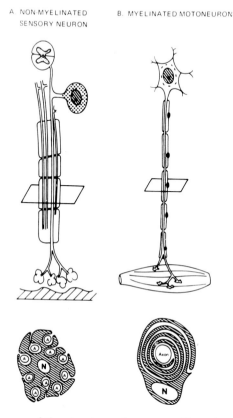

A. NON-MYELINATED   B. MYELINATED MOTONEURON
  SENSORY NEURON

FIG. 2.7. Diagram of the structure of an unmyelinated sensory neuron
and a myelinated motor neuron.

muscles (see fig. 2.7). Both have a nucleus with a prominent nucleolus. The
nucleus of the motor neuron of the anterior horn almost invariably has only
one nucleolus, but that of the posterior root ganglion may occasionally have
two or three. Both neurons have similar subcellular organelles, including
rough endoplasmic reticulum (the Nissl substance of light microscopy),
polyribosomes, Golgi apparatus, mitochondria, smooth endoplasmic reticulum, neurofilaments and neurotubules, and occasional lysosomes and
glycogen granules (fig. 2.8). The Nissl substance, which comprises a vast

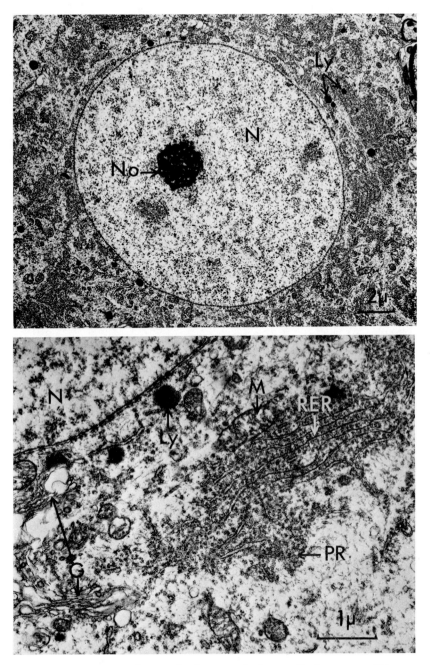

FIG. 2.8. Electron micrograph of an anterior horn cell of a mouse. *a* View of the whole nucleus (N) and cytoplasm. *b* High power of part of the cytoplasm. No—nucleolus, Ly—lysosomes, G—Golgi bodies, RER—rough endoplasmic reticulum, PR—polyribosomes, M—mitochondria.

protein factory (see page 52) is however more prominent in the anterior horn motor neuron. Each neuron is closely invested by satellite cells, which in the spinal cord are usually oligodendrocytes, and which show a close metabolic interrelationship with the perikaryon (see page 64 *et seq.*). The perikaryal cytoplasm adjacent to the origin of the axon has little or no Nissl substance, and is termed the axon hillock. The initial segment of the axon is devoid of a myelin sheath and has an area of increased electron density immediately below the axolemma similar in nature to that seen at the nodes of Ranvier. It should be remembered that the anterior horn cell lies in the central nervous system, and that the myelin sheath within the spinal cord is central in type and derived from oligodendroglial cells and not Schwann cells. This part of what is functionally the *peripheral* nervous system is therefore potentially liable to many *central* nervous system diseases.

The neurons of the anterior horn comprise two types of motoneurons, the larger α and smaller γ, as well as the interneurons. The α-motoneurons innervate the skeletal muscle, and evidence exists of at least two types that supply slow twitch fibres of histochemical type I, and fast twitch fibres of histochemical type II. No morphological or histochemical separation of 'type I' or 'type II' motoneurons has however been observed. The motoneurons are arranged in the spinal cord in longitudinally orientated columns supplying individual groups of muscles. The α-motoneurons vary considerable in size, and the reason for this variation is uncertain. It is possible that a large perikaryon may be related to a large volume of the peripheral axon. Thus the large perikarya might be supposed either to innervate a very large motor unit such as one in the proximal musculature, or a motor unit in a distal muscle where the length of the axon is long. This, however, is a supposition, and remains to be proven. The γ-motoneurons have small perikarya, and innervate the intrafusal muscle fibres of the *muscle spindles*, forming the basis of the reflex arc underlying muscle tone (see pages 43–44). Similarly the posterior root ganglia perikarya vary widely in size, and it is probable that the smaller perikarya give rise to unmyelinated axons, and the larger to myelinated nerve fibres.

Motor end-plates

After a small amount of intramuscular branching, the larger myelinated axon of an α-motoneuron loses its myelin sheath, and forms a complex ramification in gutters on the surface of an extrafusal muscle fibre (Coërs and Woolf 1959). Both the presynaptic axonal and postsynaptic sarcolemmal components of the motor end-plate show intricate specialization (fig. 2.9). The terminal expansion of the axon contains many *synaptic vesicles* of about 50 nm diameter as well as the organelles common to the axon, though there are fewer neurotubules than neurofilaments (Duchen 1971). The synaptic vesicles are spheres bounded by a single membrane. Sympathetic nerve synaptic vesicles are larger and of different structure,

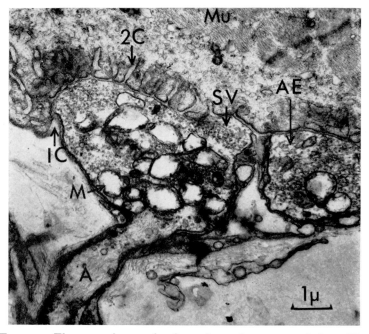

FIG. 2.9. Electron micrograph of a guinea pig motor end-plate. The axon (A) had a terminal expansion (AE) which contains mitochondria (M) and synaptic vesicles (SV). The axonal expansion lies within a primary synaptic cleft (IC) of the muscle (Mu), from which radiate the secondary synaptic clefts (2C).

with a large dense central core; in some central nervous synaptic terminals, the synaptic vesicles are oval in shape. These synaptic vesicles contain the transmitter substance for the nerve ending, which is acetylcholine in the case of the motor end-plate, as well as a number of other proteins which may be enzymes involved in the synthesis of the transmitter, proteins which bind the transmitter, or possibly substances which exert a trophic influence on the skeletal muscle fibre. The postsynaptic membrane is considerably thickened with a number of infoldings. The axon lies in the *primary synaptic cleft* or gutter, from which radiate the *secondary synaptic clefts*, with their electron-dense thickened subsarcolemmal membrane. The cholinergic receptors as well as acetylcholinesterase lie within the membrane of the secondary synaptic cleft.

In man the limb skeletal muscle fibre very rarely has more than one motor end-plate, which produces a *propagated impulse* spreading over the muscle fibre in response to a nerve stimulus. The frog slow ('tonic') muscle fibre on the other hand has many motor end-plates, each of which is capable of producing a localized depolarization of the sarcolemma, and a *localized contracture*. Mammalian extraocular muscles have motor end-plates which are of two types, *en plaque endings* of which there is usually only one per muscle fibre and which are similar in structure to the motor end-plates described above, and *en grappe endings* of which there may be more than ten per muscle fibre and which are similar in structure to the en grappe endings on tonic muscle fibres of lower vertebrates. γ-motoneurons participate in three types of motor end-plates on the striated intrafusal muscle fibres (Mathews 1964, Kennedy 1970). Some intrafusal fibres have a single en plaque ending, while others have multiple end-plates of the en grappe form. A third form is the *trail ending*. It is possible that the en grappe type ending produces a localized non-propagated contracture of the fibre in mammalian muscle spindles as they do in the frog, while the en plaque ending evokes a propagated axon potential similar to that in the extrafusal muscle fibres. The function of the trail endings is not clear.

Sensory nerve endings

Much emphasis used to be placed upon the different receptors believed to underlie the various modalities of superficial sensation. These included Krause's end-bulbs for cold, Ruffini endings for warmth, Meissner's corpuscles and Merkel's discs for touch, Pacinian corpuscles and Golgi-Mazzoni endings for pressure, and free nerve endings for pain. Each has a well-marked structure, but there are now reasons for doubting that they are essential for the reception of each modality. Hairy skin is capable of the perception of all the modalities of sensation, but has almost no receptor other than perifollicular nerve nets and free nerve endings. The corneal epithelium has only free nerve endings, but is capable of the perception of touch and temperature as well as pain. The theories of sensation are discussed on page 44 *et seq.*

The sensory nerve endings of the muscle spindle are of two main types, the primary sensory ending of the type IA afferent fibre which is distributed to the equatorial region of the intrafusal muscle fibres, and secondary sensory endings of the type II afferent fibres which are localized to the region between the equator and the poles. In the cat the primary sensory ending is annulospiral in form, while in man it is ribbon-like and branched. The secondary sensory endings resemble flower sprays.

Structure of anatomical nerve

A nerve such as the femoral nerve comprises many thousands of individual nerve fibres grouped into *fasciculi* (Sunderland 1968). Each fasciculus is surrounded by a sheath of *perineurium* consisting of three or four layers of

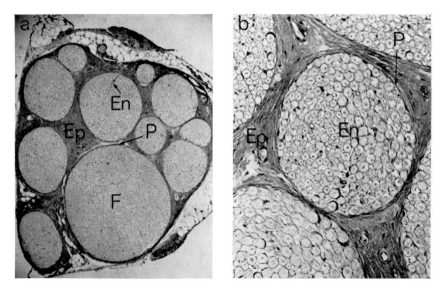

FIG. 2.10. Transverse section of rabbit nerve showing fascicular anatomy. PTAH. *a* Low power. *b* Higher power. F—fasciculus, Ep—epineurial connective tissue, P—perineurium, En—endoneurial connective tissue.

specialized cells. The perineurium constitutes a major diffusion barrier within the nerve. The walls of the blood vessels may have perineurial elements surrounding them which are in part responsible for the blood-nerve barrier. This is similar in function to the blood-brain barrier. It is present soon after birth in most animals, and prevents the access of many of the larger molecular weight substances to the nerve fibres. The perineurial cells have high levels of adenosine triphosphate (ATP) and creatine phosphate to provide energy for this barrier function. Collagen and connective tissue elements of the *epineurium* surround the fasciculi, binding them into the anatomical nerve. Within each fasciculus there is a moderate amount of *endoneurial* connective tissue (see fig. 2.10). The fasciculi constantly divide and rejoin along the length of the nerve trunk (see fig. 2.11), the function being to intermingle and redistribute the nerve fibres so that a focal lesion of one fasciculus will produce only partial denervation over the whole area supplied by the nerve, and not total denervation of any area.

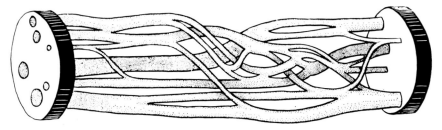

FIG. 2.11. Fascicular architecture in a 3 cm segment of human musculo-cutaneous nerve of the arm. (*From* Sunderland 1968.)

The motor nerve fibres run from the spinal cord in the *anterior root*, which runs close to the *posterior root* in the subarachnoid space until the two fuse into the *mixed spinal nerve* immediately distal to the posterior root ganglion. This usually lies lateral to the dural sheath of the spinal cord, and is invested in a fibrous root sheath, which is an extension of the dura. Thence the motor axon passes through *plexuses* and *anatomical nerves* to the skeletal muscle. Sensory nerve fibres run from the terminals through the anatomical nerves and plexuses to the posterior root ganglion, where the perikarya lie, and the central branch passes to the spinal cord in the posterior root (fig. 2.12). These constitute the anatomical basis of the monosynaptic spinal reflex.

Patterns of innervation

The nerve plexuses such as the brachial plexus (fig. 2.13) and the lumbo-sacral plexus (fig. 2.14) subserve a similar function to that of the fascicular branching in the anatomical nerve, namely protection against total denervation by a lesion of a single part of the plexus. Through them the nerve fibres from a single spinal cord segment pass to several different muscles, and

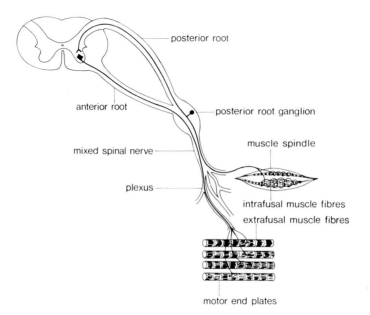

FIG. 2.12. Anatomical basis of the monosynaptic spinal reflex.

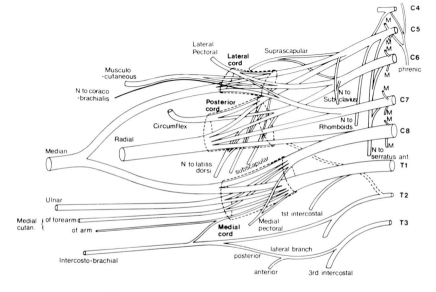

FIG. 2.13. Diagram of the brachial plexus.

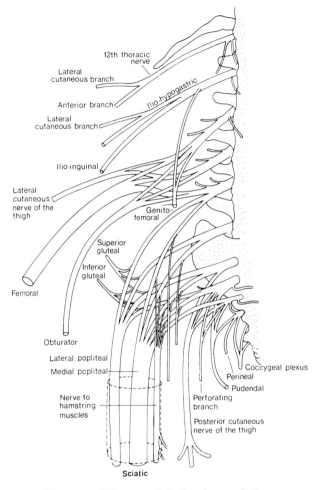

12th thoracic
nerve

Lateral
cutaneous branch

Ilio-hypogastric

Anterior branch

Lateral
cutaneous branch

Ilio-inguinal

Lateral
cutaneous
nerve of the
thigh

Genito-
femoral

Superior
gluteal

Inferior
gluteal

Femoral

Obturator

Lateral popliteal

Medial popliteal

Coccygeal plexus

Perineal

Pudendal

Nerve to
hamstring
muscles

Perforating
branch

Posterior cutaneous
nerve of the thigh

Sciatic

FIG. 2.14. Diagram of the lumbosacral plexus.

each muscle is usually innervated from more than one spinal cord segment. Similarly there is considerable overlap between the areas of skin innervated by two adjacent spinal cord segments. The area of skin innervated by a single spinal cord segment is termed a *dermatome* (fig. 2.15), and similarly the muscles supplied by a single spinal cord segment are termed a *myotome* (table 2.1). A knowledge of these segmental representations, and of the muscles and areas of skin innervated by individual nerves (table 2.2 and fig. 2.15) is essential for the elucidation of the site of any peripheral nerve injury as discussed in chapter 3.

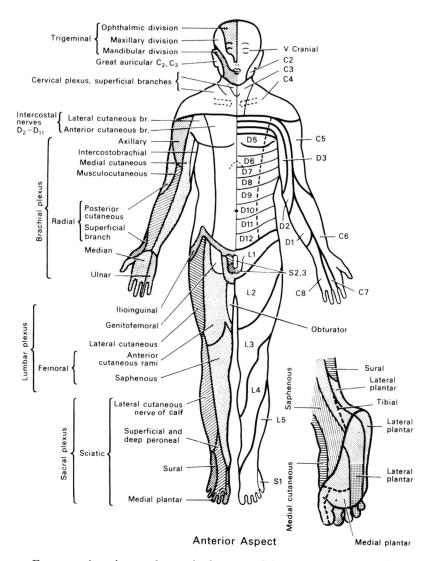

FIG. 2.15. Anterior *a* and posterior *b* aspects of the cutaneous areas of distribution of the spinal segments and the peripheral nerves. (*From* Brain and Walton 1969 *Diseases of the Nervous System,* fig. 7*a* and *b.* Oxford University Press, London.)

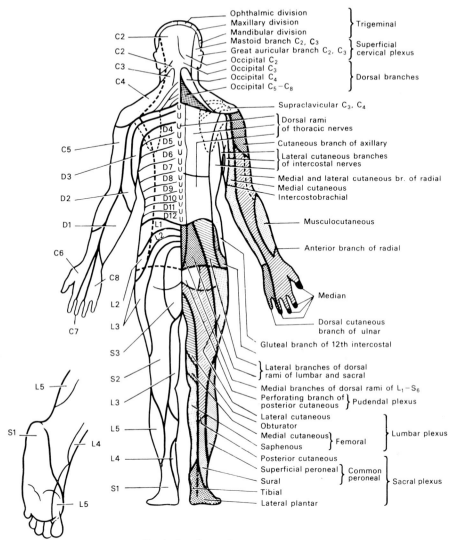

Posterior Aspect

TABLE 2.1a. Segmental innervation of the muscles of the upper extremity. (*From* Brain and Walton 1969. *Diseases of the Nervous System*, pp. 34–36. Oxford University Press, London; Modified from Bing R. 1927)

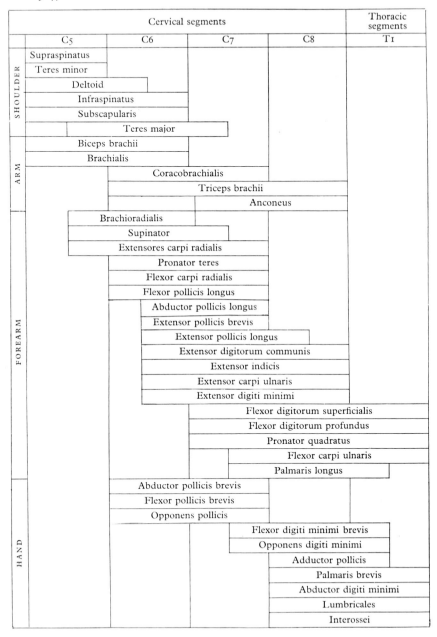

TABLE 2.1b. Segmental innervation of the trunk muscles. (*From* Brain and Walton 1969. *Diseases of the Nervous System,* pp. 34–36. Oxford University Press, London; modified from Bing R. 1927)

Segment	Muscle(s)
Cervical segments	Short deep cervical muscles; Splenius; Trapezius; Levator scapulae; Latissimus dorsi; Rhomboid; Longus capitis; Longus colli; Scaleni; Pectoralis major; Pectoralis minor; Subclavius; Serratus anterior; Diaphragm
Thoracic segments	Serratus posterior superior; Serratus posterior inferior; Long deep muscles of the back; Rectus abdominis; Obliquus externus abdominis; Transversus abdominis; Obliquus internus abdominis; Quadratus lumborum; Intercostal muscles
Lumbar segments	Quadratus lumborum
Sacral segments	Levator ani and sphincter ani, rectal muscles, coccygeus
Coccygeal segment	Levator ani and sphincter ani, rectal muscles, coccygeus

Segment columns: Cervical 1 2 3 4 5 6 7 8 — Thoracic 1 2 3 4 5 6 7 8 9 10 11 12 — Lumbar 1 2 3 4 5 — Sacral 1 2 3 4 5 — Coccygeal segment

TABLE 2.1C. Segmental innervation of the muscles of the lower extremity. (*From* Brain and Walton 1969. *Diseases of the Nervous System*, pp. 34–36. Oxford University Press, London; modified from Bing R. 1927)

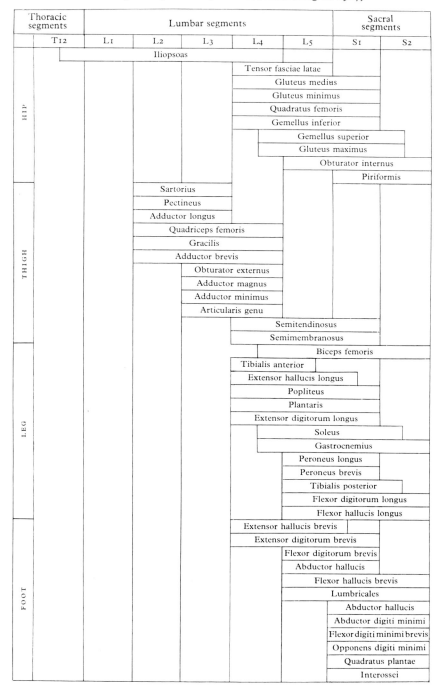

	Thoracic segments	Lumbar segments					Sacral segments	
	T12	L1	L2	L3	L4	L5	S1	S2
HIP		Iliopsoas	Iliopsoas	Iliopsoas				
					Tensor fasciae latae	Tensor fasciae latae	Tensor fasciae latae	
					Gluteus medius	Gluteus medius	Gluteus medius	
					Gluteus minimus	Gluteus minimus	Gluteus minimus	
					Quadratus femoris	Quadratus femoris	Quadratus femoris	
					Gemellus inferior	Gemellus inferior	Gemellus inferior	
						Gemellus superior	Gemellus superior	Gemellus superior
						Gluteus maximus	Gluteus maximus	Gluteus maximus
						Obturator internus	Obturator internus	Obturator internus
							Piriformis	Piriformis
THIGH			Sartorius	Sartorius				
			Pectineus	Pectineus				
			Adductor longus	Adductor longus				
			Quadriceps femoris	Quadriceps femoris	Quadriceps femoris			
			Gracilis	Gracilis	Gracilis			
			Adductor brevis	Adductor brevis	Adductor brevis			
				Obturator externus	Obturator externus			
				Adductor magnus	Adductor magnus			
				Adductor minimus	Adductor minimus			
				Articularis genu	Articularis genu			
LEG					Semitendinosus	Semitendinosus	Semitendinosus	Semitendinosus
					Semimembranosus	Semimembranosus	Semimembranosus	Semimembranosus
						Biceps femoris	Biceps femoris	Biceps femoris
				Tibialis anterior	Tibialis anterior	Tibialis anterior		
				Extensor hallucis longus	Extensor hallucis longus	Extensor hallucis longus	Extensor hallucis longus	
				Popliteus	Popliteus	Popliteus	Popliteus	
				Plantaris	Plantaris	Plantaris	Plantaris	
				Extensor digitorum longus	Extensor digitorum longus	Extensor digitorum longus	Extensor digitorum longus	
					Soleus	Soleus	Soleus	Soleus
					Gastrocnemius	Gastrocnemius	Gastrocnemius	Gastrocnemius
					Peroneus longus	Peroneus longus	Peroneus longus	
					Peroneus brevis	Peroneus brevis	Peroneus brevis	
						Tibialis posterior	Tibialis posterior	
						Flexor digitorum longus	Flexor digitorum longus	Flexor digitorum longus
						Flexor hallucis longus	Flexor hallucis longus	Flexor hallucis longus
FOOT					Extensor hallucis brevis	Extensor hallucis brevis		
					Extensor digitorum brevis	Extensor digitorum brevis	Extensor digitorum brevis	
						Flexor digitorum brevis	Flexor digitorum brevis	
						Abductor hallucis	Abductor hallucis	
						Flexor hallucis brevis	Flexor hallucis brevis	Flexor hallucis brevis
						Lumbricales	Lumbricales	Lumbricales
							Abductor hallucis	Abductor hallucis
							Abductor digiti minimi	Abductor digiti minimi
							Flexor digiti minimi brevis	Flexor digiti minimi brevis
							Opponens digiti minimi	Opponens digiti minimi
							Quadratus plantae	Quadratus plantae
							Interossei	Interossei

TABLE 2.2. Muscular supply of peripheral nerves. (*From* Brain and Walton 1969. *Diseases of the Nervous System*, pp. 31–33. Oxford University Press, London; modified from Bing R. 1927)

Plexus cervicalis (C1–C4)

Nn. cervicales	Mm. longus colli	Flexion, extension, and rotation of the neck
	Mm. scaleni	Elevation of ribs (inspiration)
N. phrenicus	Diaphragma	Inspiration

Plexus brachialis (C5–T2)

N. thoracic. ant.	M. pect. maj. et min.	Adduction and forward depression of the arm
N. thoracic. long.	M. serrat. ant.	Fixation of the scapula during elevation of the arm
N. dorsalis scap.	M. levator scapul.	Elevation of the scapula
	Mm. rhomboidei	Elevation and drawing inwards of the scapula
N. suprascap	M. supraspinatus	Elevation and external rotation of the arm
	M. infraspinatus	External rotation of the arm
N. subscapul.	M. latissimus dors. ⎫ M. teres major ⎬	⎧ Internal rotation and dorsal adduction of the arm ⎨
	M. subscapularis	Internal rotation of the arm
N. axillaris	M. deltoideus	Elevation of the arm to the horizontal
	M. teres minor	External rotation of the arm
N. musculocut.	M. biceps brach.	Flexion and supination of the forearm
	M. coracobrachialis	Flexion and adduction of the forearm
	M. brachialis	Flexion of the forearm
N. medianus	M. pronator teres	Pronation
	M. flexor carpi rad.	Flexion and radial flexion of the hand
	M. palm. long.	Flexion of the hand
	M. flex. digit. superficialis	Flexion of the middle phalanges of the fingers
	M. flex. poll. long.	Flexion of the terminal phalanx of the thumb
	M. flex. digit. (radial portion)	Flexion of the terminal phalanges of the index and middle fingers
	M. abduct. poll. brev.	Abduction of the first metacarpal

Table 2.2 (*cont.*)

	M. flex. poll. brev.	Flexion of the first phalanx of the thumb
	M. opponens poll.	Opposition of the first metacarpal
N. ulnaris	M. flexor carpi uln.	Flexion and ulnar flexion of the hand
	M. flex. digit. prof. (ulnar portion)	Flexion of the terminal phalanges of the ring and little fingers
	M. adductor poll.	Adduction of the first metacarpal
	Mm. hypothenares	Abduction, opposition, and flexion of the little finger
	Mm. lumbricales	Flexion of the first phalanges, extension of the othèrs
N. radialis	M. triceps brach.	Extension of the forearm
	M. brachioradialis	Flexion of the forearm
	M. extensor carpi rad.	Extension and radial flexion of the hand
	M. extensor digit.	Extension of the first phalanges of the fingers
	M. extensor digit. minimi	Extension of the first phalanx of the little finger
	M. extensor carpi uln.	Extension and ulnar flexion of the hand
	M. supinator brevis	Supination of the forearm
	M. abduct. poll. longus	Abduction of the first metacarpal
	M. extensor poll. brevis	Extension of the first phalanx of the thumb
	M. extensor poll. longus	Abduction of the first metacarpal and extension of the terminal phalanx of the thumb
	M. extensor indic. prop.	Extension of the first phalanx of the index finger

Nn. thoracales (T1–T12)

	Mm. thoracici et abdominales	Elevation of the ribs, expiration, compression of abdominal viscera, etc.

Plexus lumbalis (T12–L4)

N. femoralis	M. iliopsoas	Flexion of the hip
	M. sartorius	Internal rotation of the leg
	M. quadriceps	Extension of the leg

Table 2.2 (*cont.*)

N. obturatorius	M. pectineus M. adductor longus M. adductor brevis M. adductor magnus M. gracilis	} Adduction of the thigh
	M. obturator extern.	Adduction and external rotation of the thigh

Plexus sacralis (L5–S5)

N. gluteus sup.	M. gluteus med. M. gluteus min.	} Abduction and internal rotation of the thigh
	M. tens. fasciae latae	Flexion of the thigh
	M. piriformis	External rotation of the thigh
N. gluteus inf.	M. gluteus max.	Extension of the thigh
N. ischiadicus	M. obturator int. Mm. gemelli M. quadratus fem.	} External rotation of the thigh
	M. biceps femoris M. semitendinosus M. semimem- branosus	} Flexion of the leg
N. peroneus: prof.	M. tibialis ant.	Dorsal flexion and inversion of the foot
	M. extens. digit. long	Extension of the toes
	M. extens. hall. long.	Extension of the great toe
	M. extens. digit. brev.	Extension of the toes
	M. extens. hall. brev.	Extension of the great toe
superf.	Mm. peronei	Dorsal flexion and eversion of the foot
N. tibialis	M. gastrocnemius M. soleus	} Plantar flexion of the foot
	M. tibialis post.	Plantar flexion and inversion of the foot
	M. flex. digit. long.	Flexion of the terminal phalanges, II–V
	M. flex. halluc. long.	Flexion of the terminal phalanx of the great toe
	M. flex. digit. brev.	Flexion of the middle phalanges, II–V
	M. flex. halluc. brev.	Flexion of the first phalanx of the great toe
	Mm. interossei plant.	Movement of the toes
N. pudendus	Mm. perinei et sphinct.	Closure of sphincters, cooperation in sexual act

Vascular supply of nerve

The nerve has an extensive plexus of blood vessels, the *vasa nervorum*, in the epineurium. The arteries run longitudinally between the fasciculi (fig. 2.16), and many intercommunicate forming an extensive plexus. The plexus is supplied by nutrient arteries usually arising directly from the nearest large limb artery. These nutrient arteries are very variable in location. The epineurial plexus of blood vessels is so extensive that, for instance,

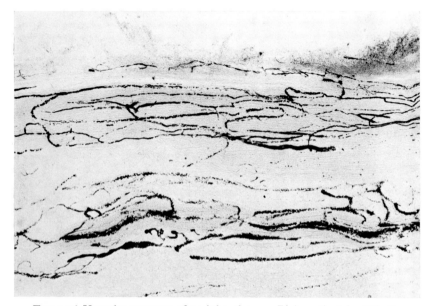

FIG 2.16. Vascular anatomy of peripheral nerve. Pickworth stain. (Kindly provided by Dr A. K. Asbury.)

the rabbit sciatic nerve can survive total occlusion of all its nutrient vessels in the thigh (Adams 1943). From the plexus arise arterioles which pierce the perineurium of each fasciculus, and join the intrafascicular capillary plexus. This again mainly runs longitudinally between the nerve fibres with transverse intercommunications.

NERVE PHYSIOLOGY
Excitable membrane

The neuron, like all cells in the body, has a membrane which is polarized, the interior having a potential of approximately -70 mV in relation to the external surface of the cell. This is due to the semipermeable character of the neuronal membrane. The permeability of protein and other intracellular anions, and of sodium is low. The resultant Donnan equilibrium results in a high concentration of potassium and a low concentration of chloride within the neuron, the *resting membrane potential* being given by the following equation:

$$Em \propto \log \frac{[K^+]_o}{[K^+]_i}$$

where *Em* is the resting membrane potential and $[K^+]_o$ and $[K^+]_i$ are the concentrations of potassium outside and inside the membrane respectively. As will be seen below, this is an oversimplification for the membrane is not totally impermeable to sodium, metabolic pumps existing to keep the $[Na^+]_i$ at low levels. Also the permeability of the membrane to potassium and chloride has certain finite limits.

The neuron has the additional specialized capability, shared with the skeletal muscle fibre of generating a propagated wave of depolarization, the *action potential*. The understanding of the events during an action potential is due largely to the work of Hodgkin and Huxley (Hodgkin 1965, Katz 1966). Graded depolarization of the membrane produces graded activation of a *sodium carrier system* which transports sodium from the outside inwards, thus tending to depolarize the membrane. There are normally two opposing influences tending to prevent this depolarization, the *sodium pump* which extrudes the entering sodium ions, and the Donnan equilibrium which tends to drive potassium out of the cell to re-establish the membrane potential. However if the graded depolarization is sufficiently rapid and above a certain threshold voltage, the activation of sodium carriers reaches explosive proportions and sufficient sodium ions enter the neuron to depolarize that section of the neuronal membrane. The membrane is now freely permeable to sodium and thus the *Em* becomes dependent on the ratio $[Na^+]_o/[Na^+]_i$. The membrane potential therefore reverses, producing an overshoot of the potential difference across the membrane beyond the isoelectric point (fig. 2.17).

This depolarized area of membrane acts as a sink for current to flow from the adjacent areas of the nerve fibre. In their turn they are depolarized beyond the critical threshold voltage, leading to complete depolarization. This depolarization spreads as an active wave in a non-decremental fashion throughout the neuron and along the axon, and constitutes the nerve action potential.

Sodium carriers which produce the explosive depolarization of the membrane have a relatively small capacity and are exhausted by the reversal of depolarization of the membrane. Also at this stage there is a marked electrochemical gradient for potassium, which leaves the cell rapidly. Finally the relatively slowly activated sodium pump now begins to extrude sodium and reaccumulate potassium. These factors combine rapidly to repolarize each area of the membrane after depolarization. After an *absolute refractory period* of about 1 ms and a *relative refractory period* of 2–3 ms, during which the sodium carriers are probably being reactivated, the nerve can again conduct a propagated action potential of full amplitude.

This description is relatively simplified, and alternative hypotheses exist. Nachmansohn (1970) believes that local release of acetylcholine from

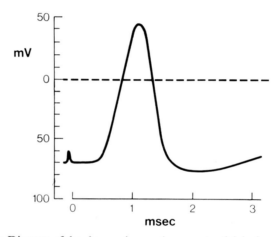

F I G. 2.17. Diagram of the changes in membrane potential during an evoked action potential.

neuronal membrane, rather than the electrotonic spread of current, depolarizes the adjacent membrane, thereby propagating the action potential. On the other hand Tasaki (1968) favours a macromolecular theory, the lipoprotein components of the axolemma having fixed charge properties, and existing in two stable states, the polarized and depolarized.

Synaptic transmission

While the transmission of a nerve impulse along a nerve fibre is an electrical phenomenon, that from the α-motoneuron to the muscle or from the upper motoneuron to the α-motoneuron is chemically mediated. The function of the motor end-plate is the best elucidated of such synaptic events. The transmitter here is *acetylcholine*, contained in membrane-bound synaptic vesicles within the axon terminal expansions. Acetylcholine is synthesized within the synaptic terminals by choline acetylase, which probably originates in the perikaryon in the spinal cord. These vesicles from time to time randomly contact the plasmalemma of the prejunctional axonal expansions and are released. The acetylcholine attaches to the postjunctional cholinergic receptors which produce a minute depolarization of the postjunctional sarcolemmal membrane of about 0·5 mV. This is termed the *miniature end-plate potential*. The amount of acetylcholine in each quantum or synaptic vesicle is probably of the order of one million molecules.

When a nerve impulse enters the prejunctional axonal expansions, there is a simultaneous release of 80–100 such vesicles which stimulate the postjunctional receptor to generate an *end-plate potential* of about 40–50 mV. This release requires the presence of a moderate concentration (2–4 mEq/l) of calcium. Higher concentrations of calcium (about 20 mEq/l), manganese in a concentration of 1 mEq/l or magnesium in a concentration of 20 mEq/l may block the release of synaptic vesicles. The sarcolemmal membrane has very similar properties to that of the neuronal membrane described above. In normal circumstances the end-plate potential produces a depolarization of about 50 mV which is suprathreshold for the induction of a propagated action potential over the muscle sarcolemma. The wave of depolarization thus spreads over the muscle fibre, and contraction of the fibre results from the events of excitation-contraction coupling.

The action of acetylcholine, which becomes attached to receptors on the postjunctional membrane, is terminated in two ways. Diffusion is probably the main event leading to the termination of the action of acetylcholine. Hydrolysis by acetylcholinesterase on the postjunctional membrane is the other event leading to the release of free choline. Much of this is taken up by the prejunctional axonal expansion, and recycled into acetylcholine. The postjunctional membrane and sarcolemma repolarize by a similar mechanism to that described for the neuronal membrane above, and after the absolute and relative refractory periods, become again susceptible to re-excitation.

Neuromuscular transmission may be blocked at a number of sites in the chain of excitation:

1 blockage of the synthesis or depletion of the synaptic content of acetylcholine, e.g. by hemicholinium;

2 blockage of the release of synaptic vesicles, e.g. by high doses of calcium or botulinum toxin;

3 blockage of cholinergic receptors by competitive inhibitors such as curare;

4 depolarization of the postjunctional receptors by depolarizing inhibitors such as decamethonium.

Stimulation of the perikarya is by a similar process to that occurring at the motor end-plate. Less is known about transmitter substances within the central nervous system, though a number of such substances have been recognized, including acetylcholine, the catecholamines nor-adrenalin, adrenalin and dopamine, 5-hydroxytryptamine and γ-amino butyric acid. The perikaryal surface is almost entirely covered by synaptic boutons. The structure of the central synapses, including those on the α-motoneuron, are similar to that of the motor end-plates, though simpler. Moreover the synaptic area is much less than that of the motor end-plate with the result that the maximum *excitatory synaptic potential* generated by the release of excitatory transmitter by a nerve action potential spreading through one synaptic bouton is insufficient to reach threshold depolarization for the induction of a neuronal action potential. The summation of several depolarizing excitatory synaptic potentials is required before the threshold is reached. Some synapses release a transmitter substance which induces hyperpolarization of the membrane (*inhibitory synaptic potential*). These inhibitory transmitters probably increase the cell permeability to chloride and potassium.

Nerve conduction velocity

In comparison with the conduction of an electrical current in a wire which occurs at the speed of light, the conduction of a nerve action potential by electrotonic and electrochemical processes is relatively slow (Erlanger and Gasser 1937). Unmyelinated nerve fibres of diameter 0·2–3 µm conduct the nerve action potential at 0·5–2·0 m/s. Myelinated nerve fibres of axonal diameter 1–15 µm have conduction velocities ranging from 3–90 m/s (Boyd and Davey 1968). Clearly therefore both axonal diameter and the presence of a myelin sheath play a part in producing the increase in conduction velocity seen in larger axons. The exact role of the myelin sheath has given rise to some debate. The *theory of saltatory conduction* proposes that the myelin sheath acts as an insulator allowing current to flow across the axolemma only at the node of Ranvier. Thus the action potential is supposed to jump from one node to the next, thereby increasing the rate of conduction along the nerve fibre. As Rushton (1951) showed, the electrical theory of saltatory conduction indicates that the observed ratio of axonal diameter to total myelinated nerve fibre diameter of about 0·6 provides the optimum safety factor for stimulation of one node by the activation of the previous one. Similarly the observed constant ratio of internodal length to external diameter for fibres of different diameters provides the optimal velocity of conduction of the nerve impulse. The theory predicts that the myelinated nerve fibre will conduct more rapidly than the unmyelinated at diameters greater than 0·2 to 1·0 μm.

However there is reason to doubt that the distance between nodes of Ranvier is the major factor leading to an increased conduction velocity. The maximum conduction velocity of a nerve which has regenerated for one or more years after a crush lesion is between 80 and 100 per cent of normal, though the internodal length of all the myelinated nerve fibres is about 0·3 mm, that is one-third of the internodal length of the normal largest myelinated nerve fibres (Vizoso and Young 1948). It seems more likely that the conduction velocity of the myelinated nerve fibre depends only on the axonal diameter and/or the myelin sheath thickness. The function of the myelin sheath may simply be to restrict ionic fluxes, and thus the metabolic demands of the sodium pump to the nodes of Ranvier. This explanation cannot be the whole story since smallest fibres have the largest surface to volume ratio, and thus the greater need for restriction of metabolic demands.

The structure of the node of Ranvier has an interesting bearing on this discussion. The presence both of the complex interdigitations of the Schwann cell nodal processes, and of the amounts of acid mucopolysaccharide 'gap substance' combine to restrict the egress of potassium ions from the axolemmal region (Langley and Landon 1968). These potassium ions are thus available for immediate reabsorption in exchange for sodium ions which are being pumped out following the passage of a nerve action potential.

Reflex arc

Strong stimulation of the skin of the flank of the dog produces scratching of that area, the reaction being termed a *reflex*. The simplest possible organization of such a reflex is shown in fig. 2.12 which depicts a monosynaptic reflex derived from the muscle spindle receptors. Such a reflex arc underlies the tendon reflexes, which are of particular value in the clinical assessment of the peripheral nervous system (chapter 3). Muscle tone and non-emergency movements from posture to posture involve an elaboration of this reflex arc into a servo loop. The tension of the intrafusal muscle fibres is 'set' by stimuli travelling from the spinal cord in the γ-motor nerve fibres which are under supraspinal control. If these induce a change in the rate of firing, the intrafusal fibre length changes, resulting in an alteration in the rate of firing of the spindle afferent nerve fibres. This induces, via the monosynaptic reflex, a change in rate of firing of the α-motoneuron. There is therefore a change in the contraction of the whole muscle until the new position 'set' by the γ-motoneuron drive is established, when the movement ceases.

Most reflexes however, including the scratch reflex, are polysynaptic. They involve several interneurons which act as computer programmes organizing the complex motor response to a simple impulse of sensory information.

Sensation

Several theories of sensation have held sway for many years. Though information continues to accumulate about sensation, the exact mechanism of perception of sensation remains to be finally clarified. The '*specific modality*' *theory* indicated that there were specific skin receptors for cold, hot, touch, pressure and pain (Sinclair 1955). In addition there were receptors for monitoring deep sensation, the specificity of which is at present not doubted. These include the muscle spindles and Golgi tendon organs, and the joint capsule receptors. Impulses from pain and temperature receptors were believed to be carried by small myelinated and unmyelinated nerve fibres, while touch, vibration and joint position senses were carried by medium and large myelinated nerve fibres. This theory appeared to fit with the experimental evidence of differing conduction velocity of impulses resulting from different stimuli. For instance pain causes a double sensation, the rapidly conducted pricking part was believed to travel by the medium-sized myelinated nerve fibres, and the unpleasant burning part in the unmyelinated nerve fibres. The theory also seemed to fit with the clinical observation that conditions causing the loss of the larger myelinated nerve fibres caused impairment of joint position and touch sensation, while relatively sparing pain and temperature sensation.

However the anatomical reasons for doubting this theory with regard to superficial sensation are outlined above (page 24). A modification has been advanced, namely that certain axon terminals in the skin, though not in specialized endings, have a lower threshold for one modality of sensation than others. They thus still show a modality specificity. Single unit recordings support their being such specificity of sensory nerve terminals.

The 'pattern' theory, which was proposed as an alternative, suggested that sensation was 'perceived' by the organism as a result of the temporospatial integration of impulses within the stimulated nerve fibres. Afferent information certainly has a great complexity from which such a pattern might be derived. Some sensory units produce only one or at the most a few nerve action potentials as a result of the application of a constant stimulus to the receptor territory. Such rapidly adapting receptors include those responding to touch and pressure. Other sensory units, including those responding to pain, and to tension in the joint capsules and tendons, continue to discharge almost indefinitely as long as a constant stimulus is applied. They are termed slow adapting receptors. This information, combined with the recognition of the position of the active nerve terminals, might be collated into an integrated picture of the sensory stimulus.

The 'gate' theory of Melzack and Wall (1965) combines some of the features of both the 'pattern' and 'specific modalities' theories with additional experimental evidence (fig. 2.18). Impulses arriving at the substantia gelatinosa in small fibres coming from receptors responding to pain and temperature, inhibit the substantia gelatinosa neurons, perhaps through a chain of interneurons. The substantia gelatinosa neurons themselves exert a presynaptic inhibitory effect on the input to the secondary sensory neuron. Thus a sensory barrage in the small nerve fibres tends to hold the gate open for all stimuli. Conversely an incoming sensory barrage predominantly in the larger fibres stimulates the substantia gelatinosa cells, thereby shutting the gate and inhibiting transmission of both large and small myelinated nerve fibre input through the substantia gelatinosa. The large fibre volley has however direct access to the central pathways via the posterior columns. Such a theory offers an explanation of the hyperalgesia of partial peripheral nerve lesions, by indicating that the decreased number of large fibres is unable to close the gate to the input of such information through the substantia gelatinosa. This input is interpreted by the organism as painful. The gate theory also offers an explanation of the marked effects of higher centres upon the sensory thresholds as a result of the efferent control of afferent impulses. It has difficulty, however, in explaining why some diseases of peripheral nerves affecting mainly the large fibres do not produce the hyperalgesia that would be predicted, and why other diseases

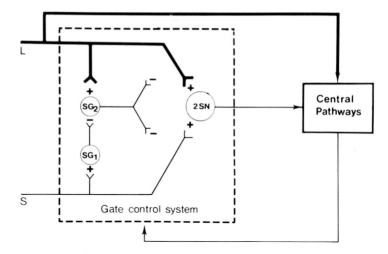

FIG. 2.18. The 'gate' theory of sensation, modified from Melzack and Wall (1965). Impulses in the large diameter fibres have direct access to central pathways, and entering the substantia gelatinosa of the spinal cord (dotted box) stimulate the neuron SG2 to produce presynaptic inhibition blocking the access of impulses to the secondary sensory neuron (2SN), that is closing the gate. Impulses entering in small diameter fibres indirectly inhibit presynaptic inhibition, facilitating the entry of impulses into the secondary sensory neurons.

affecting particularly the small fibres are associated with spontaneous pain.

COMPOUND NERVE ACTION POTENTIAL AND FIBRE COMPOSITION OF DIFFERENT NERVES

If a stimulus, which is supramaximal for every nerve fibre, is applied to a nerve trunk and the evoked *compound nerve action potential* recorded at some distance from the point of stimulation, pictures similar to those shown in fig. 2.19 are obtained. The largest myelinated nerve fibres conduct at the fastest rates, and the impulse arrives at the recording electrode first. This produces a large amplitude *A wave* which can be separated into α, β and γ components with conduction velocities of 90, 50 and 30 m/s respectively. The next potential, the *B wave*, has a conduction velocity of about 10 m/s, and is of smaller amplitude. The third wave, the *C wave*, is of the lowest amplitude, the conduction velocity being about 2 m/s.

We now have a considerable understanding of the fibre diameter spectrum of various nerves, the function of fibres of each diameter, and the correlation of the conduction velocity and compound nerve action potential. The fibre composition of mixed (that is sensorimotor) nerves can be elucidated in two ways. Firstly the nerve may be de-afferented or de-efferented in different animals by cutting the posterior or anterior roots respectively, and allowing time for fibre degeneration to occur. The remaining fibres are purely motor or sensory respectively (fig. 2.20). Secondly the function of

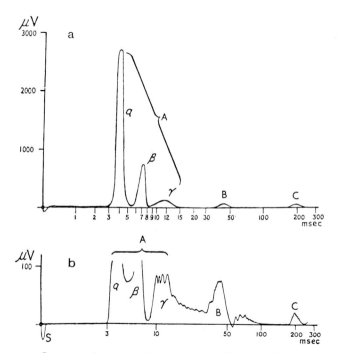

F IG. 2.19. Compound nerve action potential of frog sciatic nerve. (*From* Bell, Davidson and Scarborough 1956. *Textbook of Physiology and Biochemistry*, 3rd edn. Livingstone, Edinburgh; *after* Erlanger and Gasser 1937.)

these fibres may be investigated with single unit recording techniques, noting whether the afferent fibre responds to stimulation from the muscle spindle, pain receptor, guard hair and so on. The efferent fibres similarly may be separated into α-fibres to the extrafusal muscle fibres, and fast and slow γ-fibres to the intrafusal muscle fibres.

A signal example of such a correlative study is that of Boyd and Davey (1968). These studies have shown that the A potential is due to the largest

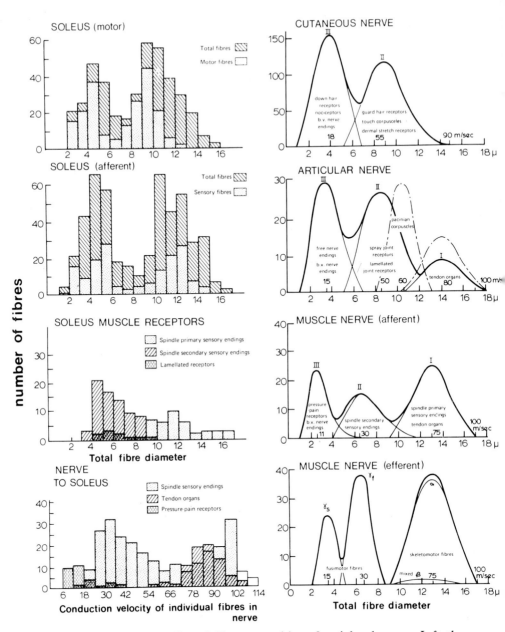

FIG. 2.20. Myelinated fibre composition of peripheral nerves. *Left*, the proportion of sensory and motor fibres in representative nerves to soleus muscle of cats, and the separation of the various sensory fibres by function, fibre diameter and conduction velocity. *Right*, typical fibre diameter spectra of a cutaneous nerve, an articular nerve, and the afferent and efferent fibres of a muscle nerve, showing the proportion of fibres of each size, their function and conduction velocity. (*After* Boyd and Davy 1968.)

myelinated nerve fibres. The α-wave is produced by α-motor nerve fibres and group Ia sensory fibres from the spindle primary sensory endings and tendon organ receptors. The nerve fibres responsible for the α-wave have a diameter range of 10–18 μm. The β-wave is produced by group II sensory fibres such as those from the Pacinian corpuscles and guard hairs, with a fibre diameter range of 6–12 μm. The γ-wave is produced by fast γ motor fibres innervating intrafusal muscle fibres, and by group II afferent fibres from spindle secondary endings, with a diameter of 4–8 μm. The B potential

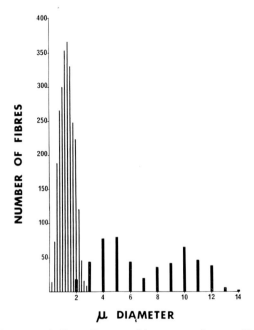

FIG. 2.21. Compound fibre diameter histogram of unmyelinated (fine bars) and myelinated (heavy bars) fibres of the normal human sural nerve. (*From* Ochoa and Mair 1969. *Acta Neuropath.* (*Berl.*) **13, 197**.)

results from small myelinated nerve fibres of a diameter 2–6 μm, which consist of slow γ motor fibres and group III sensory afferents from down hair receptors and pain receptors. The C potential is due to unmyelinated nerve fibres with a diameter of 0·2–3 μm, which are mainly group III pain afferents and postganglionic autonomic nerve fibres. The unmyelinated nerve fibres in a sensory nerve like the sural nerve outnumber myelinated nerve fibres by about four to one (fig. 2.21), though the potential generated by them is very small.

BIOCHEMISTRY OF NERVES

Neuronal fibrous proteins

As described on page 14, the axon is rich in neurotubules and neurofilaments, which are similar in structure to microtubules and microfilaments seen in many other cells, and also in flagellae and cilia. They have been suggested to have a cytoskeletal function or to play a part in subcellular and intracellular movements. Both are thought to be composed of globular subunits arranged in a helical manner. Colchicine and vinblastine have played a large part in elucidating the chemistry of these structures. Both cause loss of neurotubules and proliferation of neurofilaments. Both bind to a monomer subunit of molecular weight 60,000, which is named *neurotubular protein* (Schmitt and Samson 1968). The removal of colchicine or vinblastine allows the reformation of the neurotubules. The evidence suggests, though it does not prove, that both neurotubules and neurofilaments are composed of helical chains of dimers of this protein (fig. 2.22a and b).

Neurotubular protein has close similarities to actin from striated muscle fibres, both in its amino acid composition, and in its reaction with myosin to produce a gel. The neurotubular protein binds one molecule of guanosine triphosphate (GTP) per molecule of monomer, while actin binds one molecule of adenosine triphosphate per molecule of G-actin (molecular weight 60,000). This led to the suggestion that neurotubules might function in a similar way to actin in skeletal muscle. Substances and particles within the axon might roll along the neurotubules by a similar mechanism to that by which actin and myosin filaments slide over one another during muscle contraction (fig. 2.22c, d and e). The energy for this is believed to be derived from the splitting of high energy phosphate bonds in GTP of the neurotubular protein. In support of this hypothesis, 'myosinoid'-proteins have been isolated from axons, and ultrahigh resolution electron micrographs of axons have shown cross-bridge formations spreading from neurotubules and neurofilaments. One puzzling fact which is difficult to explain by this hypothesis is that neurotubular protein itself appears to flow from the nerve cell body down the axon.

Axoplasmic flow

Movements of particles within cells and the movements of animal cells like amoebae and vertebrate macrophages, have been seen since the earliest days

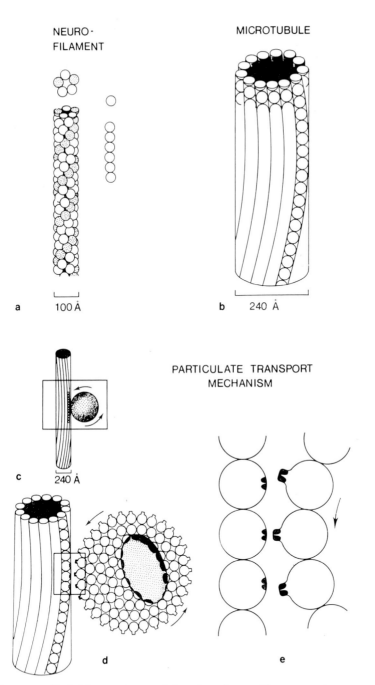

FIG. 2.22. Probable structure and function of neurofilaments and neuro-tubules. *a* Neurofilament structure. *b* Neurotubule structure. *c, d* and *e* Increasing magnification of the probable mechanism of particulate movement along the neurotubule (see text). (*After* Schmitt and Samson 1968.)

of microscopy (Jahn and Bovee 1969). Such movement of particles within neurons and axons in tissue culture have been known for many years. The major interest in such movements began when Weiss and Hiscoe (1948) placed ligatures around regenerating nerves and found that the axons became distended above the constriction. This led to the theory of the flow of axoplasm from the perikaryon down the axon. It helps to explain the very high rate of protein synthesis present in perikarya, located in the very ex-

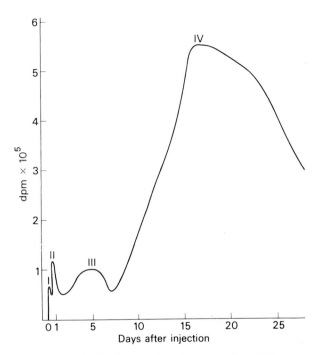

FIG. 2.23. Radioactivity in the lateral geniculate body at different intervals after intraocular injection of ^{3}H-leucine. Four peaks of radioactivity moving at different rates can be seen. (*From* Karlsson and Sjöstrand 1971. *Acta Neuropath.* (*Berl.*) Suppl. V, p. 207.)

tensive rough endoplasmic reticulum of the Nissl substance. The amount of protein exported down the axon may well be one and a half times the perikaryal volume per day.

Many explanations have been advanced for the mechanism providing the driving force behind axoplasmic flow. These include the 'secretion pressure' of the perikaryon, and the peristaltic pumping action of axons or

Schwann cells. However particle movements occur in cells without the structure or movements of axons and their Schwann cells, and neither explanation is attractive. The evidence points strongly to neurofilaments and neurotubules playing the major role in the movement of axoplasm as described above. This evidence includes the fact that in favourable situations it has been found that axoplasmic flow is localized to regions rich in neurotubules, and that dissociation of the neurotubules by colchicine blocks axoplasmic flow.

It was once thought that axoplasmic flow occurred at a rate of 1–2 mm/day. Later, more rapid movements of the order of 100 or more mm/day became recognized. The fastest rate so far reported is about 3 m/day. In some systems, moving peaks of axoplasmic constituents can be recognized (fig. 2.23), which lead to the suggestion that there were certain specific rates of flow, the 'slow' flow at 1–2 mm/day, and the 'fast' flow of 100–300 mm/day. However a considerable amount of material moves between these peaks, and intermediate rates have been recognized. In some systems the amount of material moving at the slower rates greatly exceeds the fast (fig. 2.24), while in others the amounts are nearly equal.

So far centrifugal axoplasmic flow has been mentioned, but centripetal flow also occurs simultaneously. This is in agreement with microscopic evidence of particle movements within axons which often reverse in direction and at times occur in both directions at once. The centripetal flow is probably smaller in amount than the centrifugal, though accurate quantitation has not been performed.

The function and fate of this transported material is still a matter for debate. Its role might be:
1   to provide the enzymes or precursors for the distal synthesis of transmitter substances;
2   to provide trophic factors for the effect of the nerve on the postsynaptic cell;
3   to provide for the transmission of information within the neuron which is a very long cell;
4   to provide information to or trophic effects upon the Schwann cell;
5   to provide nutrients for the distal nerve terminals.
The fate of the material exported from the perikaryon might include:
1   discharge or degradation distally;
2   discharge or degradation along the axon;
3   interchange with structural proteins along the axon;
4   reversal of the direction of flow and return to the perikaryon.

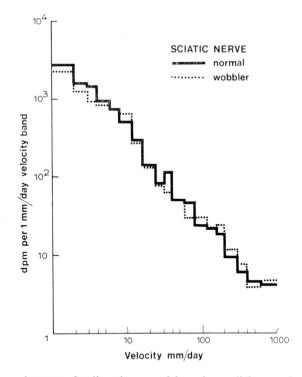

FIG. 2.24. Amount of radioactive material moving at different velocities in the sciatic nerve of mice. (*From* Bradley *et al.* 1971.)

Considerably more research is required before details of the function of axoplasmic flow will become clear, and its role in disease processes elucidated. For further details, reviews by Barondes (1967), Grafstein (1969), Dahlström (1971) and Bradley *et al.* (1971) should be consulted.

Myelin

Myelin is a complex of many different molecular species organized into a regular macromolecular structure of striking ultrastructural form. The many chemical compounds involved in its structure have been isolated and characterized. Several hypotheses attempt to explain how these compounds are interlinked in the myelin. Much however remains to be elucidated about the structure and chemistry of myelin. Only an outline of the chemical constituents and arrangements will be given. For further details the reader is referred to Davison and Peters (1970), O'Brien (1970) and biochemical texts.

Water constitutes about 40 per cent by weight of fresh myelin.

Lipids of myelin

Lipids make up about 75 per cent of the dry weight of myelin, the remainder being protein.

Cholesterol

Cholesterol makes up about 40 per cent of the total lipids of peripheral nerve myelin (expressed as molar per cent).

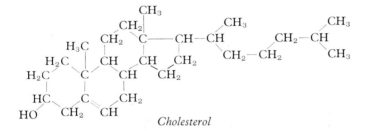

Cholesterol

The remainder of the lipids are of several complex types. They are best understood by building up their structure from their basic biochemical building blocks.

Phospholipids

These are phosphate esters either of glycerol or the base sphingosine, and their derivatives.

$$CH_2\!-\!OH \qquad\qquad HO\!-\!CH\!-\!CH\!=\!CH.(CH_2)_{12}.CH_3$$
$$CH\!-\!OH\ (\beta) \qquad\qquad CH\!-\!NH_2$$
$$CH_2\!-\!OH\ (\alpha) \qquad\qquad CH_2\!-\!OH$$

Glycerol   Sphingosine

Glycerol may be phosphorylated in the α or β position, but it is only the L-α (equivalent to D-β) form which is present in phospholipids. The other hydroxyl groups may be esterified with long chain fatty acids. These compounds, *phosphatidic acids*, are the basis of several phospholipids.

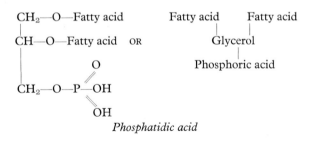

$$CH_2-O-Fatty\ acid$$
$$CH-O-Fatty\ acid \quad OR$$
$$CH_2-O-P \overset{O}{\underset{OH}{\diagup}} OH$$

Fatty acid   Fatty acid
Glycerol
Phosphoric acid

Phosphatidic acid

The phosphoric acid residue may be esterified either with *ethanolamine* producing *ethanolamine glycerophosphatide*, which constitutes about 12 per cent of the total lipids of peripheral nerve myelin; with *choline* producing *choline glycerophosphatide* which constitutes about 10 per cent of the total lipids; with *serine* making *serine glycerophosphatide*, which is about 7 per cent of the total; or with *inositol* making *inositol glycerophosphatide*, about 2 per cent of the total lipids.

$$CH_2-OH$$
$$CH_2-NH_2$$
Ethanolamine

Fatty acid   Fatty acid
Glycerol
Phosphoric acid—Ethanolamine
Ethanolamine glycerophosphatide
(Cephalin)

$$CH_2-OH$$
$$CH_2-N \overset{CH}{\underset{+}{\diagup}} CH_3$$
$$OH^- \ CH_3$$
Choline

Fatty acid   Fatty acid
Glycerol
Phosphoric acid—Choline
Choline glycerophosphatide
(Lecithin)

$$CH_2-OH$$
$$CH-NH_2$$
$$COOH$$
Serine

Fatty acid   Fatty acid
Glycerol
Phosphoric acid—Serine
Serine glycerophosphatide
(Cephalin)

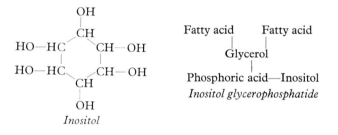

Inositol

Fatty acid   Fatty acid
Glycerol
Phosphoric acid—Inositol
Inositol glycerophosphatide

The chemical names of these compounds are sometimes given in different forms, including choline phospholipid or phosphatidylcholine.

Inositol may be phosphorylated or pyrophosphorylated, giving di- and tri-phosphoinositides respectively. The form of the association of all the inositides with myelin is unclear since they are turned over much more rapidly than other myelin lipids with the possible exception of gangliosides.

The α hydroxyl group of the glycerol residue of phosphatidic acid may be esterified with a fatty acid and the β group joined to a fatty aldehyde as a vinyl ether. These compounds esterified with ethanolamine, serine or choline are called ethanolamine *plasmalogens* or *phosphatidal ethanolomine* etc. In adult myelin, the principal plasmalogen is derived from ethanolamine.

CH_2—O—Fatty acid

CH—O—CH=CH—(CH_2)—CH_3

CH_2O——Phosphoric acid

Ethanolamine
Ethanolamine plasmalogen

Substitution of only one of the hydroxyl groups of the glycerophosphoryl bases with a fatty acid gives a series of compounds generically known as *lyso-phosphatides*.

CH_2—O—Fatty acid

CH—OH

CH_2—O—Phosphoric acid—Choline
Lysolecithin

The lysophosphatides are powerful surfactants and tend to disrupt lipid bilayers, as for instance when formed by the action of activated complement. Lysolecithin is formed, together with cholesteryl acetate, in demyelinating lesions by enzymic transfer of a fatty acid residue from lecithin to choles-terol.

In the same way that phosphatidic acid is formed from glycerol, *ceramide phosphate* is derived from sphingosine, except that the fatty acid linkage is an amide rather than an ester.

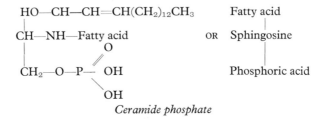

Ceramide phosphate

Esterification of ceramide phosphate with choline forms sphingomyelin, which makes up 13 per cent of the total lipids of peripheral nerve myelin.

Fatty acid
|
Sphingosine
|
Phosphoric acid—Choline
Sphingomyelin

Glycolipids

If the remaining free hydroxyl group of ceramide is linked to various car-bohydrates through a glycosidic bond, a large group of complex glycolipids is formed. The simplest members are the *cerebrosides*, which are formed by linkage with galactose or glucose, and which constitute about 11 per cent of the total lipids of peripheral nerve myelin.

Galactocerebroside, the only cerebroside found in myelin, occurs as its sulphated ester, *sulphatide*. The latter stains metachromatically with basic dyes, accumulates in oligodendroglia and Schwann cells in metachromatic leucodystrophy (see page 174), but comprises only 2 per cent of normal myelin lipids. No further compounds with galactose as the first unit are known. Several galactocerebrosides, differing only in the fatty acid residue, have been named, e.g. kerasin, phrenosin (or cerebron) and nervon.

Sphingosine—Fatty acid   Sphingosine—Fatty acid
| |
Galactose   Galactose—Sulphate
Galactocerebroside   *Sulphatide*

Glucocerebroside does not occur in myelin, but accumulates in the reticuloendothelial system in Gaucher's disease. Additions of various hexoses, amino-hexoses and sialic acids (N-acetylneuraminic acid, NANA) to glucocerebroside yield the complex glycolipids known as *gangliosides*, which constitute about 1 per cent of both central and peripheral myelin lipids. These gangliosides may have as many as eight saccharide residues with branched chain configurations. Degradation products of these containing two to six saccharide residues accumulate in nervous tissue in various inherited conditions, such as Fabry's disease and Tay-Sachs' disease. With the possible exception of the inositides, the gangliosides turn over at a faster rate than the remainder of myelin lipids, and are predominantly neuronal glycolipids.

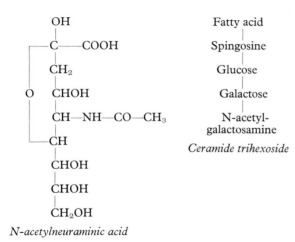

The structure of four of the major gangliosides is probably as follows:

Fatty acid	Fatty acid
Sphingosine	Sphingosine
Glucose	Glucose
Galactose—NANA	Galactose—NANA
	N-acetylgalactosamine
G_{M3}	G_{M2}

Fatty acid   Fatty acid
| |
Sphingosine   Sphingosine
| |
Glucose   Glucose
| |
Galactose—NANA   Galactose—NANA
| |
N-acetylgalactosamine   N-acetylgalactosamine
| |
Galactose   Galactose—NANA
G_{M1} G_{D1a}

Fatty acid residues of phospholipids and glycolipids

Each myelin lipid contains 15–90 different fatty acids, and ethanolamine
and serine plasmalogens also contain fatty aldehydes. Thus each different
complex lipid must be thought of as a class of compounds, each differing
from the others in its fatty acid moieties. Fatty acids of 18–24 carbon
atoms, and an even number of carbon atoms are the most common, but
α-hydroxy-fatty acids, branched chain fatty acids, unsaturated fatty acids,
and those with an odd number of carbon atoms also occur. The total number of individual molecular species of lipid in myelin may well be more than
1500. Though names are given to the fatty acids (see table 2.3), they are

TABLE 2.3. some of the more important fatty acids present in myelin

Carbon atoms	Saturated fatty acid	Mono-ethenoid fatty acid	Di-ethenoid fatty acid	Tri-ethenoid fatty acid	Tetra-ethenoid fatty acid
C_{16}	Palmitic				
C_{18}	Stearic	Oleic	Linoleic	Linolenic	
C_{20}	Arachidic				Arachidonic
C_{22}	Behenic				
C_{24}	Lignoceric	Nervonic			
C_{26}	Cerotic				

now usually defined by their carbon chain length, the number and position
of double bonds and branch chains. Thus nervonic acid is $C24:1$.

The myelin of older subjects has more longer chain fatty acids and
more unsaturated long chain fatty acids than that of younger ones. Serine,
choline and ethanolamine glycerophosphatides have mainly C16 and C18
fatty acid residues. Sphingomyelin has predominantly C22 and C24 fatty

acid residues, the proportion of longer chain and unsaturated residues up to C24 increasing with maturation. Stearic acid constitutes more than 75 per cent of the fatty acid residues of the gangliosides. On the other hand, cerebrosides contain mainly C22 and C24 fatty acids, sulphatides particularly have even longer chain fatty acids. Only cerebroside and sulphatide of the myelin lipids are substituted by α-hydroxy fatty acids, and the normal and α-hydroxy substituted galactolipids occur in approximately equal quantities.

Proteins of myelin

About 30 per cent by weight of adult human myelin is protein, though it is somewhat less in other species. The proteins of myelin are unusual in that they are extractable from homogenized tissue or from isolated myelin into various organic solvents such as petroleum ether or, more particularly, mixtures of chloroform and methanol. Some, particularly the so-called Wolfgram protein, are better extracted when the organic solvent is slightly acidified. It is clear that in such extracts the proteins are not monodisperse, but form multimolecular aggregates or micelles, in which lipids are bound with varying degrees of firmness. These organic solvent-soluble aggregates are termed proteolipids, and the strong association of some of the lipids and proteins has obvious significance for the stability of the myelin sheath. The individual proteins of the proteolipids may be dissociated from the lipids by a variety of methods, such as treatment with mineral acids and simple salts, or detergents and acid phenol, or by denaturation of the proteins under special conditions. The quantitatively important proteins fall into three groups.

Basic protein antigens

These are the most readily dissociable proteins of the proteolipid complexes, and it is sometimes difficult to make them behave as true proteolipids. Once obtained in lipid-free water-soluble form, they cannot be returned to organic solvent solution. Central myelin has only one basic protein (except in some rodent species where a second, smaller, but strongly homologous protein occurs) constituting 30–40 per cent of the total protein. The structure of this protein from several species, including man, has been determined. It has a molecular mass of about 18,000 daltons, and the high content of both arginine and lysine is noteworthy. Peripheral myelin has two basic proteins, one of which appears identical with that of central myelin (comprising approximately 5 per cent of total myelin proteins) and the other (comprising approximately 20 per cent of total protein) which is of molecular mass 12,500 daltons, but is otherwise less well characterized. Both proteins are very susceptible to enzymic digestion, for instance with trypsin.

The chief interest in these proteins is that immunization of animals with them produces allergic reactions damaging the myelin of which the protein is characteristic. Immunization with crude extracts of peripheral nerve gives rise to both peripheral and central nervous lesions.

Folch–Lees proteolipid proteins

These proteins require more vigorous treatments to free them from lipid, and are relatively easily degraded to insoluble materials which are not susceptible to enzyme digestion and which are the basis of neurokeratin. Recently the protein from central myelin has been obtained in lipid-free water-soluble form, from which it may be returned to solution in organic solvents by special two phase chromatographic techniques. The Folch-Lees proteolipid proteins of central and peripheral myelin are of molecular mass 26,000 and approximately 21,000 daltons respectively, and constitute about 50–60 per cent and less than 20 per cent of the total myelin proteins respectively. Both are reported to have relatively high sulphur and tryptophan contents.

Other proteolipid proteins

In peripheral myelin, the major component of the proteolipid protein differs from the Folch-Lees proteolipid protein in being more readily extractable by acidified, rather than neutral chloroform-methanol. This component comprises about 60 per cent of total myelin protein, has a molecular mass approximately 21,000 daltons, is digestible by trypsin, and is probably a glycoprotein. Another proteolipid protein of central myelin, often called Wolfgram protein, has an approximate molecular mass of 36,000 daltons and constitutes less than 10 per cent of the total myelin protein. Both central and peripheral proteins are poorly characterized.

Differences between peripheral and central nervous myelin

Considerable differences exist between central and peripheral myelin, though most studies have concentrated on the former. Peripheral myelin contains less glycolipid and more sphingomyelin than central myelin. The choline glycerophosphatides of peripheral myelin contain a higher proportion of polyunsaturated fatty acids, linoleic acid comprising 5·6 per cent of the total fatty acids of lecithin; in central myelin it comprises only 0·5 per cent of the total. In peripheral myelin, very long chain fatty acids (C25 and C26) make up less than 2 per cent of the whole, while in central nervous myelin they account for 5–20 per cent of the total fatty acids.

Peripheral nerve myelin contains less Folch-Lees proteolipid and more acid-soluble proteolipid than central myelin. Immunization with central nervous basic protein induces experimental allergic encephalomyelitis in which the lesions are confined to the central nervous system. Because of the two components in peripheral myelin basic protein, immunization with this agent produces changes mainly in the peripheral nervous system, but with some central lesions.

Metabolism of myelin

In the rat and mouse, Schwann cell division is most active in the first few days of postnatal life. It soon decreases to the very low level seen in adult animals. Myelination begins about the time of birth, and to judge by the incorporation of ^{14}C-acetate into lipids, is maximum at the second postnatal day. In the human foetus these stages begin about the sixteenth week of intrauterine life, and by the time of birth the peripheral nerves are already well myelinated. Further synthesis of myelin, however, continues as the increase in axonal diameter and body length produce consequent increase in myelin sheath thickness and internodal length. For further details of the biochemical events during myelination the reader is referred to Davison (1970).

In the adult, myelin is metabolically relatively stable. There is very little uptake into myelin of lipid or protein precursors, and the half-life of most of the lipid components is of the order of months or years. A small metabolically active component of myelin lipids may exist, though the subcellular localization of this is unknown. Cholesterol is largely conserved during myelin degeneration, and reutilized for new myelin synthesis. Similar conservation of the other myelin components may occur.

Myelin breakdown during segmental demyelination or axonal degeneration occurs initially in the Schwann cell and to a variable extent in macrophages which remove myelin debris from the Schwann cells. The breakdown of myelin involves activation of Schwann cells and macrophage cytoplasm, increase in oxidative and protein synthetic enzymes, as well as specific activation of catabolic enzymes. These include proteases, phosphatases, esterases and neuraminidases. Many of these are lysosomal in origin. Complete digestion of myelin is evidently not easy for the cell, residual bodies of lipofuscin often being the gravestones of membrane lipid destruction. π-granules and other laminated osmiophilic Schwann cell inclusions seen in normal nerve may be the residua of myelin remodelling during myelination.

Structural organization of myelin

Work still continues to elucidate the structure of myelin, but a considerable amount is already known (Hendler 1971). The lipid components of the membrane are arranged radially to the lamellae, and the protein components tangentially. Dark bands on electron micrographs correspond to the protein and polar hydrophilic groups of the lipids, while the clear zones result from the preparative dissolution of hydrophobic lipids. The major dense lines result from the apposition of the inner (cytoplasmic) side of the Schwann cell membranes, and the less electron-dense intraperiod line is formed from the apposition of the outer (basement membrane) side of the Schwann cell plasmalemmal membrane (see fig. 2.3). It seems probable that the basic protein antigens occupy the intraperiod line locus. The arrangement of the lipids is obviously complex. Fig. 2.25 shows one possible arrangement.

Satellite cell-neuron interrelationships

The anatomical relationship between the satellite cells and neurons in the posterior root ganglia, between the oligodendrogliocytes and anterior horn neurons in the spinal cord, and between the Schwann cells and axons in the peripheral nerves is very close. Very little plasma membrane of the neuron is exposed to the interstitial fluid other than via the cytoplasm of these cells. The Schwann cell and other satellite cells may therefore potentially play a large part in regulating the supply of oxygen, water, salts and nutrients to, and the removal of waste products from the neuron. Hydén (1967) has demonstrated a close interrelationship between the glia and neurons of the cochlear nucleus. The glial cells probably provide the neurons with high energy compounds and metabolites in addition to the substances already mentioned. Schwann and Remak cells may have a similar role in the peripheral nervous system (Singer and Salpeter 1966a and b). In myelinated nerve fibres the Schmidt-Lanterman incisures may be a route for the passage of substances from the superficial Schwann cell cytoplasm through the myelin to the axon, and the interchange of substances between the axon and Schwann cell may also occur at the paranodal regions. The locally high potassium concentration at the Schwann cell and Remak cell membranes after a train of nerve impulses must have an effect upon the

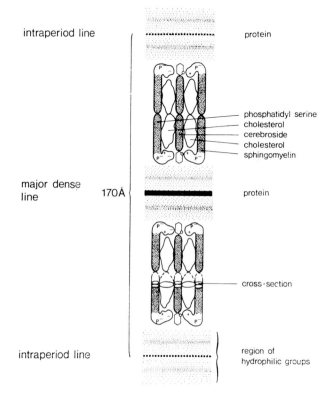

intraperiod line — protein

— phosphatidyl serine
— cholesterol
— cerebroside
— cholesterol
— sphingomyelin

major dense line   170Å — protein

— cross-section

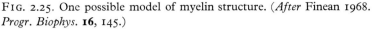

intraperiod line — region of hydrophilic groups

FIG. 2.25. One possible model of myelin structure. (*After* Finean 1968. *Progr. Biophys.* **16**, 145.)

resting membrane potential of these cells. Similarly the presence of these cellular barriers may conserve potassium, allowing rapid reaccumulation of the ion by the axon.

The neuron has a similar important influence upon the Schwann cell and other satellite cells. Activation of satellite cells of the anterior horn or posterior root ganglia is one of the earliest events following damage to the axons in the peripheral nerves. The stimulus to the Schwann cell to digest the myelin in axonal degeneration must result from some positive stimulus or the loss of some inhibitory influence of the axon upon the Schwann cell. The axon determines whether a myelin sheath is formed or not, its thickness, and the actual size of the Schwann cell, that is of the internodal length. These important relationships await further elucidation.

REFERENCES

ADAMS W.E. (1943) The blood supply of nerves. II The effects of occlusion of its regional sources of supply on the sciatic nerve of the rabbit. *J. Anat. (Lond.)* **77**, 243–250.

BARONDES S.H. ed. (1967) Axoplasmic transport. *Neurosci. Res. Prog. Bull.* **5**, 307–419.

BOYD I.A. and DAVEY M.R. (1968) *Composition of Peripheral Nerves.* Livingstone, Edinburgh.

BRADLEY W.G., MURCHISON D. and DAY M.J. (1971) The range of velocities of axoplasmic flow. A new approach, and its application to mice with genetically inherited spinal muscular atrophy. *Brain Res.* **35**, 185–197.

COËRS C. and WOOLF A.L. (1959) *The Innervation of Muscle.* Blackwell, Oxford.

DAHLSTRÖM A. (1971) Axoplasmic transport (with particular respect of adrenergic neurons). *Phil. Trans. Roy. Soc. Lond., B* **261**, 325–358.

DAVISON A.N. and PETERS A. (1970) *Myelination.* C.C.Thomas, Springfield, Illinois.

DAVISON A.N. (1970) The biochemistry of the myelin sheath. In *Myelination*, ed. Davison A.N. and Peters A., pp. 80–161. C.C.Thomas, Springfield, Illinois.

DUCHEN L.W. (1971) Electron microscopic comparison of the motor end plates of slow and fast skeletal muscle fibres of the mouse. *J. neurol. Sci.* **14**, 37–45.

ERLANGER J. and GASSER H.S. (1937) *Electrical Signs of Nervous Activity.* University of Pennsylvania Press, Philadelphia.

FRIEDE R.L. and SAMORAJSKI T. (1968) Myelin formation in the sciatic nerve of the rat. *J. Neuropath. exp. Neurol.* **27**, 546–570.

GRAFSTEIN B. (1969) Axonal transport: communication between soma and synapse. In *Advances in Biochemical Psychopharmacology*, vol. 1, ed. Costa E. and Greengard P., pp. 11–25. Raven Press, New York.

HALL S.M. and WILLIAMS P.L. (1970) Studies on the 'incisures' of Schmidt and Lanterman. *J. Cell Sci.* **6**, 767–791.

HENDLER R.W. (1971) Biological membrane ultrastructure. *Physiol. Rev.* **51**, 66–97.

HODGKIN A.L. (1965) *The Conduction of the Nervous Impulse.* Liverpool University Press, Liverpool.

HYDÉN H. (1967) Dynamic aspects of the neuron-glia relationship. In *The Neuron*, ed. Hydén H., pp. 179–219. Elsevier, Amsterdam.

JAHN T.L. and BOVEC E.C. (1969) Protoplasmic movements within cells. *Physiol. Rev.* **49**, 793–862.

KATZ B. (1966) *Nerve, Muscle and Synapse.* McGraw-Hill, New York.

KENNEDY W.R. (1970) Innervation of normal human muscle spindles. *Neurol. (Minneap.)* **20**, 463–475.

LANGLEY G.K. and LANDON D.N. (1968) A light and electron microscopic histo-chemical approach to the node of Ranvier and myelin of peripheral nerve fibres. *J. Histochem. Cytochem.* **15**, 722–731.

LANTERMAN A.J. (1877) Ueber der feineren Bau der markhaltigen Nervenfasern. *Arch. mikrosk. Anat. EntwMech.* **13**, 1–8.

MATHEWS P.B.C. (1964) Muscle spindles and their motor control. *Physiol. Rev.* **44**, 219–288.

MELZACK R. and WALL P.D. (1965) Pain mechanisms: a new theory. *Science* **150**, 971–979.

NACHMANSOHN D. (1970) Proteins in bioelectricity. In *Protein Metabolism of the Nervous System*, ed. Lajtha A, pp. 313–333. Plenum Press, New York.

O'BRIEN J.S. (1970) Chemical composition of myelinated nervous tissue. In *Handbook of Clinical Neurology*, vol. 7, ed. Vinken P.J. and Bruyn W.G., pp. 40–61. North-Holland, Amsterdam.

PETERS A., PALAY S.L. and WEBSTER H. DE F. (1970) *The Fine Structure of the Nervous System. The cells and their processes.* Hoeber Medical Division, Harper and Row, New York.

RUSHTON W.A.H. (1951) A theory of the effects of fibre size on medullated nerve. *J. Physiol. (Lond.)* **115**, 101–122.

SCHMIDT H.D. (1874) On the construction of the dark or double-bordered nerve fibre. *Mon. Microsc. J. (Lond.)* **11**, 200–221.

SCHMITT F.O. and SAMSON F.E. JR. ed. (1968) Neuronal fibrous proteins. *Neurosci. Res. Prog. Bull.* **6**, 113–219.

SINCLAIR D.C. (1955) Cutaneous sensation and the doctrine of specific energy. *Brain* **78**, 584–614.

SINGER M. and SALPETER M.M. (1966a) The transport of ^{3}H-L-histidine through the Schwann cell and myelin sheath into the axon, including a re-evaluation of myelin function. *J. Morph.* **120**, 281–315.

SINGER M. and SALPETER M.M. (1966b) Transport of tritium-labelled L-histidine through the Schwann and myelin sheaths into axons of peripheral nerve. *Nature* **210**, 1225–1227.

SUNDERLAND S. (1968) *Nerves and Nerve Injuries.* Livingstone, Edinburgh.

TASAKI I. (1968) *Nerve Excitation. A macromolecular approach.* C.C. Thomas, Springfield, Illinois.

VIZOSO A.D. (1950) The relationship between internodal length and growth in human nerves. *J. Anat. (Lond.)* **84**, 342–353.

VIZOSO A.D. and YOUNG J.Z (1948) Internode length and fibre diameter in developing and regenerating nerves. *J. Anat. (Lond.)* **82**, 110–134.

WECHSLER W. (1970) Development and structure of peripheral nerve in vertebrates. In *Handbook of Clinical Neurology*, vol. 7, ed. Vinken P.J. and Bruyn G.W., pp. 1–39. North-Holland, Amsterdam.

WEUSS P. and HISCOE H. (1948) Experiments on the mechanism of nerve growth. *J. Exp. Zool.* **107**, 315–395.

3

Clinical Features of
Peripheral Nerve Disease

The causes of peripheral nerve disease probably run into several hundreds. The clinical presentations of peripheral neuropathies are, however, much more limited. Peripheral neuropathies may be classified in six main ways:

1 *Rate of onset:* acute—usually less than one week; subacute—usually less than one month; chronic—longer than one month.

2 *Type of nerve fibre involved:* motor; sensory; autonomic; mixed.

3 *Size of nerve fibre involved:* large; small; mixed.

4 *Distribution:* proximal; distal; diffuse.

5 *Pattern:* mononeuropathy; mononeuritis multiplex; symmetrical poly-neuropathy; ganglio-radiculopathy.

6 *Pathology:* axonal degeneration; segmental demyelination; mixed.

Most of the terms used in this list are self-evident. The pathological processes are described in chapter 5. A word of explanation is required about the various patterns of neuropathies. When only one nerve, for example the median nerve or the long thoracic nerve, are involved, the term mononeuritis or *mononeuropathy* is applied. The ending *-itis* usually implies inflammation, which is not the basis in every case, and the more general ending *-pathy* is preferred. The term *mononeuropathia multiplex* is used when several different nerves are involved, either at the same time or sequentially. The more euphonious term *mononeuritis multiplex* is preferred by many. A *distal symmetrical polyneuropathy* is the commonest pattern of nerve involvement. The symptoms and signs usually begin in the toes, spreading upwards; later the fingers and hands are involved in a similar centripetal spread. Very occasionally the symptoms begin in the fingers, only later occurring in the feet. The term *ganglio-radiculopathy* is applied when the neurological symptoms and signs fit into the distribution of one or more spinal nerve roots. The lesion in these cases lies within the nerve roots and the posterior root ganglia.

Each classification has its uses in pointing towards an understanding of the basic mechanisms underlying the disease, but more particularly as an aid to diagnosis. This is discussed more fully in chapter 11 where a diagnostic synopsis is constructed.

SYMPTOMS AND SIGNS OF PERIPHERAL NERVE DISEASE

Disease of the peripheral nervous system may cause sensory, motor and autonomic dysfunction. Disease of the autonomic nervous system is a special case, and is considered separately in chapter 7. The symptoms of peripheral nerve disease may be divided into positive and negative phenomena, while the signs are almost entirely the negative ones of loss of function. The signs and symptoms may also be grouped into those due to damage to the larger myelinated nerve fibres and those due to small myelinated and unmyelinated nerve fibre damage.

Sensory abnormalities

Symptoms

The *negative phenomena* of sensation are relatively easy to understand. Loss of large myelinated nerve fibre function, as seen in tabes dorsalis and many toxic neuropathies, causes a raised threshold and, if sufficiently severe, loss of joint position and touch sensation. Patients complain of numbness, and are often unable to recognize objects with their hands when their vision is obstructed. They may feel as though their hands are wrapped in cotton wool, and that they are walking on sponge rubber. Tight band-like sensations or feelings of swelling in the limbs may also result from loss of large sensory fibre function in the peripheral nerves. More usually however these abnormal sensations are due to spinal cord posterior column lesions. Unsteadiness of gait, particularly in the dark, is a frequent complaint. Loss of small nerve fibre function causes a raised threshold and, if sufficiently severe, eventual loss of pain and temperature sensation, leading to injury and ulceration due to loss of protective reflexes. Patients may therefore develop various neuropathic disorders, including burns, ulcers, abscesses and neuropathic (Charcot) joints, which are disturbing in their appearance and systemic effects, but are painless to the individual.

Of the *positive phenomena*, pain, which arises from compression or infiltration of a nerve or pressure over a traumatic area, is relatively easily understood. These processes presumably cause direct stimulation of the afferent pain-conducting fibres. The spontaneous sensation of pins and needles (*paraesthesiae*) may also arise from the spontaneous uncoordinated discharge of larger myelinated nerve fibres. Many of the other positive sensory symptoms are however more difficult to understand. Patients with certain neuropathies complain that their feet feel as though they are burning, and the sensation may make walking difficult and hinder sleep. The neuropathies of thiamine deficiency, malabsorption, alcoholism, diabetes, uraemia and occasionally carcinoma are particularly liable to cause the sensation of *burning feet*. Patients with partially diminished sensation in many parts of the body may complain that the area feels raw. Touching the partly denervated skin may produce unpleasant pricking sensations to which the term *contact dysaesthesiae* is applied. The term *hyperalgesia* is applied when pain is perceived at an abnormally low intensity of stimulation. The pain may be felt excessively. The term *hyperpathia* is best restricted to the state where the pain threshold is raised, but when this threshold is exceeded the pain perceived is excessive. This is best seen in the thalamic syndrome, which usually follows a cerebrovascular accident affecting sensory pathways in the thalamus, but may occur in disorders of the peripheral nerve.

The patient may complain of '*restless legs*' either while sitting, or in bed at night. He may say his legs feel uncomfortable, painful, or even burning. Walking around often relieves the symptoms. 'Restless legs' occasionally occur in mild peripheral neuropathies and may also be associated with iron deficiency states. However, usually it occurs without any other disease, and the term *Ekbom's syndrome* is applied to this idiopathic condition. Chlorpromazine, diazepam or carbamazepine may relieve this symptom complex.

Lightning pains, classically seen in tabes dorsalis, are sudden, brief stabs of pain often described as like red-hot needles being suddenly thrust into the legs. They may occur in episodes, but each sensation lasts only for a fraction of a second. Patients who have any part of the limb amputated may complain of spontaneous sensations coming from the part which is no longer present. Sometimes this is due to an amputation neuroma, and an exquisitely tender area will be found on compression of the scar. On other occasions the *phantom pains* must be presumed to have a central origin, and may at times be partly suppressed by psychotherapeutic agents. Following partial traumatic lesions, usually of the median or sciatic nerves, patients may suffer severe spontaneous diffuse burning pain in the limb, which is made worse by contact and many psychological factors. This pain has been termed *causalgia*, and is discussed more fully on page 152.

Signs

The clinical examination of the sensory system is designed to give objective evidence of sensory loss. Each modality of sensation is systematically examined over the whole body. Care is taken that the patient does not receive additional clues, for instance by surreptitiously having his eyes open, or by hearing the rustle of the examiner's clothes with each stimulus. Sensory loss may be total or partial, and thus the examination is divided into two parts, the first designed to demonstrate areas of *total loss of sensation*. The patient is provided with the option of a positive or negative response. In testing pain sensation, he is stimulated randomly with the sharp point or the blunt head of the pin, and asked to tell which he feels. Similarly in testing vibration sensation, the tuning fork applied to bony points is randomly arranged to be either vibrating or not, and the patient is asked to tell whether he feels it vibrating or not. The testing of temperature sensation with a hot or cold object also provides the patient with an alternative choice. In touch sensation he responds when he feels the cotton wool or remains silent if he does not perceive it. In testing joint position sensation he is asked to say when he feels the movement, and remains silent if he misses it. In all these tests, total loss of sensation is recorded when his responses are no better than chance, that is when the proportion of correct responses falls to 50 per cent. The boundaries of such loss of touch, pain or temperature sensation must be accurately outlined, systematically progressing from the abnormal area into the normal. The testing object is advanced from the anaesthetic area until the patient first perceives the stimulus, and this is marked as the boundary of total loss. Attempts to find the boundary by proceeding from the area of normal sensation into the abnormal are more inaccurate because the patient finds it difficult to state where sensation *just* disappears.

The second stage of the clinical examination of sensation is to outline *areas of partial loss* of the sensation of touch, pain and temperature. This is more difficult, requiring a more subjective response on the part of the patient. The stimulus is advanced from the abnormal area into the normal, the patient states when he feels the sensation normally, and this is marked as the boundary of the partial loss of sensation. He is also asked to describe the aberrant sensation. The boundaries of partial loss of sensation are usually indistinct.

Unfortunately the clinical examination of the sensory system as described here depends both on the stimulus applied by the examiner and the response of the subject, and both are subject to considerable variability.

Subject variability

The mental state of the patient will profoundly affect the sensory examination. The sensory threshold in a drowsy patient or one whose attention rapidly wanders such as a child, will vary greatly from moment to moment, and his attention has constantly to be redirected for the results to be reliable. Anxiety will lower the threshold for pain and raise that for other modalities. Sedation usually raises the threshold for all modalities, though barbiturates tend to lower that for pain. Every effort should therefore be made to reassure the patient, to explain to him carefully what is wanted, and to avoid fatigue.

Stimulus variability

The object is to make the series of sensory stimuli applied to the patient as constant as possible, and to have a thorough knowledge of the range of perception of such stimuli in normal individuals. Thus it is important to know that a light touch of cotton wool is felt more exquisitely over hairy skin than over glabrous skin such as the fingertip; that a pin-prick is less keenly felt on the thicker skin of the palmar surface of the digits than of the dorsum; that the skin of the back is much less sensitive than of the chest or abdomen; and that the threshold for perception of joint movement of the terminal interphalangeal joint of the hallux is perhaps 10°, while that of the ankle is only 2°. It is similarly important to recognize that the value of the threshold for a given stimulus varies with age. The threshold may begin to rise in early adult life, but is markedly higher in those over 60 years of age.

Several attempts have been made to apply reproducible test stimuli to the sensory examination. The simplest for everyday clinical practice is the tuning fork for testing vibration sensation. This should be of 128 cycles per second or less, and the patient is asked to say as soon as he can no longer appreciate vibration. The fork is immediately transferred to the similar site on the examiner. Assuming the latter is of similar age to the patient and 'normal', the degree of impairment of vibration may be measured by how long the examiner continues to perceive vibration. The next most useful method is two-point discrimination. The patient with his eyes closed is told that he may feel one point or two, and a series of ten or twenty tests is made touching the selected area with the separation of the two points just above the expected threshold. If the patient scores more than 50 per cent correct, the distance between the points is decreased slightly and the series repeated. The threshold for distinguishing two points is the minimum distance at which more than 50 per cent of the responses are correct. The joint position sense may similarly be measured using accurately limited angles of displacement.

Touch-pressure sensation has been accurately measured by a number of methods. The earliest was von Frey's series of hairs of graded stiffness. Each hair bent when the pressure exceeded its critical value, and the first hair which could reproducibly be perceived gave the value of the touch-pressure threshold. A variety of different stimuli, some mechanically applied, have since been developed and quantitative data obtained. Even within an area of skin, there are points with higher or lower threshold, and it is best to scan the area testing at constant grid positions. Comparison between results with different test machines requires that the parameters of stimulation including the area of the stylus and the wave form, duration and frequency of stimulation be exactly reproduced. Absolute values of touch-pressure threshold cannot therefore be given, even for a standard area of skin.

Temperature sensation is usually studied clinically with vials of water at 5–10°C above or below the skin temperature. Time should be allowed for the exposed skin temperature to equilibrate in a room at about 32°C. The ability to recognize hot and cold can be judged by the proportion of correct responses, but this gives no indication of the threshold for temperature discrimination. This may be measured with thermostatically controllable hot and cold thermodes applied randomly. The discriminatory threshold is the minimum temperature difference between the skin temperature and that of the thermode at which the proportion of correct responses exceeds 50 per cent. This is approximately 0·5°C in the most sensitive areas of normal individuals, though radiant heat changes of as little as 0·001 to 0·004°C per second may in fact be appreciated.

Various algesiometers or dolorimeters have been designed for the measurement of the pain threshold. These include a sharp pin which is applied mechanically, the pressure required to produce pain being recorded, and instruments applying radiant heat to an accurately determined area of skin at a set distance from the source. Pain sensation has two parts, the early pricking pain, probably carried by small myelinated nerve fibres of about 3 μm diameter, and the late burning pain, probably carried by un-myelinated nerve fibres. Reproducible results with the dolorimeter require that the first pricking pain sensation be reported. With a radiant heat dolorimeter the threshold for pricking pain on the dorsum of the foot is about 3000 mcal/cm^2/s.

Deep pain sensation may be tested where appropriate, but has not been quantitated. A moderate squeeze applied to the tendo Achilles or testicle produces an unpleasant sickly pain. This is characteristically absent in tabes dorsalis, and other conditions causing impairment of the access to higher centres of afferent impulses in the larger myelinated nerve fibres.

Despite the care required for the examination of the sensory nervous system, rarely are the signs elicited truly objective, because the patient's response is required. Neuropathic ulcers and joints (Charcot joints) result-ing from the loss of pain sensation, and the incoordination with the eyes shut due to loss of joint position sensation (*sensory ataxia*) may perhaps be taken as objective evidence of sensory impairment. Two objective tests of the sensory pathways are however available. The first depends on recording electrical events occurring in sensory pathways during sensory nerve stimulation. The *sensory nerve action potential* may be recorded after electri-cal stimulation of the nerve some distance away (see page 88). Similarly the *cortical evoked action potential* can be recorded by averaging techniques applied to the electroencephalogram after stimulation of the sensory nerve. In both the rate of conduction and amplitude of the action potential can be measured, though in the case of the cortical evoked action potential central pathways are also involved. Secondly the *axon reflex* (fig. 3.1) may be used to demonstrate the presence of peripheral sensory nerve fibres. The triple response to scratching an area of skin consists firstly of local vasodilatation, and secondly of local oedema, both due predominantly to histamine release, and thirdly of the surrounding vasodilatation, the flare. The latter results from impulses which run from the damaged area in a sensory nerve fibre, and pass in a retrograde fashion down another branch of that fibre to an adjacent area of undamaged skin. There they release chemical substances causing vasodilatation. A similar spreading flare follows the intradermal injection of 0·01 ml containing about 5 μg of histamine. The flare response is particularly useful for separating lesions of the posterior roots, from those of the more peripheral parts of the primary sensory neuron (see page 255).

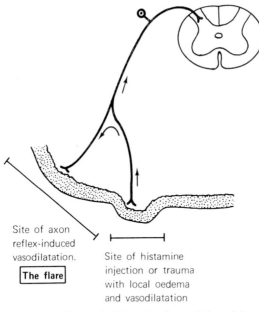

Site of axon
reflex-induced
vasodilatation.

The flare

Site of histamine
injection or trauma
with local oedema
and vasodilatation

FIG. 3.1. Axon reflex underlying the flare of the triple response.

Motor abnormalities

Symptoms

The patients usually complain of difficulty in performing certain manoeuvres, or of rapidly fatiguing while attempting them. Complaints often
include tripping over kerbs, difficulty in walking or climbing stairs, in
opening bottles or lifting the arms up to do the hair. These symptoms
should be analysed to elucidate which muscles are likely to be affected.
With insidious diseases, the patient may unconsciously adopt trick movements, and thus have severe weakness before presenting for medical advice. The patient may complain that his muscles are wasted, and may
occasionally note twitching (*fasciculation*) of muscles, which is often a
feature of anterior horn cell disease. Cramps may occasionally be a presenting complaint.

Signs

Muscle wasting may be obvious, but minor degrees may be difficult to
assess. The bulk of a muscle must be assessed against the general muscular
development of the patient. Excessive subcutaneous fat may hide the wast-

ing. Asymmetrical muscle atrophy is the most easily recognized. *Fasciculation* of groups of muscle fibres may be seen as fine irregular twitches of small parts of the muscle, which are involuntary and occur with the muscle at rest. They may sometimes be precipitated by tapping the muscle briskly and observing for half a minute thereafter. On electromyography these fasciculations are seen as single motor unit potentials, which are described as fasciculation potentials. These must be distinguished from fibrillation potentials which are usually di- or tri-phasic, and of lower amplitude and shorter duration (see page 104).

The maximum power of the individual muscle groups throughout the body is then systematically tested. This involves a subjective element depending as it does upon the degree of effort exerted by the patient. Contraction of antagonists, and marked fluctuation in power of the muscle under test when the patient is asked to produce a maximum contraction indicates a functional (psychogenic) element to the observed weakness.

The power of a muscle or muscle group is best graded according to the Medical Research Council (1943) scale:
0   No contraction;
1   Flicker or trace of contraction;
2   Active movements possible with gravity eliminated;
3   Active movements possible against gravity but not against resistance;
4   Active movements possible against both gravity and resistance;
5   Normal power.

Grade 4 involves a wide range of weakness, and it is helpful to subdivide it into grade 4+ and grade 4. It is possible to measure the maximum power of each muscle group, but assessment of this requires a knowledge of the range of normal values for patients of the same age and sex.

The aim of the examination of the motor system is to assess the power and bulk of each muscle group in the body. The muscles tested should include the trapezius, rhomboid, serratus anterior, supraspinatus, infraspinatus, latissimus dorsi, deltoid, biceps, brachioradialis, triceps, extensors of the wrist and fingers, flexor carpi ulnaris, flexor carpi radialis, flexor digitorum sublimis and flexor digitorum profundus, the lumbricals, interosseii, abductor digiti minimi, abductor pollicis brevis, long flexors and long extensors of the neck and trunk, the flexors, extensors, abductors and adductors of the hip, quadriceps femoris, hamstrings, triceps surae (gastrocnemius and soleus), invertors, evertors and dorsiflexors of the foot. An accurate charting of the bulk and power of these muscles may take an experienced clinician 10 or 15 minutes, but this data combined with a sound knowledge of the spinal segments and nerves supplying the muscles (see page 26 *et seq.*) is of vital importance to the diagnosis of peripheral nerve disease. The testing of the individual muscles is outside the range of this book, and the reader is referred to the Medical Research Council War Memorandum (1943), DeJong (1967), and Gardner-Medwin and Walton (1969).

Tendon reflexes

The tendon reflexes require the function of the γ-motor neuron, the intra-fusal fibres of the muscle spindles, the spindle sensory nerve fibres, the α-motor neuron and the extrafusal muscle fibres (fig. 2.12). Thus the knee-jerk, elicited by a sharp tap on the ligamentum patellae, requires that there be a resting tension in the quadriceps femoris muscle maintained by the activity of the γ- and α-motor fibres. The tap on the ligamentum patellae then stretches the quadriceps femoris muscle and its spindles, eliciting a volley in the group Ia afferent fibres from the spindles, which stimulates a discharge of the α-motoneurons in the cord related to the quadriceps femoris muscle, producing a twitch of the extrafusal muscle fibres. The spinal segments subserving the tendon reflexes which are usually elicited in the clinical examination are given in table 3.1.

TABLE 3.1. Spinal segments and nerves involved in the tendon reflexes commonly elicited in clinical practice

Reflex	Spinal segment	Peripheral nerve
Biceps reflex	C5–6	musculocutaneous
Supinator, brachioradialis or radial reflex	C5–6	radial
Triceps reflex	C6–7	radial
Finger reflex	C7–8	median or ulnar
Knee reflex	L2–4	femoral
Hamstring reflex	L5–S1	sciatic
Ankle reflex	S1–2	sciatic

The tendon reflexes are depressed or lost in any disease of these structures. In peripheral nerve disease, however, the reflexes may commonly be lost while the power and bulk of the muscle is relatively normal. By comparison, the reflexes are generally lost relatively late in primary muscle disease, though this rule is not invariable. An added complexity is that in some apparently normal individuals, and in those with the Holmes-Adie syndrome, the reflexes may be absent, while in anxious patients the tendon reflexes may be excessively brisk. In the *Holmes-Adie syndrome*, in addition to areflexia, one or both pupils are moderately dilated and are unresponsive to light. On accommodation, a response is very delayed, but may in fact exceed the normal range of pupillary contraction. Upper motoneuron lesions cause exaggerated tendon reflexes. The tendon reflexes are a relatively objective test of the afferent and efferent parts of the peripheral nervous system, and are thus of particular value in patients with a functional overlay.

SITE OF LESION

When examining a patient with sensorimotor complaints, it is important to keep in the forefront of one's mind the problem of localization of the lesion. It might be in the *psyche*, in the sensory and motor pathways of the *central nervous system*, in the *peripheral nervous system*, or in the *muscle*. The science of the neurological examination is outlined above. To apply such an examination to a patient may take many hours, and fatigue may vitiate the results. The art of the neurological examination is to recognize the deficit, and to concentrate on defining its site of origin. This may at times involve short cuts, which are often deprecated. Nevertheless it is a joy to see an expert quickly decipher the site of a lesion by testing a few crucial points. By comparison, the tyro's careful examination gets lost in a morass of signs of 'partially weak' muscles or 'slight' sensory impairment.

Some of the clinical points which aid in the identification of the site of the lesion are outlined below. They are not always absolute, and may require amplification and confirmation by the investigations described in chapter 4. The whole clinical picture must be taken into account rather than basing the conclusion of the site of the lesion upon the result of one test or one abnormality in the clinical examination.

Psyche

With neurological complaints of psychological origin, the symptoms are often vaguely described, diffuse and variable. There are no *objective* neurological abnormalities such as areflexia or muscle wasting. Sensory loss usually has an ill-defined border, or is patchy and varies from one examination to another. In most cases all modalities are equally involved. The muscle weakness is diffuse and variable. Distraction or encouragement may briefly produce normal power. The contraction of antagonists, and excessive associated movements may be a clue to the psychogenic origin.

Hysteria may produce more florid neurological symptoms and signs mimicking all forms of neurological disease. There may be total paralysis of one or more limbs, though the tone and tendon reflexes are normal. There may be total anaesthesia and analgesia of a part of the body. This is usually sharply demarcated from the 'normal' area, with no gradation. All modalities are typically involved, and the distribution fails to conform to any anatomical pattern. Vibration sense may appear to be lost on the affected side of the skull and sternum. Smell, hearing, facial and palatal sensation may appear to be lost on the affected side. A glove and stocking sensory loss may at times be seen, but the very sharp boundaries differentiate it from that usually seen in a distal sensory polyneuropathy. The symptoms and signs may sometimes be shown to be spurious by various tricks. For instance, a person may appear to have absolutely no power of dorsiflexion of the foot while lying in the bed, but can walk without a foot drop. The symptoms and signs may also be susceptible to suggestion, particularly that they are more severe than originally appeared.

Though the pattern of the deficit may suggest a functional or hysterical origin, one must always be wary of being satisfied with such a diagnosis. One needs to search for the reason for the hysterical manifestations. A very common diagnostic catch is an organic disease, the signs of which are immersed in a gross functional or hysterical overlay.

Central nervous system

The symptoms of central nervous disease may be indistinguishable from those of psychological origin, but the crucial separation rests upon the finding of abnormal physical signs in the former condition. There may be signs of exaggeration of the tendon reflexes due to an upper motor neuron lesion, or of sensory loss corresponding to central anatomical pathways.

Similarly the sensory and motor symptoms of a central nervous disease like multiple sclerosis may be indistinguishable from those of peripheral nerve lesions. The separation depends upon the physical signs which accompany these symptoms. The finding of weakness without wasting, of the predominance of weakness in the extensors of the arm and flexors of the leg, and the presence of exaggerated tendon reflexes and extensor plantar responses indicate that the defect lies in the central nervous system. Muscle wasting, loss of tendon reflexes, and sensory loss in a distribution corresponding to that of one or more peripheral nerves indicate the presence of peripheral nerve disease.

The involvement of certain modalities of sensation with sparing of others is not necessarily of help in separating central from peripheral nervous system damage. The modalities of sensation form two groups, that of pain and temperature, which are carried by the unmyelinated and small myelinated nerve fibres of the peripheral nerves, and the spinothalamic tracts in the central nervous system, and joint position, vibration and touch sensation, which are carried by the large myelinated fibres in the peripheral nerves, and by the posterior columns of the spinal cord. Involvement of one group of modalities with complete sparing of the other may therefore arise either from the specific involvement of either the larger or smaller fibres in the peripheral nerves, or of the individual tracts within the central nervous system.

Combined signs of both central and peripheral nervous lesions may arise in a number of diseases such as vitamin B_{12} deficiency, syphilis, sarcoidosis and the leucodystrophies. They may also result from focal lesions such as a neurofibroma of the spinal nerve root damaging both the nerve roots and the spinal cord.

Peripheral nervous system

The loss of tendon reflexes, and the restriction of motor and sensory loss to the distribution of a myotome, dermatome or peripheral nerve are characteristic of peripheral nerve disease. Symptoms and signs, which start peripherally in the digits of the feet and hands, spreading centrally, strongly suggest peripheral nerve disease. There are several sites at which peripheral nerve lesions may lie, depicted in fig. 3.2. On the motor side the function of the lower motoneuron may be impaired at any of the following points:

1 Anterior horn cells, e.g. acute anterior poliomyelitis and motor neuron disease;
2 Anterior root, e.g. arachnoiditis and neurofibromo;
3 Peripheral nerve, e.g. trauma or diphtheritic neuropathy;
4 Motor nerve terminals, e.g. toxic neuropathies of the 'dying back' type;
5 Neuromuscular junction, e.g. myasthenia gravis and botulism.

On the sensory side the primary sensory neuron may likewise be damaged at any of the following points:

1 Within the spinal cord, e.g. multiple sclerosis and spinal cord tumour;
2 Root entry zone, e.g. perhaps tabes dorsalis;
3 Posterior root, e.g. arachnoiditis, neurofibroma and probably tabes dorsalis;
4 Posterior root ganglion neurons, e.g. sensory neuropathies of the familial type or those associated with carcinoma;
5 Peripheral nerve, e.g. trauma and diphtheritic neuropathy;
6 Sensory nerve terminals, e.g. toxic neuropathies of the 'dying back' type.

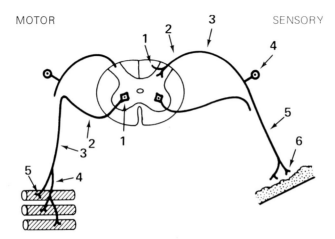

FIG. 3.2. The various sites on the motor and sensory nerves at which damage may occur leading to weakness and sensory loss respectively.

It is important to realize that two parts of the nerve cells which constitute the peripheral nervous system lie within the central nervous system. These are the anterior horn cell and the first part of its axon, and the central part of the primary sensory neuron. Focal damage to these, such as by infarction of the spinal cord, almost invariably leads to combined central and peripheral nervous signs.

A pure motor deficit may result from anterior horn cell disease, damage to the anterior roots, a peripheral neuropathy affecting purely the motor nerves, a disorder of neuromuscular transmission, or a primary muscle disease. Fasciculation is especially frequent in anterior horn cell disease. A radicular distribution suggests an anterior root lesion. Marked fatiguability and involvement of extraocular, bulbar and proximal muscles suggests myasthenia gravis. The problem of the diagnosis of a pure motor deficit is discussed further on page 283 *et seq.*

A pure sensory deficit may result from a lesion of the posterior root or ganglion, or a peripheral neuropathy affecting purely the sensory nerve fibres. Again a radicular distribution indicates root or ganglion disease, and radicular ('girdle') pain suggests a focal compressive radiculopathy.

A mixed motor and sensory deficit of peripheral nerve type may arise either from a sensorimotor degeneration or from focal damage to a mixed motor nerve. The question which must be asked is: Could the signs be due to a focal lesion of one peripheral nerve? The answer requires a knowledge of the bare bones of neuroanatomy outlined on page 26 *et seq.* The art of the neurological examination is to apply this knowledge during the examination, rather than to test everything and try to fit the picture together afterwards. The expert will immediately recognize that weakness of the triceps and extensors of the wrist and fingers cannot be due to a C7–8 root lesion but must be due to a radial nerve palsy because the brachioradialis is also involved. He sees the sparing of the abductor pollicis brevis muscle of the thenar eminence in a patient with small muscle wasting of the hand and says that this must be due to a lesion of the deep branch of the ulnar nerve and not to a radiculopathy of the first thoracic root. In another case he will notice the Horner's syndrome associated with wasting of the small muscles of one hand and diagnose a Pancoast tumour of the apex of the lung. Only experience, combined with a careful neuroanatomical consideration of every case will produce ease with these problems.

Lesions of the cauda equina may cause considerable diagnostic difficulties. The anatomical arrangement is such that a focal lesion such as a prolapsed intervertebral disc or a neurofibroma may compress many nerve roots, producing an extensive sensory and motor deficit. The resultant picture may be indistinguishable from that of an extensive process such as an ependymoma of the filum terminale or arachnoiditis.

In many patients the symptoms and signs are in a glove and stocking distal distribution, and cannot be due to any focal nerve or root lesion. This pattern always suggests a peripheral neuropathy. At present the cause of this pattern is not certain (see page 136), though it must have a basis in the unusual length of nerve cells.

REFERENCES

DEJONG R. N. (1967) *The Neurologic Examination*, 3rd edn. Hoeber, New York.

DYCK P. J., LAMBERT E. H. and NICHOLS P. C. (1971) Quantitative measurement of sensation related to compound action potential and number and sizes of myelinated and unmyelinated fibers of sural nerve in health, Friedreich's ataxia, hereditary sensory neuropathy, and tabes dorsalis. *Handbook of Electroencephalography and Clinical Neurophysiology* **9**, 9–83–9–118.

DYCK P. J., SCHULTZ, P. W. and O'BRIEN P. C. (1972) Quantitation of touch-pressure sensation. *Arch. Neurol. (Chic.)* **26**, 465–473.

GARDNER-MEDWIN D. and WALTON J. N. (1969) A classification of the neuromuscular disorders and a note on the clinical examination of the voluntary muscles. In *Disorders of Voluntary Muscle*, ed. Walton J. N., pp. 411–453. Churchill, London.

MEDICAL RESEARCH COUNCIL WAR MEMORANDUM (1943) No. 7, revised 2nd edn. HMSO, London.

4

Investigation of Patients with Peripheral Nerve Disease

The investigation of patients with peripheral nerve disease is aimed at learning more about the condition and discovering the cause of the disease. These investigations require to be aimed with thought rather than applied as a diagnostic blunderbuss. Before investigations are instituted a full history (chapter 11), a careful examination (chapter 3), and a diagnostic formulation both of site (chapter 3) and of aetiology (chapter 11) should be attempted. This is the classical teaching in all disease, and certainly applies to peripheral nerve disease. The clinician must know something of the techniques and limitations of the various investigations in order to interpret them intelligently. The investigator must know something of the clinical picture and the results of other investigations to interpret his findings. This is the field *par excellence* for close teamwork.

The special investigations fall into three main categories: electrophysiological, structural and biochemical. A large number of other investigations may also be required to rule out diseases of other parts of the nervous system which may be confused with peripheral nerve disease, to look for other diseases which may be causing the peripheral nerve damage, and to look for associated abnormalities which may be of diagnostic help. For want of a better word, these are grouped under the term *clinical*. Tests of autonomic nerve function are described in chapter 7.

CLINICAL INVESTIGATIONS

The number of these investigations is very large, and it is only intended to provide an outline here. Further consideration of tests of diagnostic significance are found in the consideration of each disease in chapter 6. A full blood count is required in all patients. Anaemia may be associated with

84

many diseases ranging from carcinoma and uraemia to vitamin B_{12} deficiency. The blood film and red cell indices may show macrocytosis indicative of the latter. The serum vitamin B_{12} level should be measured in the many conditions which are not clinically typical of vitamin B_{12} deficiency, since the presentation may be atypical and is readily treatable. Acanthocytes may be seen in Bassen-Kornzweig disease, or atypical white cells may be seen in infectious mononucleosis or leukaemia. The erythrocyte sedimentation rate (ESR) is a useful screening indication of generalized disease, and where abnormal points to further examination of plasma proteins. Blood sugar studies are required where diabetes mellitus or hypoglycaemia are under consideration. Blood urea, electrolytes and liver function tests may reveal unsuspected renal or liver disease. The serum levels of calcium, magnesium and phosphate should be examined whenever neuromuscular transmission is at fault. Increased urinary excretion of various porphyrins and their precursors should be sought in suspected porphyria. Aminoaciduria may occur in a number of different diseases. Specific toxins such as drugs, arsenic, thallium, and heavy metals like lead and mercury may be detected in the urine.

Serological tests for syphilis should be performed in all patients. Syphilis used to be called the 'Great Imitator', and though tabes dorsalis is the only common condition in which it damages the peripheral nerve (posterior root) it should always be considered. Specific tests like the Treponema pallidum immobilization test (TPI) and the fluorescent antibody tests may be needed in suspected tabes where the other serological reactions may have reverted to normal by the time of presentation.

The cerebrospinal fluid may be abnormal in peripheral nerve disease, though it is more frequently abnormal in central nervous disease. The picture of albumino-cytologic dissociation is characteristic of the Guillain-Barré-Strohl syndrome, but may also be caused by meningiomata, neurofibromata and spinal block. The Lange curve abnormalities and the rise in γ-globulin and immunoglobulins in the C.S.F. which occur in neurosyphilis are also found in multiple sclerosis. An increased number of cells in the C.S.F. may be found in the chronic meningitides, granulomatous conditions such as sarcoidosis, and arachnoiditis. Myelography may sometimes be required to investigate patients with radicular syndromes. Other radiological studies include chest x-ray and gastrointestinal studies looking for an underlying carcinoma, and x-rays of the site of peripheral nerve compression looking for bony abnormalities.

ELECTROPHYSIOLOGICAL INVESTIGATIONS

The electrical signs of nervous activity play a large part in investigating neurological disease, and this is particularly true of diseases of the neuro-muscular apparatus. The clinically useful investigations include a study of the conduction velocity and nerve action potentials in the sensory and mixed nerves, of the features of neuromuscular transmission, and of electromyography.

Nerve conduction studies

Motor conduction

The principle of these studies is simple and is illustrated in fig. 4.1 for the median nerve. The nerve is stimulated at a convenient (usually superficial)

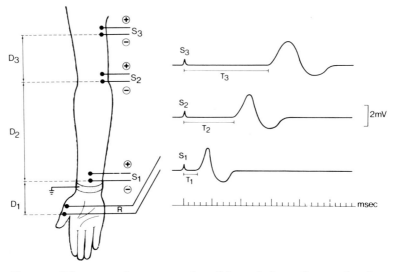

FIG. 4.1. Diagrammatic representation of the technique of measuring the maximum motor conduction velocity in the median nerve.

site by bipolar electrodes, which may be either metal balls, saline-soaked pads or needles. Contact is facilitated by cleaning the skin with ether, and applying a conductive medium like saline, or electrode jelly between each electrode and the skin. The evoked muscle action potential (MAP) is re-corded either with surface electrodes, one over the belly and one over the tendon of the muscle, or with intramuscular needle electrodes. A large earth lead lies between the stimulating and recording electrodes to reduce the stimulus artifact on recording. The recording apparatus consists of a cathode ray oscilloscope and pre-amplifiers, and some means of producing a permanent record of the results. This system should be capable of accur-ately responding to 5–10,000 cycles per second, and of amplitudes from 1 μV to 20 mV. The stimulus is derived from a constant voltage isolated stimulator, capable of providing square wave pulses of 0·01–10 ms dura-tion and of voltage up to 200 volts. A stimulus duration of 0·1 ms is usually used. The applied voltage is slowly increased until an evoked MAP is ob-tained. The site at which the stimulating electrode produces an evoked MAP of greatest amplitude is obtained. The stimulating voltage is increased to obtain the maximum evoked MAP. To ensure that the stimulus is supramaximal, it is then increased by a further 30 per cent.

The stimulus to the median nerve is first applied at the wrist (S_1) and the conduction time between the stimulus and the first deflection from the baseline of the evoked MAP is measured from the oscillograph record (T_1). The distance between the stimulating cathode and the proximal recording electrode (D_1) is also measured. The procedure is repeated with stimula-tion in the anticubital fossa (S_2), and axilla (S_3), and the appropriate con-duction times measured $(T_2$ and $T_3)$. The distance between the cathodal sites for S_1 and S_2 (D_2), and S_2 and S_3 (D_3) are also measured. The maxi-mum motor conduction velocity (MMCV) is given by the equations:

$$\text{MMCV (elbow-wrist) in m/s} = \frac{D_2 \text{ in mm}}{T_2 - T_1 \text{ in ms}}$$

$$\text{MMCV (axilla-elbow) in m/s} = \frac{D_3 \text{ in mm}}{T_3 - T_2 \text{ in ms}}$$

T_1 is the terminal latency expressed as 'X ms for Y cm'. The latency clearly depends upon the distance from the stimulating to the recording electrode. It comprises the time for conduction of nervous impulse to the synapses, the synaptic delay, and the time of conduction of the muscle action potential to the recording electrodes. It is also worth taking note of the amplitude and duration of the evoked MAP with each stimulus, and of the maximal stimulus voltage which is an admittedly rather inaccurate in-dex of the sensitivity of the nerve to electrical stimulation.

Sensory conduction

A similar principle applies to sensory conduction studies. Purely sensory nerves can be studied by stimulating digital (sensory) nerves, and recording from the mixed nerves (orthodromic stimulation) as shown in fig. 4.2, or by stimulating mixed nerves and recording from the digital nerves (antidromic stimulation). The arrangement of the stimulating electrodes is the same as in motor nerve conduction studies but ring electrodes around the digit are used for recording. The sensory nerve action potential (NAP) is however of

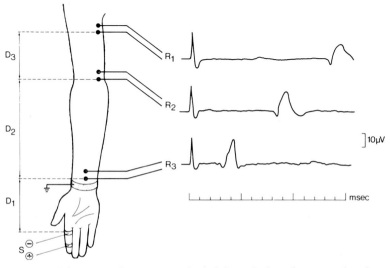

FIG. 4.2. Diagrammatic representation of the technique for measuring the maximum sensory conduction velocity in the median nerve by orthodromic stimulation.

much smaller amplitude than the MAP, being only of the order of 10–50 μV, and averaging techniques are often required. Needle recording electrodes near the nerve may increase the amplitude of the sensory NAP. It was originally customary to record the conduction times T_1, T_2 and T_3 from the beginning of the stimulus to the peak of the sensory NAP of appropriate records R_1, R_2, R_3, since the peak was the most easily identified part of the potential. Averaging techniques now allow a clearer picture of the sensory NAP, and thus the recording of the maximum sensory conduction velocity, calculated in a similar manner to that for the motor velocity.

Values for individual nerves

The nerves most commonly studied in clinical practice are the median as described above, the ulnar and lateral popliteal nerves (see Kaeser 1970). Techniques are, however, well described to study at least motor conduction velocity in the radial (Trojaborg and Sindrup 1969), phrenic (Newsom Davis 1967), femoral (Chopra and Hurwitz 1968), sciatic and medial popliteal nerves (Yap and Hirota 1967). In fact almost any nerve in the body accessible to needle electrodes can be studied. The conduction velocity in most nerves is of the order of 50–70 m/s. The values of the conduction velocity determined are however subject to a number of variables which need to be understood. *Age* has an important effect (Thomas and Lambert 1960). The MMCV in newborn infants is only 20–30 m/s, and it rises with age to reach the adult range at about 3–5 years. There is also a fall again after the thirtieth year of about 10 per cent by the eightieth year. *Temperature* is also important, the MMCV falling by about 2·4 m/s for each 1°C drop in temperature (Abramson *et al.* 1966). The slower conduction velocity in the distal parts of the limbs compared with the proximal part is partly due to this. Wasted limbs are particularly liable to be cold, and it is important that the temperature of the electrophysiology laboratory be about 30°C, that 15 min be allowed for equilibration, and that the skin temperature be measured at the recording site. The *stimulus amplitude* influences the conduction time. This is because the site of initiation of the

TABLE 4.1. Normal range of motor and sensory nerve conduction velocities in median and ulnar nerves (elbow-wrist) and lateral popliteal nerve (knee-ankle) and terminal latency

Nerve	Motor maximum conduction velocity (m/s)	Motor terminal latency (ms)	Evoked muscle action potential (mV)	Sensory maximum conduction velocity (m/s)	Sensory terminal latency (ms)
Median	49–68	2·0–4·5	4·4–14·5	60–70	1·8–3·6
Ulnar	49–66	1·8–3·6	4·3–15	60–70	1·8–3·4
Common peroneal (lateral popliteal)	45–57	3·4–6·8	7·7	45–70	

nerve impulse spreads from the stimulus electrode towards the recording electrode with increased voltage. The use of standardized supramaximal stimuli is important. *Measurement* induces further errors. The greatest difficulty is in accurately measuring the length of the nerve under study, for the distance between the skin marks may be inaccurate by up to 2 cm. Mispositioning of the electrodes, and anomalies of the paths of the nerves may add to this problem. As a result a normal day-to-day variation of at least ± 5 per cent can be expected in measurements of conduction velocity. *Technique* including whether surface or needle electrodes are used, and *apparatus* also play a part in these variables and it is important that each electrophysiology laboratory obtains its own normal values.

Table 4.1 gives the range of values for the three commonly studied nerves taken from studies quoted by Kaeser (1970) to which reference should be made for further details.

Range of conduction velocities

The methods described above measure only the conduction velocity of the few fastest and probably therefore largest nerve fibres, and take no account of the very large majority of smaller myelinated and unmyelinated nerve fibres. If a nerve is damaged in such a way that a few of the largest myelinated nerve fibres remain, though the rest of the fibres have degenerated, then the maximum conduction velocity may be normal, and at the most there may be a decrease in amplitude of the evoked action potential. There are several ways of eliciting information about the slower conducting nerve fibres.

Dispersion of evoked action potential

Whether the action potential is obtained from nerve or muscle, the dispersion is an index of the range of conduction velocity. This dispersion is magnified at greater distances from the point of stimulation. Thus the ratio of the duration of proximally and distally evoked action potentials is greater where the range of conduction velocity is greater.

Single nerve fibre studies

These have been performed in man by Knutsson and Widén (1967) and Bergmans (1970). Only a few single nerve fibres can be studied in each nerve, and they probably are usually though not necessarily the largest ones.

Blocking techniques

These have been developed to study the slower conducting nerve fibres. The principle of these methods is that two stimuli are applied at distant points along a nerve in rapid succession. The nerve action potential pro-

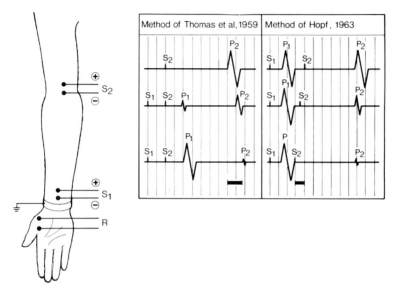

FIG. 4.3. Diagram of two methods of estimating the range of nerve fibre conduction velocities in man. The black bars show the range of conduction times which in the method of Thomas et al. is the interval between the beginning of the maximum and minimum P_2 response, and in the method of Hopf is the interval between the time of S_2 which just produces a minimum response and that which just produces a maximum response (see text).

duced by one stimulus arrives at the site of the second stimulus during the refractory period of some of the fibres. The conduction in these fibres is therefore blocked, and the conduction of the other more slowly conducting fibres can therefore be studied. Two methods are diagrammatically represented in fig. 4.3. The *method of Thomas et al.* (1959) is to apply a supramaximal test stimulus (S_2) at the elbow a few milliseconds after a variable blocking stimulus (S_1) at the wrist, recording in the hand. The fastest conduction time (latency) is determined in the usual way with the amplitude of S_1 at zero, by measuring the interval between S_2 and the first displacement of the evoked muscle action potential (P_2). As the intensity of the blocking stimulus (S_1) is increased, more and more fibres at the wrist are stimulated, and thus are refractory when the action potential of the test stimulus S_2 arrives at the wrist. The impulses coming from the elbow in the slower conducting fibres will however reach the wrist after the refractory period has passed, and will thus get through the 'block'. The interval between S_2 and the first displacement of P_2 is thus increased. If the intensity of S_1 is increased to the stage that it almost abolishes P_2, the latency of the evoked MAP is that of the slowest conducting nerve fibres. The range of velocity is thus given by the equation:

$$\text{Range} = \frac{\text{Longest latency} - \text{shortest latency}}{\text{Shortest latency}} \times 100 \text{ per cent}$$

The *method of Hopf* (1963) differs in that S_1 and S_2 are both supramaximal, the interval between the stimuli being variable. If the interval is long, the refractory period in all the fibres at the wrist following S_1 will have passed by the time S_2 is applied. As the interval shortens, the slowest conducting fibres will still be in their refractory period following S_1 when S_2 test volley arrives, and therefore P_2 begins to decrease in amplitude. As the interval between S_1 and S_2 is decreased further, eventually *all* the fibres are in the refractory period when the S_2 test volley arrives, and P_2 is therefore abolished. The range of velocities is given by the equation:

$$\text{Range} = \frac{\text{Interval for maximal } P_2 - \text{interval for minimal } P_2}{\text{Latency of first displacement of maximal } P_2} \times 100 \text{ per cent}$$

By the method of Thomas *et al.* (1959), most fibres conduct with a velocity of more than 85 per cent of the fastest fibres, though in a few the conduction velocity is about 40 per cent less than that of the fastest. By the method of Hopf (1963) the range of conduction velocities is about 88–100 per cent of the fastest.

Nerve conduction in vitro

This has been studied in sural nerve biopsies in man by Dyck and Lambert (1966). By this method it is possible to demonstrate the complete compound nerve action potential with A, B and C peaks. The A peak is due to large myelinated nerve fibres conducting at about 70 m/s, the B being due to small myelinated nerve fibres conducting at about 10 m/s, and the C potential due to unmyelinated nerve fibres conducting at about 2 m/s (see page 46 *et seq.*). It is therefore clear that the blocking techniques described above study only a very small part of the true range of conduction of fibres in a peripheral nerve.

Late waves

When a motor nerve is stimulated electrically, an evoked nerve action potential travels to the muscle producing an electrical response, the M wave. The latency of this response is short, the conduction velocity usually being 50–70 m/s as described above. In suitable situations, evoked muscle action potentials may appear with a greater latency. Two main types of late wave are recognized, the H reflex and the F wave. The impulses for both initially travel towards the spinal cord only to return later to the muscle. The H reflex was originally elicited from leg muscles, especially the soleus, while the F wave is particularly found in the small hand muscles. Under suitable circumstances however both may be elicited from a wide variety of muscles.

H reflex

As the stimulus current is slowly increased from subliminal values, the first evoked muscle action potential is the H reflex, having a long latency (fig. 4.4). The H wave is best elicited from the more distal leg muscles. As the stimulus intensity is increased, the direct M wave is elicited, and gradually the amplitude of the H wave falls. If the stimulation site is moved distally, the interval between the M and H waves gradually increases suggesting that the H reflex travels centrally. The latency indicates that it travels by a monosynaptic path through the spinal cord.

Other late waves

These include the F wave, and may take a similar antidromic course to the H reflex, but return to the muscle via an axon reflex without invading the spinal cord.

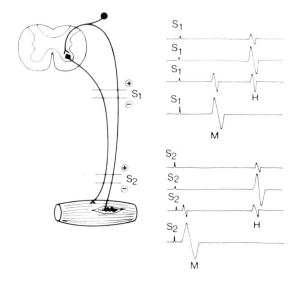

FIG. 4.4. The H reflex. As the stimulus strength is increased at each stimulus site (from above downwards) the H wave appears, becomes maximal, and then gradually disappears as the M wave reaches maximum. As the stimulus is moved towards the muscle (S_2) the interval between the M and H waves increase.

Conduction velocity in disease states

Following transection of a nerve

Though transection abolishes the transmission of a nerve impulse across the break in the nerve, the fibres in the distal part of the nerve remain electrically excitable for 72 to 96 hours after transection. Many fibres however begin to break down well before this (see page 130 *et seq.*), and by 48 hours the amplitude of the evoked nerve action potential has fallen by 90 per cent of normal due to loss of fibres. The conduction velocity remain within 20 per cent of the normal right up to the time of cessation of conduction. If the nerve is allowed to regenerate after a crush, nerve conduction once more becomes re-established. Initially the newly regenerated axons are of abnormally small diameter, and the newly formed myelin sheath abnormally thin. Both result in a very slow rate of conduction.

Both parameters recover almost to normal in the next 12 to 24 months and the maximum nerve conduction velocity continues to rise to 60 to

95 per cent of normal with increasing maturation of the axon and myelin sheath diameter (Berry *et al.* 1944, Sanders and Whitteridge 1946). However the myelinated nerve fibres in such a regenerated nerve have internodes which are all about 0·3 mm long compared to the previous internodal length of the largest fibres of about 1·5 mm (see page 118). It is therefore clear that the internodal length does not govern the conduction velocity (Cragg and Thomas 1957) (see page 43).

Neuropathies with axonal degeneration

In axonal neuropathies (see page 135), there is patchy degeneration of axons. However providing some large myelinated nerve fibres are unaffected, the maximum conduction velocity may be normal despite a very severe neuropathy. The loss of fibres will be indicated by the fall in the amplitude of the evoked NAP, and the amplitude of the sensory NAP may fall below the threshold for the method and become unrecordable. In 'dying back neuropathies' (see page 136), the terminal latency may be abnormally slowed, while the proximal nerve conduction velocity may be normal.

Neuropathies with segmental demyelination

In these there is a loss of the myelin sheaths, extending from widening of the node of Ranvier to total demyelination of internodes in a patchy fashion throughout the nerve (see page 137 *et seq.*). This process leads to a blockage of conduction in many nerve fibres, and to profound slowing of conduction in others. In experimental diphtheritic neuropathy, the rate may drop to 20 m/s, and in chronic hypertrophic neuropathies in man conduction velocities of as little as 3 m/s have been recorded. Similarly the mixed NAP may fall to only 5 per cent of normal and the sensory NAP is often decreased to below the sensitivity of the methods, becoming unrecordable.

There is a remarkable capacity of the central nervous system to adapt to delayed conduction of impulses in the peripheral nervous system. In experimental diphtheritic neuropathy, clinical recovery of the animals may occur despite continuing low motor nerve conduction velocities (Morgan-Hughes 1968), and in chronic hypertrophic neuropathies in man, the patients may have no complaints despite a maximum conduction velocity which is only 12 per cent of normal (Bradley and Aguayo 1969).

Nerve entrapment or compression

Nerve compression leads first to local segmental demyelination and decreased axonal diameter, and later to progressive axonal degeneration (see page 152 *et seq.*). The site of compression can readily be localized by electrophysiological studies, for there is focal slowing of the maximum nerve conduction velocity across the site of compression. In ulnar nerve entrapment at the elbow for instance, the conduction velocity from the axilla to above the elbow and from below the elbow to the wrist may be 60 m/s, while the conduction across the short segment of the elbow may only be 15 m/s.

Drawbacks of nerve conduction measurements

The major drawback of the usual clinical investigations of nerve conduction is the total lack of information concerning other than the largest myelinated nerve fibres. For instance in amyloid neuropathy, the patient may have profound analgesia resulting in severe burns and abscess formation with perfectly normal maximum conduction velocity studies. Another pitfall is that a proximal demyelinating lesion such as that in the nerve roots in the Guillain-Barré-Strohl syndrome, may block nerve conduction to and from the spinal cord, yet leave distal nerve conduction velocities entirely normal. The use of the H reflex may help circumvent this pitfall, for it will tend to be depressed or abolished by such a proximal demyelinating lesion. A significant symptomatic neuropathy may be present and yet the decrease in the number of the largest myelinated nerve fibres may be insufficient to be detectable by a fall in the amplitude of evoked NAP. It is therefore wrong to conclude that the peripheral nerves are normal because the peripheral maximum nerve conduction velocity studies are normal. In a mixed neuropathy, the effect of segmental demyelination in slowing nerve conduction will predominate, and a major degree of axonal degeneration may not be recognized by nerve conduction studies alone. All of these drawbacks must be recognized when interpreting nerve conduction studies.

Motor unit counts

The motor unit is defined as the anterior horn cell, its branched axon and the muscle fibres which it innervates. The number of muscle fibres in a motor unit in different muscles has been estimated by dividing the total number of muscle fibres in a muscle by the total number of anterior horn cells and motor nerves supplying that muscle. This number varies from about ten in the extraocular muscles to several thousand in the larger limb muscles. McComas has developed a method for analysing the total number of motor units in the extensor digitorum brevis muscle of man *in vivo* (McComas *et al.* 1971). The technique is diagrammatically represented in fig. 4.5. The nerve to the extensor digitorum brevis muscle is stimulated at the ankle, and the evoked MAP recorded with surface electrodes extending over the end-plate zone of the muscle. The nerve stimulus is gradually increased from subliminal values until a threshold evoked MAP is obtained. This has all-or-none characteristics, and is the first evoked motor unit. With gradually increasing stimulus strength, a second, third, and further motor unit action potentials can be evoked in a stepwise manner. The mean

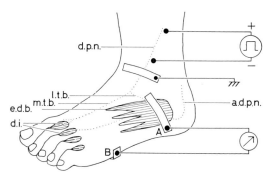

FIG. 4.5. Technique for estimating the motor unit count in the extensor digitorum brevis muscle. (*From* McComas *et al.* 1971.)

amplitude of these initial motor units can be calculated. If a supramaximal stimulus is now applied, the amplitude of the maximum evoked MAP is the sum of the amplitude of each motor unit action potential. The estimated number of motor units in the muscle is given by the formula:

$$\text{Estimated motor unit count} = \frac{\text{Amplitude of maximal evoked muscle action potential}}{\text{Mean amplitude of initial single evoked motor unit potentials}}$$

The mean number of motor units in the extensor digitorum brevis muscle of normal individuals of age 4 to 58 years was 199 ± 60, and the lowest value accepted as normal was 120. The method has potential application to the small muscles of the hands, but regrettably it is not applicable to larger limb muscles. The method depends on the end-plates lying within an equal distance of the recording electrode. It makes the assumption that the degree of branching in the motor axons is the same in all individuals, and in all diseases studied. If branching normally produces two axons at the ankle from one anterior horn cell in the spinal cord, the estimated motor unit count will be *twice* the true number of motor units. If for some reason in any condition no branching occurred then the estimate will be the *true* number of motor units, and if twice the normal amount of branching occurred, then the estimate would be four times the true number of motor units. No way exists of estimating the degree of branching.

Neuromuscular transmission

The major part of our understanding of synaptic transmission emanates from studies using microelectrodes implanted into muscle fibres at the end-plate zone. Such studies are however not possible for routine clinical practice. The methods available for clinical assessment of neuromuscular transmission are repetitive nerve stimulation, and the study of agents acting upon neuromuscular transmission.

Repetitive nerve stimulation

Neuromuscular transmission in a normal individual will tolerate repetitive stimulation of up to 40 per second with less than a 30 per cent decrement of the evoked MAP in 10 seconds. In patients with myasthenia gravis (see page 270 *et seq.*) if two single stimuli to the motor nerves are applied at an interval which may range from 20 ms to 2 s, the second evoked muscle action potential may be significantly smaller than the first. Repetitive stimulation at as little as 3 per second produces a rapidly decremental response. The amplitude may fall to 50 per cent of the first response within a few seconds (Desmedt and Borenstein 1970) (see fig. 4.6). A maximum voluntary effort will similarly cause decrement of the evoked MAP. This failure of neuromuscular transmission is the physiological accompaniment of the clinically observed easy fatiguability in myasthenia gravis. Unfortunately the response is not necessarily seen in every muscle in myasthenia gravis, and therefore the absence of a decremental response in the small hand muscles does not exclude the diagnosis.

In the myasthenic syndrome of Eaton and Lambert (see page 273), the clinical complaint is of weakness, but the diagnostic sign is of facilitation of power with repeated effort. Electrophysiologically this is seen as an abnormally small first evoked muscle action potential, followed by an *incremental* response of more than 50 per cent with stimuli applied at 10–30 per second.

Substances acting upon neuromuscular transmission

Classically neuromuscular transmission in myasthenia gravis is enhanced by anticholinesterases, and worsened dramatically by competitive blocking agents like curare. Diagnostic tests are based upon these effects.

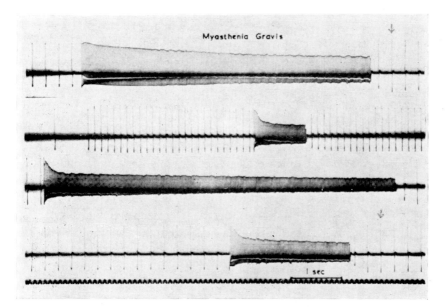

FIG. 4.6. Four examples of the decremental response of the evoked muscle action potential to rapid repetitive nerve stimulation in patients with myasthenia gravis. (*From* Simpson J.A. 1960. *Scottish Medical Journal* **5**, 419.)

Anticholinesterase tests

Edrophonium is a short-acting anticholinesterase, and is useful in the diagnosis of myasthenia gravis. A clinically involved muscle is fatigued to the point of maximum weakness; an extraocular muscle is often particularly useful for this. An intravenous injection of edrophonium is then given, leading to an immediate rise in the concentration of acetylcholine at the motor end-plates, and thus to facilitation of neuromuscular transmission. The injection is fractionated, 0·5–1 mg being given initially, followed by a further 1–2 mg 2 min later if there is no response. The remaining 7 mg may be given after a further 2 min if normal power is not restored. This fractionation is important because a few individuals may be unduly sensitive to anticholinesterases, and thus develop cardiac arrest or go into cholinergic block with the full dose of 10 mg of edrophonium.

The usual result of the edrophonium test is a dramatic increase in muscle strength within ½–2 min of the injection, and the power of the fatigued muscle may return to normal. This response may be followed electrophysiologically during repetitive nerve stimulation. Neostigmine 1·5 mg with 0·6 mg of atropine sulphate may be administered intramuscularly as a diagnostic test if edrophonium fails. The latency of its effect is about 15 min.

Neuromuscular blocking agents

Any test using neuromuscular blocking agents must only be undertaken with the help of an anaesthetist and with full facilities for intubation and artificial respiration. Patients with myasthenia gravis are unusually resistant to depolarizing neuromuscular blocking agents such as decamethonium iodide. They may have little effect from 2–5 mg of this compound which will produce paralysis in a normal person. On the other hand they are exquisitely sensitive to the effects of competitive neuromuscular blocking agents such as d-tubocurarine. This is unlike the situation in the myasthenic syndrome, where this differential sensitivity is not present. An intravenous injection of d-tubocurarine at a dose of 3 mg/40 lb body weight will paralyse a normal individual. Two to 5 per cent of this dose is normally without any effect, but will severely weaken or even completely paralyse a patient with myasthenia gravis. The response may be followed electrophysiologically with repetitive nerve stimulation.

Neither the decamethonium nor the d-tubocurarine test are entirely safe, and a regional curare sensitivity test has been developed by Foldes *et al.* (1968). After the arm has been elevated for one minute, the arterial and venous supplies to the hand are occluded by a sphygmomanometer cuff at above systolic pressure applied to the arm. An intravenous injection of 0·2 mg of d-tubocurarine is given into a vein below the cuff. Five and a half minutes later the cuff is released, and the grip strength measured at 7, 11 and 16 min after injection. In normal individuals and patients with purely

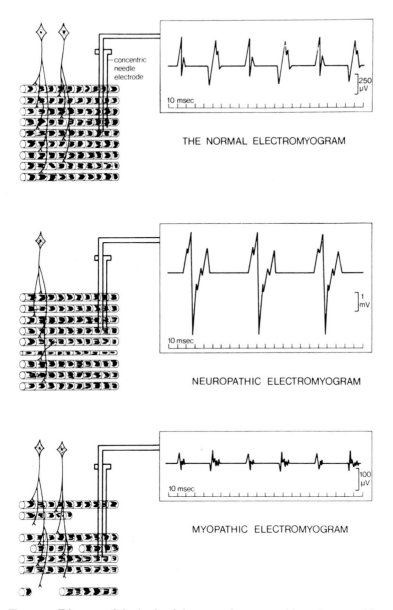

FIG. 4.7. Diagram of the basis of the normal, neuropathic and myopathic electromyogram during weak voluntary contraction.

ocular myasthenia, the grip fell by 10·0 ± 3·9 per cent, while in those with generalized myasthenia gravis it fell by 67·9 ± 7·0 per cent.

Electromyography

The principle of electromyography is illustrated in fig. 4.7. The recording electrode is a needle, usually with a concentric insulated wire in the middle.

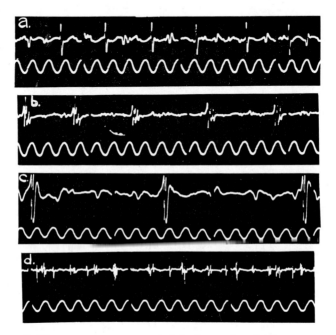

FIG. 4.8. Electromyograms recorded during weak voluntary contraction. *a* Normal motor unit potentials. *b* Long duration neuropathic polyphasic motor unit potentials. *c* Large amplitude long duration neuropathic motor unit potentials. *d* Small amplitude myopathic polyphasic potentials. Calibration 50 cycles at 300 μV. (*From* Richardson and Barwick 1969.)

Only the tip of this wire is free of insulation, the outer part of the needle acting as the second electrode. Such a needle records the electrical events occurring in the muscle fibres only in the region of the tip of the needle, and this activity may be amplified and recorded by a cathode ray oscilloscope (Richardson and Barwick 1969, Lenman and Ritchie 1970).

Normal electromyogram

At rest, when the needle is inserted, there is a brief discharge from injured muscle fibres of less than 0·5 s, and then electrical silence. *Weak contraction* evokes isolated muscle action potentials (MAP) usually of 8–12 ms duration and 200–800 μV amplitude (figs. 4.7 and 4.8). The exact values depend on the muscle under test. Each muscle action potential is the summation of the electrical events occurring in the muscle fibres of a single motor unit. It

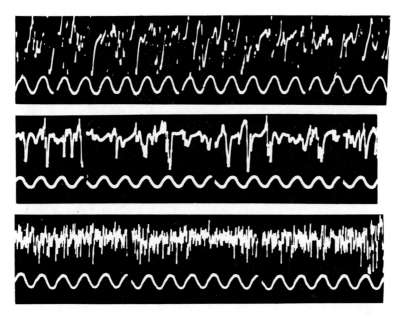

FIG. 4.9. Electromyograms recorded during maximal voluntary contraction. *Upper,* normal full interference pattern. *Middle,* neuropathic incomplete interference pattern. *Lower,* myopathic full interference pattern of low amplitude. (*From* Richardson and Barwick 1969.)

is however irregular in outline because the electrical events in the individual muscle fibres of the motor unit do not reach the recording unit in a smoothly synchronized fashion. This is because of the varying distance which the nerve impulse travels at about 60 m/s along the intramuscular nerves, and the varying distance along the muscle fibres that the muscle action potential travels at about 4 m/s from the motor end-plates to the recording electrode. The usual muscle action potential has a maximum of three phases crossing the baseline. A *mild contraction* elicits a few more MAPs. With *maximum voluntary effort* the superimposition of a large number of MAPs completely obliterates the baseline. This is called a *full interference pattern* (fig. 4.9).

Electromyogram in neuropathic disorders

In disorders of the α-motoneuron and peripheral motor nerves, there is atrophy of some muscle fibres and reinnervation of others by surviving motoneurons. *At rest, fibrillation potentials* may be seen. These perhaps result from supersensitivity of single denervated fibres to circulating acetylcholine, or from the spontaneous discharge of single presynaptic terminals of degenerating motor nerves. They are usually of 1–2 phases, 0·5–2 ms in duration and 30–150 μV amplitude. *Weak contraction* produces isolated MAPs which are much larger than normal because each motor unit has many more muscle fibres, and which are longer and more polyphasic than normal because of sprouting of the intramuscular nerves producing considerable delay in intramuscular conduction (figs. 4.7 and 4.8). Because of the fall-out of motor units, on *maximum voluntary effort* individual MAPs can still be recognized and the baseline is not completely obliterated (fig. 4.9). This is termed an *incomplete interference pattern*. Because of intramuscular nerve sprouting, and the decreased number of motor units, the size and spread within the muscle of surviving motor units is increased. This can be demonstrated either by a multi-electrode with many recording points on a single needle, or with two needles at a distance. Normally synchronization of MAPs does not occur if the needles are more than 0·5 cm apart, but with increased intramuscular sprouting synchronization may be seen with the needles more than 2 cm apart.

Electromyogram in myopathies

The patchy loss of whole or parts of individual muscle fibres produces a characteristic picture. *At rest*, the muscle is silent in most myopathies, though in polymyositis there is a marked increase in insertional activity. *Weak contraction* elicits MAPs which are of lower amplitude than normal due to the loss of muscle fibres. They are more polyphasic than normal since this loss of fibres prevents the smoothing effect of summation of a large number of individual muscle fibre potentials. They are shorter than normal because the smaller individual muscle fibre action potentials are not recorded (figs. 4.7 and 4.8). *Mild contraction* produces a full interference pattern because all the motor units must be contracted in the weakened muscle to produce even a mild contraction. *Maximum voluntary effort* produces a full interference pattern with a very decreased maximum amplitude compared with normal (fig. 4.9).

Fibrillation potentials are not specific for neuropathic disorders. They may be profuse in polymyositis perhaps due to involvement of the motor nerve terminals, or perhaps as a result of an area of necrosis effectively denervating the parts of the muscle fibre away from the innervation zone. Recent evidence suggests that regenerating fibres may be the site of fibrillation potentials. A similar explanation may be applied to the muscular dystrophies where fibrillation potentials may often be elicited. Mixed neuropathies and myopathies are obviously difficult to separate. Mild early and severe late neuropathies and myopathies may not be easy to diagnose because so few muscle fibres remain and secondary changes of the muscle and nerve may occur. Like all investigations, electrophysiological studies must be considered together with the clinical picture and the results of all the other studies.

STRUCTURAL STUDIES

Peripheral nerve

Biopsy examination of the peripheral nervous system is possible if care is taken in the selection of the nerve. Removal of a length of the nerve will denervate a part of the body and thought must be given to which nerve will produce the least neurological deficit while revealing the maximum information. It is also important to be certain that the information which can be expected from the biopsy is sufficient to justify the procedure, and cannot be obtained in some other way (see also Thomas 1970). In most cases very little information can be gleaned from the simple haematoxylin and eosin-stained section, which is all that is studied in many routine pathological laboratories. Quantitative, single fibre, and ultrastructural studies are required completely to elucidate the nature of the disease. The proper study of a nerve biopsy is therefore a lengthy process. It may also be somewhat frustrating due to the structure of the nerve. The lesion may be proximal to the site of the biopsy, and all that is seen is axonal degeneration secondary to this lesion, which cannot itself be identified. In particular many degenerations of the peripheral nervous system are due to changes in the perikarya, which are unfortunately not susceptible to biopsy.

These difficulties obviously do not exist in the autopsy investigation of the peripheral nervous system. Here the whole nerve may be studied from the anterior horn cell and posterior root ganglion neuron to the sensory and motor terminations, but the sheer extent of the study may be daunting. Moreover changes begin soon after death which make study difficult. The ultrastructure of the cells deteriorate within an hour of death. Though much information can be obtained at the light microscopic level, swelling of the Schmidt-Lanterman clefts and separation of the myelin lamellae begins to cause difficulty after about 12 hours.

This section will outline the procedures involved in the study of the peripheral nerve. The technical details of the stains and procedures employed are given in the Appendix.

Choice of nerve

Optimally the clinical and electrophysiological studies define the site of the lesion and this is biopsied. More commonly the level of the lesion cannot be defined or is diffuse. The choice is then of which nerve and where to take a sample.

Sensory nerve

In a pure sensory neuropathy a sensory nerve such as the sural may be biopsied. The loss of sensation which results is frequently small due to the overlap from adjacent nerves, and usually disappears within a few months with regeneration of nerve fibres. However where regeneration is impaired, this recovery may be delayed. Some people are bothered by painful dysaesthesiae during recovery of sensation. For this reason Dyck advises restricting the procedure to the removal of only one fascicle of the nerve, the remainder of which is left intact (Dyck and Lofgren 1968). This rarely results in significant sensory loss or late dysaesthesiae. Clearly the procedure must not endanger sensation of important structures like the fingers, but within these restrictions any sensory nerve accessible to the surgeon may be biopsied. As may be seen below, optimally 8–10 cm of nerve are required, which limits the choice of nerve.

Motor nerve

Only in the anterior roots and intramuscular nerve terminals may motor fibres be separated from sensory fibres. The investigation of a pure motor neuropathy is thus difficult. The intramuscular nerve endings may be studied by methylene blue preparations of motor point biopsies (see page 120 et seq.). Anterior nerve root biopsy is not feasible. All other nerves including muscular nerves are mixed, at least 50 per cent of the fibres being sensory. Few muscular or mixed nerves can be taken in toto because of the resultant muscle paralysis. Exceptions include the nerve to the extensor digitorum brevis muscle in the foot, to the peroneus tertius muscle in the shin and to the palmaris longus muscle in the forearm. None is however an easy dissection, and considerable experience of the anatomy of these nerves in the cadaver is required before attempting a biopsy. Fascicular biopsy of any mixed nerve may be performed, but fear of the production of significant paralysis usually limits this procedure.

Nerve biopsy procedure

The technique of sural nerve biopsy will be described. Modification is required for fascicular biopsies and other nerves.

Operation

The nerve may be removed under general or local anaesthesia. Care must be taken to avoid damaging the nerve throughout the operation. Infiltration with local anaesthetics, and touching the nerve during the procedure should particularly be avoided. Application of a tourniquet to the leg to allow operation in a bloodless field is not recommended if the nerve is required for electron microscopy. The site of the nerve is shown in fig. 4.10. A 10 cm length of the nerve is freed, grasped at one end only, and cut from the body with sharp scissors.

Histological preparation

Immediately after removal, the nerve is laid on dental wax and cut into five pieces 2 cm in length with razor blades. These are treated as shown in fig. 4.10 and table 4.2. Technical details are given in the Appendix. Unless the nerve is fixed under tension, the nerve fibres take up a wavy course, making good orientation impossible. Fixation with a weight hanging on one end is the best procedure, though alternatively the nerve may be stretched on a piece of card prior to fixation. The threads for hanging the weights must be tied to the nerve or threaded through it with a fine needle. Penetration with Flemming's solution is slow, and more prolonged fixation or

TABLE 4.2. An outline of the histological techniques used in the preparation of nerve biopsies (for technical details see Appendix)

Segment	Fixation	Post-fixation	Embedding medium	Section thickness	Stains
1	Susa for 4–8 h		Paraffin wax or Pertefi's double embedding method	5–8 μm	H and E. Solochrome cyanin. Silver stains such as Glees and Marsland or Palmgren for axons
2	Flemming's solution for 24 h		Paraffin wax or Pertifi's double embedding method	5–8 μm	Weigert-Pal for myelin sheaths
3	3·6% glutaraldehyde in 0·1 M phosphate buffer at pH 7·4 for 2 h at 4°C	2% osmic acid in same buffer for 2 h at 4°C	Araldite	Semi-thin 1–2 μm. Ultra-thin for electron micrography	Semi-thin: toluidine blue. Ultra-thin: uranyl acetate and lead citrate
4	Formol-calcium solution for 24 h	1% osmic acid in same buffer for 24 h. Maceration in 30%, 60% and 100% glycerol over 3 days			(For teasing single nerve fibres)
5	Formol-calcium or none		Frozen	10–20 μm	(For histochemical techniques, metachromatic stains etc.)

prior dissection of individual fasciculi is required for nerves any thicker than the sural nerve.

It is difficult to obtain first class fixation of nerve for *electron microscopy*. Penetration of glutaraldehyde is relatively slow, the perineurium being a barrier. Any attempt to cut the nerve into smaller fragments produces extensive damage to the myelin sheaths. It is better to fix the whole sural nerve in glutaraldehyde for 1 hour under tension, and then to cut it longitudinally into pieces about 1–2 mm in diameter and then to continue fixation under tension for a further 1 hour. The nerve is further cut into pieces

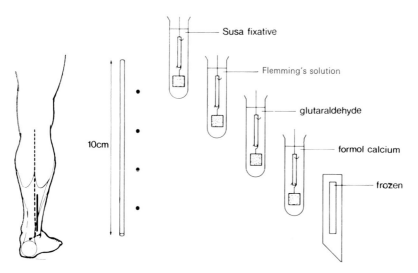

FIG. 4.10. Surface markings of the sural nerve, and division of the biopsy into five pieces (see text).

1 mm in diameter prior to osmic acid post-fixation. Alternatively small twigs or fasciculi may be dissected before fixation. The terminal 3 mm at either end of each piece must be discarded after fixation to eliminate the major crush artefacts which appear as myelin rosettes (Haftek and Thomas 1968). Transverse and longitudinal sections embedded in plastic and stained with toluidine blue are useful for viewing the structure of the nerve at the light microscopic level. Appropriate ultrathin sections are examined under the electron microscope. Axonal degeneration (fig. 4.11), myelin fragmentation and segmental demyelination (fig. 4.12), the abnormally thin

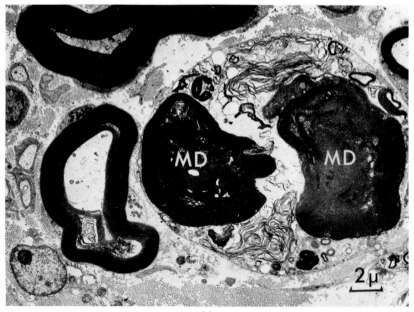

(a)

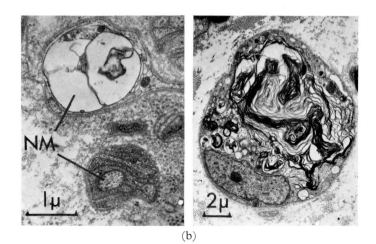

(b)

FIG. 4.11. Electron micrographs of axonal degeneration. *a* Large myelinated fibre in which the axon has been lost and the myelin completely
broken down to debris (MD). *b Left*, vacuolated swollen unmyelinated
nerve fibre above and normal unmyelinated nerve fibre below (NM).
Right, small nerve fibre in which the myelin sheath has broken down,
though the Schwann cell nucleus is preserved and active.

myelin sheath which indicates remyelination after segmental demyelination (fig. 4.13), and onion bulb formation (fig. 4.13) are easily recognized
under the electron microscope. Myelin debris in macrophages and Schwann
cells indicates myelin breakdown. The electron microscopy of nerve,
however, is not an easy field. There are many artefacts and 'abnormalities',
and a thorough knowledge of the range of appearances in normal nerve is
of the utmost importance. In a few conditions, specific pathological
changes are recognized, and these are described in chapter 6.

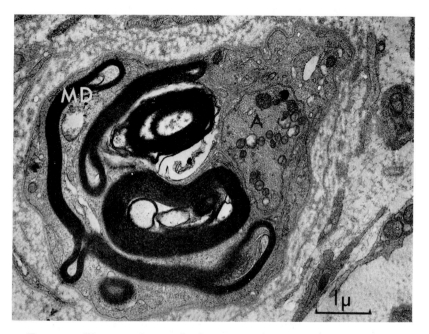

FIG. 4.12. Electron micrograph of a nerve undergoing segmental demyelination. The axon (A) is denuded of myelin, and shows minor structural
alterations. The debris of the myelin sheath (MD) is undergoing digestion on one side of the Schwann cell cytoplasm.

The *Susa-fixed material* is mounted in paraffin wax to provide a longitudinal and transverse section. Better preservation is obtained by methacrylate embedding (Rindell 1967). Haematoxylin and esoin staining shows
the general cellular structure. Solochrome cyanin stains the neurokeratin of
the myelin, the protein net-like matrix remaining after removal of lipids
during processing. The appearance is very different from myelin *in vivo* or

with the Weigert-Pal stain. All the silver stains for axons are fickle; the rarely achieved object is to obtain specific staining of axons with no major staining of the connective tissue. The method of Palmgren is perhaps the most reliable. The axons are much better examined under the electron microscope.

On haematoxylin and eosin-stained sections, cellular infiltration, blood vessel changes, thickening of the perineurium and fibrosis can be assessed.

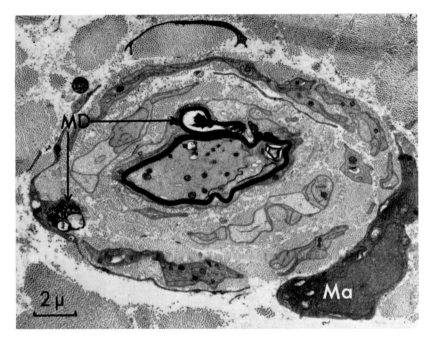

FIG. 4.13. Electron micrograph of a thinly remyelinated axon lying in the centre of an 'onion bulb'. Myelin debris (MD) lies in the cytoplasm both of the central Schwann cell and of a peripheral Schwann cell lamella. Ma, macrophage.

The density of the Schwann cells, which increases in most chronic neuropathies, particularly those with segmental demyelination, can be assessed and measured. Axonal degeneration can often be recognized by the presence of myelin digestion chambers (fig. 4.14). Rarely is the differential staining of axons and neurokeratin sufficient to allow the study of these structures. Solochrome cyanin allows study of the myelin sheaths, and is particularly useful for the demonstration of myelin ovoids resulting from the fragmentation and digestion of the myelin sheaths in axonal degeneration and of Schmidt-Lanterman clefts. Silver stains, when reliable, allow an assessment of the density of axons and their size. Fragmentation and axon spirals may be seen in axonal degeneration.

The *Flemming-fixed material* is also orientated to provide longitudinal and transverse sections and stained by the Weigert-Pal method to show the myelin sheaths. The loss of myelinated nerve fibres and particularly the size of fibre affected may be assessed by eye, though it is more accurately judged by the method of measurement described below. Active axonal degeneration is signalled by chains of myelin ovoids (fig. 4.15). A Weigert-Pal/Van Gieson stain is particularly useful for searching for onion bulb formation under the light microscope (see pages 141 and 188 *et seq.*).

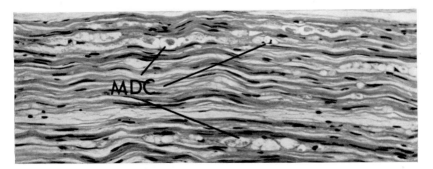

FIG. 4.14. Longitudinal section of sural nerve in polyarteritis nodosa showing axonal degeneration with myelin digestion chambers (MDC). H & E × 120.

For measuring the transverse diameter spectrum, the transverse section should be as accurately orientated as possible. Individual transversely cut fasciculi are photographed and printed at × 1000 magnification for measurement of the total number of myelinated nerve fibres, and the transverse diameter spectrum. The outer myelin sheath diameter of each myelinated nerve fibre may be measured with a ruler, or more rapidly by matching a template with holes of 1–30 mm (equivalent to 1–30 μm in the original nerve) against the photograph and counting on a semiautomatic device (Espir and Harding 1961). Various other semiautomatic particle size analysers such as the Zeiss TGZ3 may be adapted for this purpose (Romero and Skoghund 1965). Automatic devices have so far proved unable to recognize individual nerve fibres or separate these from debris, blood vessels and other structures. If the nerve is not accurately orientated, obliquely cut fibres appear as ovals with one axis artefactually larger than normal (Dyck *et al.* 1968). Allowance can be made for this by measuring only the maximum minor axis diameter. The fibres within a fasciculus which is artefactually flattened during fixation are also ovals, and for this reason fixation on a card for fibre diameter spectrum measurement is not recommended. There are always some fibres which run obliquely in fasciculi, but the block must be orientated so that as many as possible of the myelin sheaths appear as circular profiles.

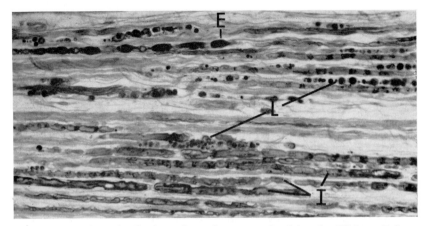

FIG. 4.15. Longitudinal section of nerve stained by the Weigert Pal method showing various stages of axonal degeneration in a patient with vincristine neuropathy. Fibres showing early breakdown of the myelin sheaths (E), and the late stage of fragmentation into myelin ovoids (L), stand out from the intact myelin sheaths (I). × 120.

All the fibres in one or more fasciculi are measured and counted. The optimal number of fibres to be counted is about 1000 for each nerve. The total cross-sectional area of the fasciculi which have been counted may be measured with a planimeter on a low-power photographic print of known magnification. From these measurements can be calculated the myelinated nerve fibre density expressed as myelinated nerve fibres/mm². If a whole sural nerve biopsy is under study, the total number of myelinated nerve fibres in the whole nerve may be calculated by multiplying the total number of fibres in the counted fasciculi by the fraction:

$$\frac{\text{Total fascicular area of the nerve}}{\text{Total area of fasciculi counted}}$$

The fascicular area depends upon preparative methods, all of which lead to considerable shrinkage of the nerve. Table 4.3 shows the degree of

TABLE 4.3. Amount of shrinkage resulting from fixation of the sural nerve in various solutions. The total transverse fascicular area after fixation and embedding in paraffin wax is expressed as a percentage of the cryostat section (unfixed) transverse fascicular area. For details of fixatives see Appendix

Fixative	Time (hours)	Total fascicular area %
Flemming's solution	24	80
2·5% glutaraldehyde in 0·1M phosphate buffer	4	70
5% glutaraldehyde in 0·1M phosphate buffer	4	69
5% formol-calcium	24	58
10% formol-calcium	24	56
5% formol-saline★	24	76
10% formol-saline★	24	62
Susa solution	4	66

★ 5 and 10% concentrated formaldehyde solution (36%) in 0·9% sodium chloride solution.

shrinkage produced by various fixatives, and it can be seen that the transverse fascicular area of the Flemming's-fixed sural nerve is reduced to 80 per cent of the area of the unfixed frozen section. Because of the variable shrinkage occurring during preparation, the fibre density depends upon the method of fixation. For this reason whole sural nerves are often preferred to fascicular biopsies for the estimation of the preservation of myelinated nerve fibres.

The myelinated nerve fibre diameter spectrum of the normal sural nerve is bimodal with peaks at 4 and 11 µm (see fig. 2.21). In young adults, the total number of myelinated nerve fibres in the whole sural nerve is 4000–12,000, and the density ranges from 6000–10,000 fibres per mm^2 of fascicular area (Dyck et al. 1968, O'Sullivan and Swallow 1968, Ochoa and Mair 1969a, Gutrecht and Dyck 1970). The number of unmyelinated nerve fibres obtained by measuring electron micrographs is approximately four

times that of the myelinated nerve fibres in the sural nerve, the axonal diameter ranging from 0·2–2·8 μm with a mode at 0·8–1·2 μm (Ochoa and
Mair, 1968a; Dyck *et al.* 1971). In order to provide a better comparison of
the diameter of the unmyelinated and myelinated nerve fibres, axonal dia-

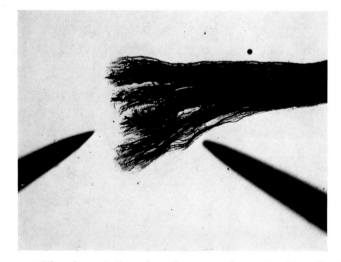

FIG. 4.16. View through dissecting microscope of nerve fascicle stained for
teasing, and dissecting needles.

meters of both should be measured on electron micrographs, though this is
a lengthy process.

Teased single nerve fibres. The portion of the nerve fixed in formol calcium is used after osmic acid staining and glycerol maceration for the dissection of single myelinated nerve fibres. Dissecting needles, a dissecting

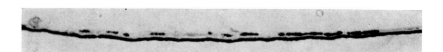

FIG. 4.17. Pair of teased nerve fibres, one of which is intact and the other
undergoing axonal degeneration with fragmentation into myelin ovoids.

microscope, a steady hand and a great deal of patience are the only apparatus required (see fig. 4.16). Fibres undergoing axonal degeneration with
fragmentation into myelin ovoids (fig. 4.17), and those showing segmental

demyelination (fig. 4.18) can readily be recognized. Quantitative studies are performed on fibres which are intact for more than five internodes. The internodal length of an individual fibre is plotted against the maximum

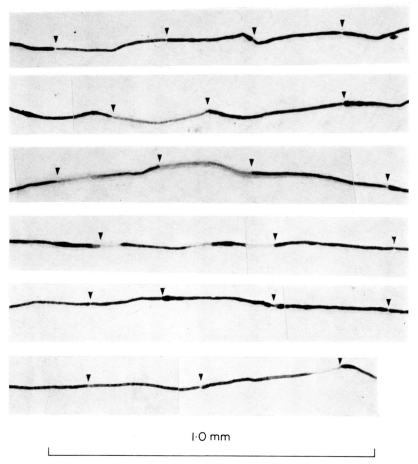

1·0 mm

FIG. 4.18. Single teased nerve fibre showing active paranodal demyelination, segmental demyelination, and intercallated internodes. Arrowheads mark nodes of Ranvier. Consecutive lengths of the fibre have been mounted below one another for convenience. Normal internodal length of a fibre of this diameter is 1·0 mm.

myelin sheath diameter as described by Fullerton *et al.* (1965) (fig. 4.19). Normally there is little variation between individual internodal lengths in a single fibre, the average internodal length increasing with increasing fibre diameter. Fibres which have undergone axonal degeneration with regeneration have internodal lengths of approximately 0·3 mm irrespective of the fibre diameter. Those which have undergone segmental demyelination and remyelination show an abnormal variation in internodal length.

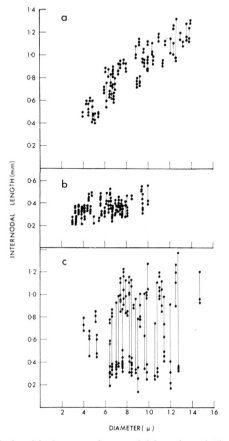

FIG. 4.19. Relationship between internodal length and fibre diameter in single teased nerve fibres from (*a*) a normal nerve, (*b*) a nerve which has recovered from axonal degeneration, and (*c*) a nerve which has recovered from segmental demyelination. Individual values of internodal length for each fibre are joined by a vertical line. (*From* Fullerton *et al.* 1965.)

Different nerves show different slopes of the line relating axonal diameter to internodal length. For instance, the slope for the facial nerve is much less steep than that for limb nerves such as the sural nerve (fig. 2.4). Similarly in the nerves of very young children, the slope is shallow, the internodal length being approximately 0·3 mm for all diameters (see chapter 2). Electron microscopy may be undertaken on single teased nerve fibres (Spencer and Thomas 1970, Dyck and Lais 1970).

Frozen sections are used for the demonstration of myelin breakdown products with oil red O and Sudan black, and for metachromatic material with toluidine blue or cresyl fast violet (see page 174, and frontispiece). Histochemical stains may also be applied.

Drawbacks of structural studies of nerve

It may take several weeks to obtain information about the number of axons of each size range which are present in the nerve. Providing segmental demyelination is not prominent, a study of the compound nerve action potential of the sural nerve *in vitro* may provide this information within a few minutes of the biopsy (see above, page 92). Segmental demyelination, however, vitiates this *in vitro* electrophysiological study.

The other problem about the anatomical studies is their exact interpretation. Fibres which are undergoing axonal degeneration and fragmentation may appear almost normal in Weigert-Pal transverse sections, and be counted in fibre diameter and total myelinated nerve fibre studies. Fibres which have totally degenerated leave no mark, and the decrease in the total number of myelinated nerve fibres may not be sufficient to allow recognition of this loss. On the other hand, fibres which have undergone segmental demyelination remain. Thus single teased nerve fibre studies overestimate the proportion of segmental demyelination in relation to axonal degeneration occurring in a disease. If demyelinated segments are extensive, many intact axons will have no myelin sheaths in the transverse section, and thus the total number of myelinated nerve fibres (in fact myelin sheaths) will be falsely low. Only counts on electron micrographs can avoid this error. Even in these, the shrinkage of the diameter of demyelinated segments of axons may complicate the interpretation.

If nerves from normal subjects or control animals are examined, a few fibres will be found undergoing axonal degeneration or segmental demyelination. The proportion is greater in the distal parts of the nerve and in older subjects. For this reason it is important to compare the pathological nerve under study with controls matched for age and site of nerve biopsy.

Despite these drawbacks the interpretation of nerve biopsy findings is generally not difficult providing the problems are borne in mind. Thus fig. 4.20 shows quantitative data on a patient with hypertrophic neuropathy with onion bulb formation (see fig. 4.13). The total number of myelinated

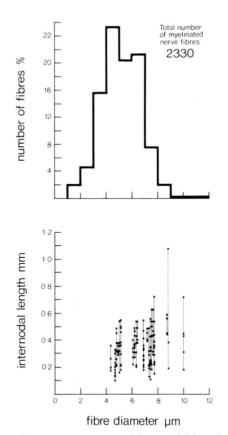

FIG. 4.20. Fibre diameter spectrum and internodal length spectrum of a sural nerve biopsy from a patient with hypertrophic neuropathy of the Dejerine-Sottas type. The total myelinated nerve fibre count is reduced to about a third of normal, the loss of the largest myelinated nerve fibres being the most marked. The internodal length spectrum shows gross segmental demyelination with remyelination.

nerve fibres, particularly those of the larger diameters, is greatly decreased. This loss may, however, be due to the excessive degree of segmental demyelination (see fig. 4.18). The loss of the larger fibres is probably due to the specific involvement of these fibres, perhaps magnified by shrinkage of the demyelinated and remyelinated axons.

Skeletal muscle

Choice of muscle

Any superficial skeletal muscle may be biopsied. For practical purposes the procedure is restricted to relatively large muscles such as the deltoid, biceps, triceps, quadriceps, anterior tibial and gastrocnemius muscles where removal of a small amount of tissue is readily replaced by regeneration, or to relatively unimportant small muscles like the palmaris longus or peroneus tertius. The selection of the site of biopsy in patients with muscle wasting is of considerable importance. Muscle which has undergone needle electromyography in the last three months should be avoided because of the consequent fibre damage. Severely affected muscle should be avoided because the degeneration is so severe that diagnosis is impossible. An attempt should be made to select mildly affected muscles.

Muscle biopsy procedure

The procedure described here has been developed in the Muscular Dystrophy Group Research Laboratories in Newcastle upon Tyne and found to produce the best histological preservation.

Operation

The biopsy may be taken under local or general anaesthesia, and the same restrictions as mentioned on page 107 apply. The muscle is exposed by an incision about 5–7 cm long running in the direction of the fibres. Groups of fasciculi about 8 mm across are separated by sharp dissection as far as possible along the natural lines of cleavage. The group is taken into a clamp made by cutting open a standard pair of ovarian forceps (fig. 4.21). The group of fibres is thus clamped at both ends at the *in vivo* length and may be cut from the body and fixed without subsequent change in length. A smaller specimen about 2 mm across may be taken in smaller clamps for electron microscopy.

In order to obtain information about the intramuscular nerves as well as the muscle, the biopsy is taken at the motor point. This is located by stimulating the intramuscular nerves with pulses of 0·1–0·5 ms duration, and determining the site of minimum threshold voltage. The incision is made at this spot, and the procedure repeated on the exposed muscle so that the biopsy is taken at the site where the motor nerve fibres are most abundant. The technique of demonstrating intramuscular nerve fibres by supravital methylene blue staining is described in the Appendix.

If the conditions permit, four pieces of muscle of about $50 \times 8 \times 8$ mm are taken, two on special clamps and two free, and treated as follows.

Histological preparation

Piece 1: for paraffin embedding, one of the clamped specimens is fixed either in 5–10 per cent formalin in 0·1 molar of phosphate buffer at pH 7·4 at room temperature for 24 hours, or in Susa fixative for 4–6 hours. Sections are cut at 5 μm and stained with haematoxylin and eosin, phosphotungstic acid-haematoxylin, and Picro-Mallory trichrome methods. Myopathic

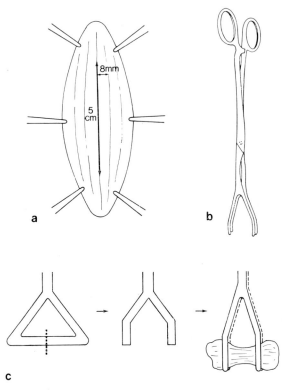

FIG. 4.21. Technique of muscle biopsy in clamps. *a* Exposure of the muscle along the line of the fasciculi. *b* Opened ovarian forceps used as muscle clamps (at different magnification from *a* and *c*). *c* Method of production of the muscle clamp from the ovarian forceps.

changes may be divided into those which are acute, including muscle fibre necrosis, phagocytosis and regeneration, and those which are chronic, including excessive variation of fibre size, internal nuclei and fibrosis. These chronic changes however may be seen in a variety of diseases including chronic denervation. In polymyositis there is often inflammatory cell infiltration, sometimes perivascular, consisting predominantly of lympho-cytes, plasmacytes and some macrophages together with acute necrotizing change in the muscle fibres.

The changes of denervation are classically groups of atrophic fibres which may sometimes be reduced to tiny bags of atrophic pyknotic nuclei with almost no myofibrils. Groups of hypertrophic fibres may indicate re-innervation. Further details of muscle histological changes may be found in Bethlem (1970).

Piece 2: for electron microscopy, small fasciculi 2 mm in diameter on special clamps are fixed in 3·6 per cent glutaraldehyde in 0·1 molar phos-phate buffer at pH 7·4 at 4°C for 1 hour, and then are cut longitudinally

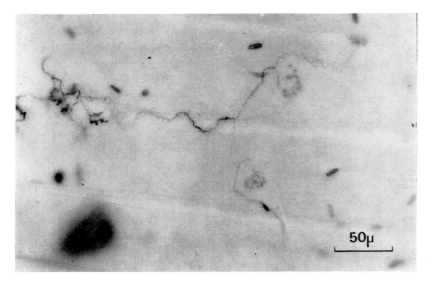

50μ

FIG. 4.22. Intramuscular nerve stained by the methylene blue method showing a single axon innervating at least seven motor end-plates (from a patient with hypertrophic neuropathy of the Dejerine-Sottas type). × 320. (*From* Coërs, Telerman-Toppet and Gérard 1973. *Arch. Neurol. (Chic.)* **29**, 215; kindly provided by Dr. C. Coërs.)

into 1 mm diameter fragments and fixed for a further hour. Further treat-ment is described in the Appendix. Another part of this piece is taken for *methylene blue preparations of intramuscular nerves*. The portion is injected *in vitro* as rapidly as possible after removal with methylene blue solution until it reaches the maximum degree of blueness. The further preparation is described in the Appendix. The intramuscular axons are seen as fine blue filaments, and the terminal ramifications in the end-plates may be identified. Occasionally degenerating axons may be seen indicating a denervating process. A small degree of branching of the nerve fibres before the end-plates (pre-terminal branching) is often seen, though excessive degrees of branching, the innervation of muscle fibre by two different axons, and axon branches arising from the terminal axon ramifications in the end-plates and running to another end-plate (ultraterminal branching) indicate reinnervation (see fig. 4.22). For further details of the intramuscular nerves the reader is referred to Coërs and Woolf (1959).

Piece 3: for cryostat sections and histochemistry, one piece of the muscle about $20 \times 8 \times 8$ mm is rapidly frozen in isopentane cooled in liquid nitrogen. Sections at 10 μm are stained by haematoxylin and eosin and for NADH diaphorase, myosin ATPase, phosphorylase and other enzymes as indicated. Fibre type grouping (see figs. 4.23 and 4.24) stands out in sharp contrast to the normal chequerboard pattern, and indicates reinnervation after previous denervation.

Piece 4: for biochemical studies, this piece is rapidly frozen as described for piece 3, and used for biochemical studies as indicated.

BIOCHEMICAL INVESTIGATIONS

In addition to the various biochemical and haematological tests described above (pages 84–85), a number of specific biochemical investigations may be indicated where certain diseases are suspected. In general these are research procedures, or at the best are undertaken only in specialized laboratories.

The plasma level of various vitamins, including vitamins B_{12} and B_1, may be required in suspected cases of malabsorption or undernutrition. The blood pyruvate level and its response to a glucose load may indicate some abnormality of vitamin B_1 metabolism (Hockaday et al. 1966). There may be an inhibitor of transketolase in uraemic patients (see pages 171–172). The fatty acids of the blood and tissues may be examined where Refsum's disease (page 190) is suspected, looking for high levels of phytanic acid. α-lipoprotein is absent from the serum in Tangier disease (page 174), and β-lipoprotein is absent in Bassen-Kornzweig disease. Measurement of the plasma levels of potentially neurotoxic drugs like isoniazid may be required. In metachromatic leukodystrophy, aryl sulphatase A activity is markedly decreased in white blood cells and tissues.

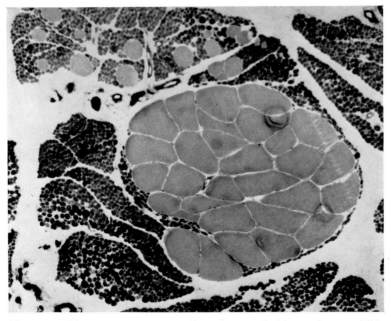

FIG. 4.23. Transverse cryostat section of a muscle biopsy from a child with infantile spinal muscular atrophy stained for myosin ATPase. The fasciculi of tiny atrophic denervated fibres are clearly seen, surrounding a fasciculus of reinnervated type I fibres. × 128.

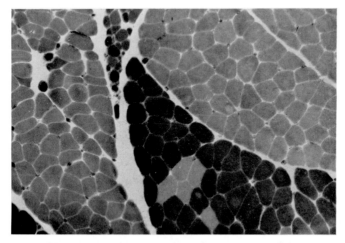

FIG. 4.24. Transverse cryostat section of an extensor digitorum brevis muscle of an adult showing fibre type grouping. Myosin ATPase. × 50. (Kindly provided by Dr Margaret Johnson.)

Autopsy or biopsy specimens of nerve may be used for the analysis of myelin and measurements of various enzymes. Gas–liquid chromatography has been applied arbitrarily to a wide range of neuropathies by Appenzeller with interesting preliminary results (Appenzeller and MacGee 1968). The accumulation of ceramide trihexoside in Fabry's disease is due to a deficiency of trihexosidase (page 174). The accumulation of ceramide hexosides and ceramide hexoside sulphates has been reported in Dejerine-Sottas disease (page 188 et seq.).

For the accurate assessment of the chemistry of myelin, it is important that levels be related to the total amount of myelin, and it would be best if these levels were estimated in purified myelin. The Folch-Lees and basic proteins may be extracted and assayed (see pages 61–62). The level of various enzymes may be measured either on homogenates or histochemically on frozen nerve sections or single teased nerve fibres. Very many enzymes may thus be studied including acid phosphatase, esterases, oxidative enzymes and proteases. The study of axoplasmic flow, which may yet prove of importance in the axonal neuropathies, is at present only suitable for use in experimental animals (see pages 50 et seq. and 136–137).

REFERENCES

ABRAMSON D. I., CHU L. S. W., TUCK S. JR, LEE S. W., RICHARDSON G. and LEVIN M. (1966) Effect of tissue temperatures and blood flow on motor nerve conduction velocity. J. Amer. med. Ass. **198**, 1082–1088.

APPENZELLER O. and MACGEE J. (1968) Gas-liquid chromatographic analysis of sural nerves in peripheral neuropathies. J. neurol. Sci. **7**, 581–592.

BERGMANS J. (1970) The Physiology of Single Human Nerve Fibres. Vander, Louvain.

BERRY C. M., GRUNDFEST H. and HINSEY J. C. (1944) The electrical activity of re-generating nerves in the cat. J. Neurophysiol. **7**, 103–115

BETHLEM J. (1970) Muscle Pathology. Introduction and atlas. North-Holland, Amsterdam.

BRADLEY W. G. and AGUAYO A. (1969) Hereditary chronic polyneuropathy. Electrophysiological studies in an affected family. J. neurol. Sci. **9**, 131–154.

CHOPRA J. S. and HURWITZ L. J. (1968) Femoral nerve conduction in diabetes and chronic occlusive vascular disease. J. Neurol. Neurosurg. Psychiat. **31**, 28–33.

COËRS C. and WOOLF A. L. (1959) The Innervation of Muscle. A biopsy study. Blackwell, Oxford.

CRAGG B. G. and THOMAS P. K. (1957) The relationship between conduction velocity and diameter and internodal length of peripheral nerve fibres. J. Physiol. (Lond.) **136**, 606–614.

DESMEDT J.E. and BORENSTEIN S. (1970) The testing of neuromuscular transmission. In *Handbook of Clinical Neurology*, ed. Vinken P.J. and Bruyn G.W., Vol. 7, pp. 104–115. North-Holland, Amsterdam.

DYCK P.J., GUTRECHT J.A., BASTRON J.A., KARNES W.E. and DALE A.J.D. (1968) Histologic and teased-fibre measurements of sural nerve in disorders of lower motor and primary sensory neurons. *Proc. Mayo Clin.* **43**, 81–123.

DYCK P.J. and LAIS A.C. (1970) Electron microscopy of teased nerve fibers: method permitting examination of repeating structures of the same fiber. *Brain Res.* **23**, 418–424.

DYCK P.J. and LAMBERT E.H. (1966) Numbers and diameters of nerve fibers and compound action potential of sural nerve: controls and hereditary neuromuscular disorders. *Trans. Amer. neurol. Ass.* **91**, 214–217.

DYCK P.J., LAMBERT E.H. and NICHOLS P.C. (1971) Quantitative measurement of sensation related to compound action potential and number and sizes of myelinated and unmyelinated fibres of sural nerve in health, Friedreich's ataxia, hereditary sensory neuropathy and tabes dorsalis. In *Handbook of Electroencephalography and Clinical Neurophysiology*, vol. 9, pp. 83–118. Elsevier, Amsterdam.

DYCK P.J. and LOFGREN E.P. (1968) Nerve biopsy. Choice of nerve, method, symptoms and usefulness. *Med. Clin. N. Amer.* **52**, 885–893.

ESPIR M.L.E. and HARDING D.T.C. (1961) Apparatus for measuring and counting myelinated nerve fibres. *J. Neurol. Neurosurg. Psychiat.* **24**, 287–290.

FOLDES F.F., KLONYMUS D.H., MAISEL W. and OSSERMAN K.E. (1968) A new curare test for the diagnosis of myasthenia gravis. *J. Amer. med. Ass.* **203**, 649–653.

FULLERTON P.M., GILLIATT R.W., LASCELLES R.G. and MORGAN-HUGHES J.A. (1965) Relation between fibre diameter and internodal length in chronic neuropathy. *J. Physiol. (Lond.)* **178**, 26P–28P.

GUTRECHT J.A. and DYCK P.J. (1970) Quantitative teased-fiber and histologic studies of human sural nerve during postnatal development. *J. Comp. Neurol.* **138**, 117–130.

HAFTEK J. and THOMAS P.K. (1968) Electron-microscope observations on the effects of localized crush injuries on the connective tissues of peripheral nerve. *J. Anat.* **103**, 233–243.

HOCKADAY T.D.R., HOCKADAY J.M. and RUSHWORTH G. (1966) Motor neuropathy associated with abnormal pyruvate metabolism unaffected by thiamine. *J. Neurol. Neurosurg. Psychiat.* **29**, 119–128.

HOPF H.C. (1963) Electromyographic study on so-called mononeuritis. *Arch. Neurol. (Chic.)* **9**, 307–312.

KAESER H.E. (1970) Nerve conduction velocity measurements. In *Handbook of Clinical Neurology*, vol. 7, ed. Vinken P.J. and Bruyn G.W., pp. 116–196. North-Holland, Amsterdam.

KNUTTSON E. and WIDÉN L. (1967) Impulses from single nerve fibres recorded in man using microelectrodes. *Nature (Lond.)* **213**, 606–607.

LENMAN J.A.R. and RITCHIE A.E. (1970) *Clinical Electromyography*. Pitman, London.

McComas A.J., Fawcett P.R.W., Campbell M.J. and Sica R.E.P. (1971) Electrophysiological estimation of the number of motor units within a human muscle. *J. Neurol. Neurosurg. Psychiat.* **34**, 121–131.

Morgan-Hughes J.A. (1968) Experimental diphtheritic neuropathy. A pathological and electrophysiological study. *J. neurol. Sci.* **7**, 157–175.

Newsom Davis J. (1967) Phrenic nerve conduction in man. *J. Neurol. Neurosurg. Psychiat.* **30**, 420–426.

Ochoa J. and Mair W.G.P. (1969a) The normal sural nerve in man. I: Ultrastructure and numbers of fibres and cells. *Acta Neuropath. (Berl.)* **13**, 197–216.

O'Sullivan D.J. and Swallow M. (1968) The fibre size and content of the radial and sural nerves. *J. Neurol. Neurosurg. Psychiat.* **31**, 464–470.

Richardson A.T. and Barwick D.D. (1969) Clinical electromyography. In *Disorders of Voluntary Muscle*, 2nd edn, ed. Walton J.N., pp. 813–842. Churchill, London.

Romero C. and Skoglund S. (1965) Methodological studies of the technique in measuring nerve fibre diameters. *Acta Morphol. Neerl. Scand.* **6**, 107–114.

Sanders F.K. and Whitteridge D. (1946) Conduction velocity and myelin thickness in regenerating nerve fibres. *J. Physiol. (Lond.)* **105**, 152–174.

Spencer P.S. and Thomas P.K. (1970) The examination of isolated nerve fibres by light and electron microscopy with observations on demyelination proximal to neuromas. *Acta neuropath. (Berl.)* **16**, 177–186.

Thomas P.K. (1970) The quantitation of nerve biopsy findings. *J. neurol. Sci.* **11**, 285–295.

Thomas J.E. and Lambert E.H. (1960) Ulnar nerve conduction velocity and H-reflex in infants and children. *J. applied Physiol.* **15**, 1–9.

Thomas P.K., Sears T.A. and Gilliatt R.W. (1959) The range of conduction velocity in normal motor nerve fibres to the small muscles of the hand and foot. *J. Neurol. Neurosurg. Psychiat.* **22**, 175–181.

Trojaborg W. and Sindrup E.H. (1969) Motor and sensory conduction in different segments of the radial nerve of normal subjects. *J. Neurol. Neurosurg. Psychiat.* **32**, 354–359.

Yap C.-B. and Hirota T. (1967) Sciatic nerve motor conduction velocity study. *J. Neurol. Neurosurg. Psychiat.* **30**, 233–239.

5

Basic Disease Processes in the Peripheral Nerve

Two main types of nerve fibre degeneration are recognized (see fig. 5.1):

1 *Axonal degeneration*, in which axon death leads to secondary breakdown of the myelin sheath. The injury causing axonal death may act either upon the perikaryon as in poliomyelitis or a spinal cord infarct, or upon the

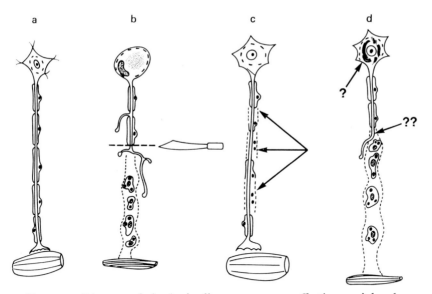

FIG. 5.1. Diagram of the basic disease processes affecting peripheral nerves. *a* Normal. *b* In Wallerian degeneration a focal lesion causes central chromatolysis of the perikaryon and distal degeneration of the axon. *c* In segmental demyelination individual myelin sheaths or Schwann cells are patchily damaged. *d* In axonal neuropathy the disease may affect either the cell body or peripheral axon causing axonal breakdown. In both forms of axonal degeneration the muscle atrophies.

peripheral axons. Where the cause is focal trauma to the peripheral nerve the term *Wallerian degeneration* is applied after Waller (1850), who first clearly described the changes following nerve section. Where axonal degeneration occurs due to diseases other than trauma, the term *axonal neuropathy* is best applied. In some of these the distal terminals of the largest fibres appear most affected. The term *'dying back' neuropathy* has been applied to diseases with this pattern. To understand the changes in axonal degeneration one needs to consider the primary and secondary changes occurring in the nerve cell body which are discussed in chapter 8.

2   *Segmental demyelination*, where the Schwann cell and myelin sheath are damaged. The axon basically remains intact, though conduction of the nerve action potential may be blocked. The process is normally patchy, damaging some Schwann cells and sparing others.

These two processes are described more fully in the next two sections.

AXONAL DEGENERATION

Wallerian degeneration

When a nerve is crushed, continuity of the axon is broken. As in all cells, the part of the cytoplasm separated from the nucleus thereafter gradually degenerates. If the basement membranes of the Schwann cells remain intact, the axons may regenerate within their own Schwann cell tubes, and reinnervation is efficient and accurate. Nerve section causes loss of continuity of the Schwann cell tubes, and regeneration is more haphazard. The changes occurring following a nerve crush are briefly described below, and for a more complete review the reader should consult Bradley and Thomas (1973).

Within 2 min of crushing the nerve there is retraction of myelin from the nodes of Ranvier, and dilatation of Schmidt-Lanterman clefts for up to 5 mm distal to the crush in all fibres (Williams and Hall 1971). The changes gradually spread distally to affect first the smaller and then the larger myelinated fibres over the next 6 hours. Histochemistry demonstrates an immediate loss of enzymes in the injured Schwann cell cytoplasm and an increase in lysosomal and oxidative enzyme activity in adjacent Schwann cells, which gradually spreads to involve all the distal Schwann cells (Morgan-Hughes and Engel 1968). By 1 hour the proximal and distal axoplasm adjacent to the crush develops into spirals and balls, a process which gradually spreads in both directions for up to 2 mm within the next 24 hours. Within 1 hour, there is an increased synthesis of organic phosphates throughout the distal part of the nerve.

By 12 hours after the crush, the distal axons begin to show signs of degeneration with the paranodal accumulation of mitochondria (Ballin and Thomas 1969). The unmyelinated fibres begin to swell (Bray et al. 1972) and undergo beading.

By 24 hours axoplasmic degeneration distal to the crush becomes obvious, with increased electron-density of the axoplasm, and fragmentation of the neurofilaments, neurotubules and endoplasmic reticulum (Ballin and Thomas 1969). The rate of degeneration is somewhat variable, though in general it is inversely proportional to the fibre diameter. Degeneration of the unmyelinated fibres is quite extensive by 24 hours (Roth and Richardson 1969).

By 24 hours degeneration of the myelin sheaths has begun in most of the myelinated fibres. The myelin splits at the intraperiod line and lamellae peel off at the nodes (Ballin and Thomas 1969), the Schwann cell processes expanding to cover the nodes of Ranvier. Protein synthesis increases in the Schwann cells of the distal part of the nerve, and their nuclei begin to divide 24 hours after the crush, the peak rate of division being from the third to ninth days.

The maximum number of Schwann cells in the distal nerve is seen at about 15–25 days after the crush (Abercrombie and Johnson 1946). The rate and extent of Schwann cell division is greatest in nerves composed of large myelinated fibres, and is much less in nerves with only unmyelinated fibres (Thomas 1948, Joseph 1950).

By 48 hours marked signs of degeneration in the myelin sheaths appear distal to the crush. There is loosening of the myelin lamellae and swelling of the fibre. At 48 hours the conduction velocity distal to the crush is still approximately 80 per cent of normal, conveyed in the few remaining intact myelinated fibres, though the amplitude has fallen to less than 10 per cent of normal because most of the fibres have degenerated by this time (see page 94). Nerve conduction fails by the fourth day.

By 3 days there is extensive breakdown of myelin within the Schwann cell cytoplasm and macrophages derived from the blood stream enter the nerve to remove the myelin debris. The myelin becomes broken into large ovoids, which may be seen as 'myelin digestion chambers' in paraffin-embedded preparations, or as osmiophilic inclusions within the Schwann

TIME

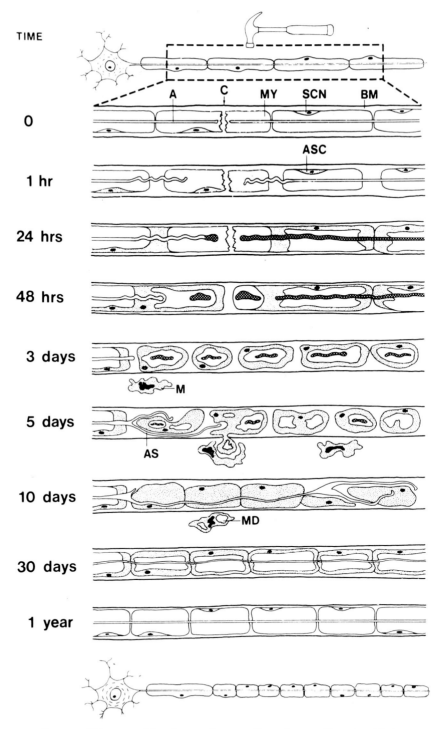

0

1 hr

24 hrs

48 hrs

3 days

5 days

10 days

30 days

1 year

FIG. 5.2. Diagram of the changes in a myelinated nerve fibre at and below the level at various times after a crush lesion.

cell in electron micrographs (see chapter 4). Despite earlier arguments, there is now no doubt that most of the digestion of myelin occurs in the Schwann cell cytoplasm, the debris then being discharged into macrophages.

By the sixteenth day most of the myelin sheaths have been removed, though some foamy macrophages containing myelin debris may still be seen 3 months after nerve section. A large part of the cholesterol of the digested myelin is reutilized for the synthesis of new myelin (Rawlins *et al.* 1970). Regenerating axon sprouts appear at about the fifth day. Those derived from myelinated fibres tend to grow within the tubes derived from Schwann cell basement membrane. Unmyelinated nerve fibres are not so restricted, and may regrow in a haphazard fashion (Thomas 1966). The axons gradually mature and become surrounded by Schwann cell cytoplasm and myelin. Over the next 12–24 months there is a gradual return towards normal of the axon diameter and myelin sheath thickness. The division of Schwann cells induced by myelin breakdown results in there being many more Schwann cells per unit length of axon. Internodes become about 0·3 mm in length in fibres of all diameters (see page 118). The changes during Wallerian degeneration are illustrated in fig. 5.2, and the changes after recovery from Wallerian degeneration in fig. 5.3.

A number of changes occur immediately proximal to the crush, including retrograde degeneration extending back for one or two nodes, a decrease in axon diameter, and occasionally segmental demyelination and remyelination. Repeated episodes of axonal degeneration and regeneration following nerve crush produce extensive nerve fibre clusters composed of several myelinated and unmyelinated nerve fibres and collagen similar to those in chronic neuropathies with axonal degeneration and regeneration (fig. 5.4). 'Onion-bulb' formation, however, does not occur with repeated nerve crushes.

A number of very important changes occur in the perikaryon following nerve section. A signal for the induction of these changes travels to the perikaryon from the site of the axonal lesion at rates of about 5 or more millimetres per day. The nature of this signal has been discussed by Cragg (1970) and Watson (1970). Retrograde axoplasmic flow transporting information from the sensory and motor nerve terminals seems the most likely candidate for this signal. The morphological changes in the perikaryon are loss of Nissl substance, swelling of the perikaryon by up to 20 per cent, and a temporary increase in nuclear size with migration of the nucleus to the periphery of the cytoplasm. The overall change is described as *central chromatolysis* (Barr and Hamilton 1948). The loss of Nissl substance is due to dispersion of polyribosomes from the stacks of rough endoplasmic reticulum (Pannese 1963), and is associated with an increased synthesis of ribonucleic acid, starting in the nucleolus and later occurring in the cytoplasm. This begins within 8 hours of nerve crush, and reaches a maximum by about the third day (Watson 1965). The rate of ribonucleic

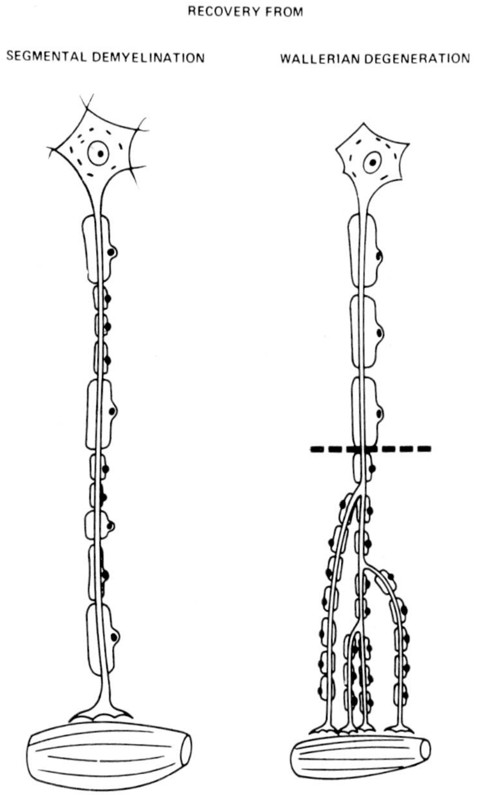

RECOVERY FROM

SEGMENTAL DEMYELINATION   WALLERIAN DEGENERATION

FIG. 5.3. Diagram of the changes in internodal length following recovery from segmental demyelination and Wallerian degeneration.

acid synthesis later falls, and protein synthesis by this time is markedly increased to produce the new axoplasm required for regeneration. At this time there appears to be a decrease in the enzymes of the Krebs and glycolytic pathways, and an increase in the pentose shunt pathways (Nandy 1968). Satellite cells around the perikarya become activated and divide within 3 days of nerve section (Kreutzberg 1968). These cells comprise all elements of the glial group, particularly microglia. Following the re-establishment of the connection between the axon and its site of innervation distally, the changes of central chromatolysis regress and disappear. A number of perikarya die, particularly if the lesion is very proximal (Cavanaugh 1951).

Axonal neuropathies

When axons suffer a focal lesion other than trauma they degenerate in a manner essentially identical to Wallerian degeneration. An infarct due to

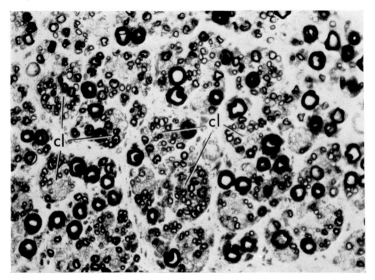

FIG. 5.4. Cluster (cl) formation in a chronic peripheral neuropathy with axonal degeneration, regeneration and sprouting. Kultschitsky's haema-toxylin. × 270. (*From* Bradley and Thomas 1973.)

polyarteritis nodosa, or an area of damage due to the injection of a toxin such as phenol, are two of the many types of focal lesion. In many other conditions axonal degeneration and secondary myelin breakdown occur though there is no focal damage. These might be termed parenchymatous axonal neuropathies, and the site of primary damage remains to be identi-fied. The argument, which centres around whether the damage is primarily of the axon or perikaryon (see fig. 5.1), is made more complex by the inter-play between these two parts of the neuron. Thus death of the perikarya causes axonal degeneration, while a focal lesion of the peripheral nerve causes central chromatolysis of the perikaryon. If the axonal lesion is very proximal the perikaryon dies, and the net result is the same as in a primary lesion of the perikaryon. As discussed in the section below, it is possible that distal degeneration of the axons ('dying back' neuropathy) may result from metabolic change in the perikaryon. Finally it is possible that the noxious agent is attacking both the axon and the perikaryon.

The importance of separating axonal from perikaryal disease is that the mechanism of damage must be very different in the two processes, and may therefore require different treatment.

'Dying-back' neuropathies

Since the end of the nineteenth century, neuropathologists have recognized that degeneration may be concentrated in the parts of nerve fibres furthest from the perikarya. This is particularly striking in Friedreich's ataxia and amyotrophic lateral sclerosis, and has also been recognized in a number of neuropathies including those of vitamin B_1 deficiency, acrylamide neuropathy and TOCP neuropathy (see chapter 6). In others, for instance acute intermittent porphyria, the distal parts of all the larger fibres appear to degenerate irrespective of the length of the axons.

A distal symmetrical polyneuropathy might theoretically result from multiple small lesions scattered diffusely throughout the nerves. The summation of these lesions would result in proportionately more damage to the longest fibres. Almost certainly, this is the explanation of the symmetrical distal polyneuropathy of collagen-vascular diseases like polyarteritis nodosa (see page 193 et seq.). Alternatively, the distribution of pathological damage in such neuropathies might indicate that the terminal parts of the axons die back from their peripheral connections, perhaps due to impairment of the supply of their metabolic requirements by the perikarya. Cavanagh and Chen (1971) found an initial inhibition of protein synthesis in the perikarya prior to the appearance of distal degeneration in a toxic neuropathy. This hypothesis is attractive, but as shown in fig. 5.5, the same pattern of degeneration would result from a total loss of the perikarya and axons of the longest fibres. These are few in number compared with the whole population of anterior horn cells and axons in the proximal parts of the main nerve trunks and very careful search would be required to detect their degeneration. Hopkins (1970) showed that acrylamide neuropathy was 'dying back' in type, distal degeneration being seen in the recurrent laryngeal nerve where the fibres run from one end to the other without significant branching or loss of fibres to proximal areas. A few isolated fibres were intact proximally and undergoing axonal degeneration distally (fig. 5.6). No other study to date has proved the 'dying back' hypothesis so rigorously.

It is possible that impairment of the axoplasmic flow of protein (see page 50 et seq.) might be responsible for the axons dying back, though we have been unable to find a gross decrease in flow in toxic and inherited axonal degenerations (Bradley and Williams 1973, Bradley and Jaros 1973). Possibly impairment of the flow of some other substance or of a small subfraction of axonal protein is responsible for the distal degeneration.

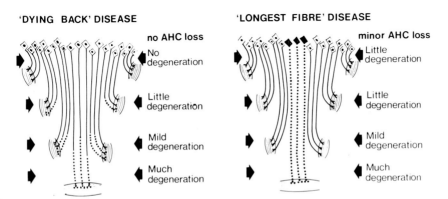

FIG. 5.5 Diagram showing the very similar gross pathological change at different levels of the peripheral nerve in a true 'dying back' disease, and one which causes total death of the longest nerve fibres. (*From* Bradley and Thomas 1973.)

SEGMENTAL DEMYELINATION

Diphtheritic neuropathy

In comparison with Wallerian degeneration, segmental demyelination is a much more variable process, affecting some Schwann cells, sparing others and very largely sparing the axons. The archetype of segmental demyelination is diphtheritic neuropathy. The mechanism by which diphtheria toxin damages Schwann cells is not clear. It causes inhibition of protein synthesis (Collier and Papenheimer 1964a and b) and particularly of the synthesis of proteolipid and basic protein of mylein during myelination (Pleasure et al. 1973). However, it is difficult to believe that this is the mode of action upon

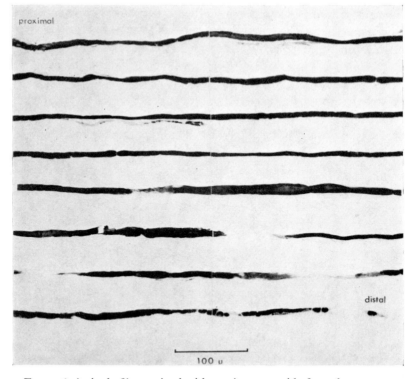

proximal

distal

100 u

FIG. 5.6. A single fibre stained with osmium tetroxide from the nerve to
extensor digitorum brevis muscle of a baboon intoxicated with acrylamide.
Successive lengths of the fibre are mounted below each other. The fibre is
intact proximally, but distally is undergoing axonal degeneration. (*From*
Hopkins 1970.)

the Schwann cells, for there are many cells in the body with more active
protein synthesis which are not specifically sensitive to diphtheria toxin.

The toxin becomes fixed within 1 hour, and is not then susceptible to
neutralization by antitoxin. Prior to the onset of symptoms and signs of a
neuropathy there is however a delay of 5–12 days for the local neuropathy
and 30–50 days for the involvement of the spinal nerves in patients with
diphtheritic pharyngitis, and of 4–7 days in animals following injection of
toxin. The delay seems to be inversely proportional to the dose of neurotoxin. What is occurring during this delay period is not known.

Different parts of the peripheral nervous system are affected in different
species, dependent upon the inherent level of the blood-nerve barrier. The
nerve roots are particularly involved in man, the cat and the rabbit, whose

blood–nerve barrier does not extend to the roots (Fisher and Adams 1955, Waksman *et al.* 1957). In the guinea pig, which has no generalized blood–nerve barrier, the peripheral nerves in general are damaged.

The earliest change is an increased irregularity of the myelin sheaths, followed by a widening of the nodal gap (Cavanagh and Jacobs 1964), the small fibres being affected before the large ones. At this stage there is no effect on the conduction velocity. Myelin in the affected internodes then begins to break down starting at the Schmidt-Lanterman clefts and the paranodal region. Demyelination may remain paranodal or involve the whole internode. Myelin breakdown occurs mainly within the Schwann cell cytoplasm, with activation of lysosomes. Macrophages remove much of the myelin debris. There is usually little or no axonal damage, though the axoplasm may show increased osmiophilia suggesting some impairment in its nutrition.

The timing of the stages of degeneration in diphtheritic neuropathy can best be followed by intraneural injection of the toxin (Jacobs *et al.* 1967, Allt and Cavanagh 1969). As in Wallerian degeneration, the smallest fibres are more susceptible, myelin breakdown occurring by the third day, while that in the large fibres does not begin until the fifth day. The outer lamellae of the myelin sheaths peel back from the nodes producing measurable widening of the node of Ranvier by the sixth day, and myelin ovoids by the seventh day (fig. 5.7). Macrophages begin to infiltrate the nerve at this stage.

A few Schwann cells die as a result of intoxication, but most become stimulated to divide from the third day onwards, the peak of activity being about the seventh day. Non-compact thin myelin sheaths begin to reform from the tenth day. In segments where damage has been limited to the paranodal region, the new myelin sheath grows in from the intact residual sheath. Where the whole of an internode has been demyelinated, the area originally invested by one Schwann cell becomes the responsibility of two or more newly divided Schwann cells. These *intercalated Schwann cells* cause a decrease in the internodal length of these areas, and therefore an increased variability of internodal length (figs. 4.19 and 5.3). Fig. 5.8 illustrates the pattern of changes in segmental demyelination.

The physiological and functional effects of these changes are intriguing. Clinical signs appear and the conduction velocity falls at the stage when there is breakdown of many of the myelin sheaths. Clinical recovery begins from the third week, though there are now extensive intercalated internodes, and the conduction velocity may still be markedly depressed (see page 95).

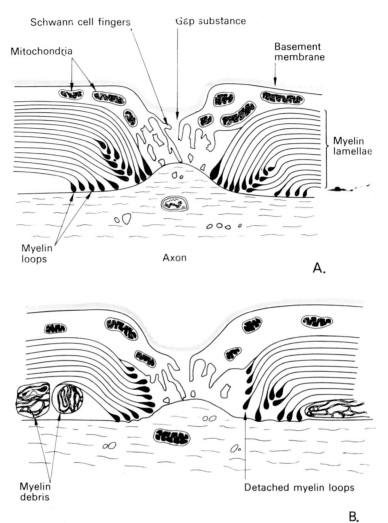

FIG. 5.7. Diagram of the changes at the nodes of Ranvier after local injection of diphtheria toxin into right sciatic nerve. *a* Normal node of Ranvier. *b* At 3 days, outer myelin loops are detached from the axolemma and inner lamellae are disorganized. *c* At 7 days, the node is widened, Schwann cell 'fingers' and gap substance are absent, and the gap is replaced by swollen Schwann cell cytoplasm. *d* At 10 days, there is marked nodal widening; there is much myelin debris within the Schwann cell processes and the axon is bare of Schwann cell covering in places. Severed terminal myelin loops are still present attached to the axolemma. (*From* Allt and Cavanagh 1969.)

Enlarged nodal Schwann cells

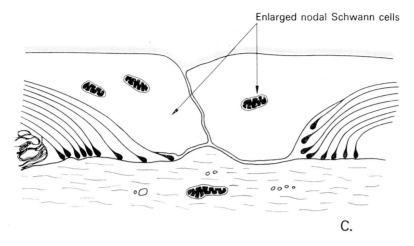

C.

Myelin debris

Bare axon

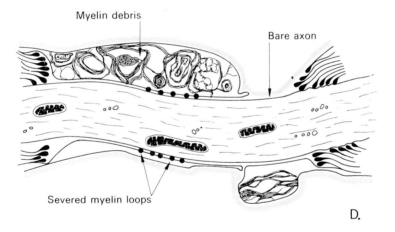

Severed myelin loops

D.

Hypertrophic neuropathy

In a number of chronic neuropathies where segmental demyelination is extensive, 'onion-bulb' formation may be seen. 'Onion-bulbs' are systems consisting of a central axon with its investing Schwann cell and usually myelin sheath, and surrounding imbricate plates of Schwann cell processes, some of which may contain non-myelinated axons (fig. 4.13).

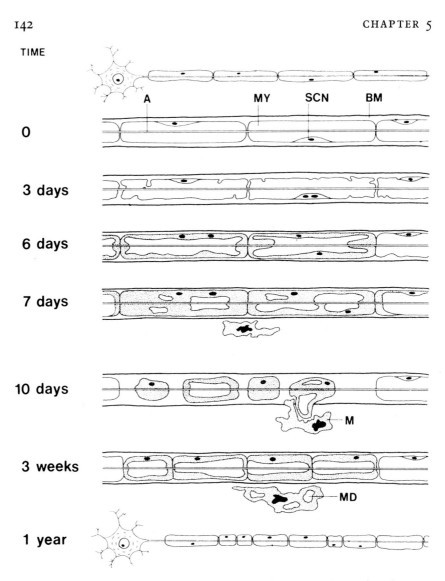

FIG. 5.8. Diagram of the pattern of changes in a nerve fibre undergoing segmental demyelination at various times after the intraneural injection of diphtheria toxin.

Experimentally these have been produced by the chronic application of agents causing segmental demyelination (Weller and Das Gupta 1968). Each episode of demyelination of an internode causes the Schwann cell to divide into two (fig. 5.9). Initially these two become the nuclei of the two new

shortened internodes termed *intercalated segments*. The repeated demyelination and division produces new Schwann cells which are unable to find a
place on the axon. These redundant Schwann cells become divested from
the axon, and form a thin plate around it. Repetition of the process as
shown in fig. 5.10 can lead to 'onion-bulb' formation.

'Onion-bulbs' are not seen with repeated Wallerian degeneration and
regeneration, presumably because the axon is not present *in continuo* during

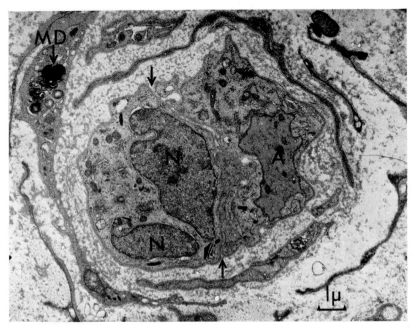

FIG. 5.9. Electron micrograph of an axon (A) in the centre of a small
onion bulb which has undergone segmental demyelination. The nucleus
(N) of the Schwann cell investing this axon has recently undergone
division, and the cytoplasm is now separating into two parts at the arrows.
One of the redundant Schwann cell processes contains myelin debris (MD).

the process, so that all the Schwann cell processes become disorientated.
Repeated episodes of damage to the nerve cause an increase in collagen, and
it is the increase in this rather than an increase in cells which causes the
hypertrophy of the nerves. Such hypertrophy may be demonstrable only by
the measured increase in the fascicular area (page 113 *et seq.*), or it may be
palpable clinically. In rare instances hypertrophied nerves may reach a size
sufficient to compress adjacent structures.

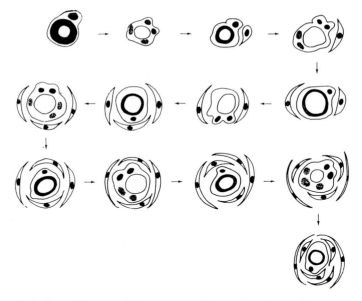

FIG. 5.10. Diagram of the process of formation of an onion bulb.

PATHOLOGY OF CLINICAL NEUROPATHIES

Most clinical neuropathies are of mixed pathology, both axonal degeneration and segmental demyelination occurring to a varying degree together.
Usually one process is predominant; diabetic polyneuropathy is *predominantly* a demyelination disease, while that of acute porphyria is *predominantly* axonal in type. However it is not easy to quantitate this predominance
accurately and, as discussed on page 119, single fibre preparations tend to
overestimate the extent of segmental demyelination, while myelinated nerve
fibre counts usually overestimate the axonal loss.

The simplest explanation for the combined presence of axonal degeneration and segmental demyelination is that the disease process attacks both
the Schwann cells and the axons. Other possibilities must however be considered. As discussed on page 64 *et seq.*, the Schwann cell may play a
part in the metabolic support of the axon, and death of the Schwann cell
may perhaps lead to axonal death (*secondary axonal degeneration*). On the
other hand the axons have a significant role in determining the metabolism
of the Schwann cells, and an abnormality of the axons might give rise to
secondary segmental demyelination. This is suggested in disease states such

as uraemia by the finding of some fibres with extensive segmental demyelination in the presence of others which show no change (Jennekens *et al.* 1969).

In a number of diseases, the pathological changes in the peripheral nerves may be diagnostic. These include leprosy, the familial amyloidoses, metachromatic leucodystrophy, the Guillain-Barré-Strohl syndrome and polyarteritis nodosa. These are described in chapter 6. Occasionally the presence of vascular changes as in diabetes, or the chance finding of carcinomatous infiltration may cast light upon the aetiology of the neuropathy. Usually however the pathological changes in the nerve help understand the nature of the condition, but are of lesser help in pointing to the aetiology. Electrophysiological studies may provide a quicker indication of the pathological nature of the condition, though as outlined on page 96, they are subject to a number of drawbacks in many disease states. Prineas (1970) suggested that the changes in degenerating axons in thiamine deficiency, TOCP and acrylamide intoxications may be different. Such differences require further investigation for they offer the possibility of extending the range of aetiological diagnosis possible from biopsy studies, though such a hope is a long way from fruition at present.

Further reviews of the field of peripheral nerve pathology are provided by McDonald (1967), Bots (1970) and Thomas (1971).

REFERENCES

ABERCROMBIE M. and JOHNSON M.L. (1946) Quantitative histology of Wallerian degeneration. I: Nuclear population in rabbit sciatic nerve. *J. Anat. (Lond.)* **80**, 37–50.

ALLT G. and CAVANAGH J.B. (1969) Ultrastructural changes in the region of the node of Ranvier in the rat caused by diphtheria toxin. *Brain* **92**, 459–468.

BALLIN R.H.M. and THOMAS P.K. (1969) Changes at the nodes of Ranvier during Wallerian degeneration: an electron microscopic study. *Acta neuropath. (Berl.)* **14**, 237–249.

BARR M.L. and HAMILTON J.D. (1948) A quantitative study of certain morphological changes in spinal motor neurons during axonal reaction. *J. Comp. Neurol.* **89**, 93–121.

BOTS G.Th.A.M. (1970) Pathology of nerves. In *Handbook of Clinical Neurology*, ed. Vinken P.J. and Bruyn G.W., vol. 7, pp. 197–243. North-Holland, Amsterdam.

BRADLEY W.G. and JAROS E. (1973) Axoplasmic flow in axonal neuropathies. II: Axoplasmic flow in mice with motor neuron disease and muscular dystrophy. *Brain,* **96**, 247–258.

BRADLEY W. G. and THOMAS P. K. (1973) The pathology of peripheral nerve disease. In *Disorders of Voluntary Muscle*, ed. Walton J. N. Churchill-Livingstone, Edinburgh.

BRADLEY W. G. and WILLIAMS M. H. (1973) Axoplasmic flow in axonal neuropathies. I: Axoplasmic flow in cats with toxic neuropathies. *Brain*, 96, 235–246.

BRAY G. M., PEYRONNARD J. M. and AGUAYO, A. J. (1972) An ultrastructural study of degeneration and regeneration of unmyelinated nerve fibres. *J. Neuropath. exp. Neurol.* 31, 197–198

CAVANAGH J. B. and CHEN F. C. K. (1971) Amino acid incorporation into protein during the 'silent phase' before organo-mercury and pBPAU neuropathy in the rat. *Acta neuropath. (Berl.)* 19, 216–224.

CAVANAGH J. B. and JACOBS J. M. (1964) Some quantitative aspects of diphtheritic neuropathy. *Br. J. exp. Path.* 45, 309–322.

CAVANAUGH M. W. (1951) Quantitative effects of the peripheral innervation area of nerves and spinal ganglion cells. *J. Comp. Neurol.* 94, 181–219.

COLLIER R. J. and PAPPENHEIMER A. M. JR. (1964a) Studies on the mode of action of diphtheria toxin. I: Phosphorylated intermediates in normal and intoxicated HeLa cells. *J. exp. Med.* 120, 1007–1018.

COLLIER R. J. and PAPPENHEIMER A. M. JR. (1964b) Studies on the mode of action of diphtheria toxin. II: Effect of toxin on amino acid incorporation in cell-free systems. *J. exp. Med.* 120, 1019–1039.

CRAGG B. G. (1970) What is the signal for chromatolysis? *Brain Res.* 23, 1–21.

FISHER C. M. and ADAMS R. D. (1955) Diphtheritic polyneuritis: a pathological study. *J. Neuropath. exp. Neurol.* 15, 243–268.

HOPKINS A. P. (1970) The effect of acrylamide on the peripheral nervous system of the baboon. *J. Neurol. Neurosurg. Psychiat.* 33, 805–816.

JACOBS J. M., CAVANAGH J. B. and MELLICK R. S. (1967) Intraneural injection of diphtheria toxin. *Brit. J. exp. Path.* 48, 204–216.

JENNEKENS F. G. I., VAN SPIJK D. VAN DER MOST and DORHOUT MEES E. J. (1969) Nerve fibre degeneration in uraemic polyneuropathy. *Proc. Europ. Dial. Trans. Ass.* 6, 191–197.

JOSEPH J. (1950) Further studies in changes in nuclear population in degenerating non-myelinated and finely myelinated nerves. *Acta Anat.* 9, 279–288.

KREUTZBERG G. W. (1968) Über perineurale Mikrogliazellen (Autoradiographische Untersuchungen). *Acta neuropath. (Berl.)* Suppl. IV, 141–145.

McDONALD W. I. (1967) Structural and functional changes in human and experimental neuropathy. In *Modern Trends in Neurology*, ed. Williams W., pp. 145–164. Butterworth, London.

MORGAN-HUGHES J. A. and ENGEL W. K. (1968) Structural and histochemical changes in the axons following nerve crush. *Arch. Neurol. (Chic.)* 19, 598–612.

NANDY K. (1968) Histochemical study on chromatolytic neurons. *Arch. Neurol. (Chic.)* 18, 425–434.

PANNESE E. (1963) Investigations of the ultrastructural changes of the spinal ganglion neurons in the course of axon regeneration and cell hypertrophy. I: Changes during axon regeneration. *Zeitschr. f. Zellforsch.* 60, 711–740.

PLEASURE D. E., FELDMANN B. and PROCKOP D. J. (1973) Diphtheria toxin inhibits the synthesis of myelin proteolipid and basic proteins by peripheral nerve *in vitro. J. Neurochem.* **20**, 81–90.

PRINEAS J. (1970) Peripheral nerve changes in thiamine-deficient rats. An electron microscopic study. *Arch. Neurol. (Chic.)* **23**, 541–548.

RAWLINS F.A., HEDLEY-WHYTE E.T., VILLEGAS G. and UZMAN, B.G. (1970) Re-utilization of cholesterol-1,2-H^3 in the regeneration of peripheral nerve. *Lab. Invest.* **23**, 237–240.

ROTH C.D. and RICHARDSON K.C. (1969) Electron microscopical studies on axonal degeneration in the rat iris following ganglionectomy. *Amer. J. Anat.* **124**, 341–360.

THOMAS G.A. (1948) Quantitative histology of Wallerian degeneration. II: Nuclear population in two nerves of different fibre spectrum. *J. Anat. (Lond.)* **82**, 135–145.

THOMAS P.K. (1966) The cellular response to nerve injury. I: The cellular outgrowth from the distal stump of transected nerve. *J. Anat. (Lond.)* **100**, 287–303.

THOMAS P.K. (1971) The morphological basis for alterations in nerve conduction in peripheral neuropathy. *Proc. roy. Soc. Med.* **64**, 295–298.

WAKSMAN B.H., ADAMS R.D. and MANSMANN H.C. JR. (1957) Experimental study of diphtheritic polyneuritis in the rabbit and guinea pig. Part I (immunologic and histopathologic observations). *J. exp. Med.* **105**, 591–614.

WALLER A.V. (1850) Experiments on the section of the glossopharyngeal and hypoglossal nerves of the frog, and observations of the alterations produced thereby in their primitive fibres. *Phil. Trans. roy. Soc. (Lond.)* B **140**, 423–429.

WATSON W.E. (1965) An autoradiographic study of the incorporation of nucleic acid precursors by neurons and glia during nerve regeneration. *J. Physiol. (Lond.)* **180**, 741–753.

WATSON W.E. (1970) Some metabolic responses of axonotomized neurones to contact between their axons and denervated muscle. *J. Physiol. (Lond.)* **210**, 321–343.

WELLER R.O. and DAS GUPTA T.K. (1968) Experimental hypertrophic neuropathy. An electron microscopic study. *J. Neurol. Neurosurg. Psychiat.* **31**, 34–42.

WILLIAMS P.L. and HALL S.M. (1971) Prolonged *in vivo* observations of normal peripheral nerve fibres and their acute reactions to crush and deliberate trauma. *J. Anat. (Lond.)* **108**, 397–408.

6

Diseases Causing Peripheral Nerve Damage

A peripheral neuropathy may be defined as a disease which causes disordered structure and/or function of the peripheral nerve. Since the causes of peripheral neuropathies include several hundred diseases, only the major groups can be considered here. The choice of order is arbitrary, and a list of the groups of conditions to be considered is given in table 6.1. The first two conditions discussed are trauma and diphtheritic neuropathy since these are the archetypes of the two main pathological processes occurring in nerve, axonal degeneration and segmental demyelination respectively (see chapter 5). Leprosy, diabetes mellitus, ageing and vitamin deficiency follow as probably the commonest causes of peripheral nerve disease in the world today, the exact order and frequency depending upon the country under consideration.

Traumatic nerve lesions

Direct nerve compression

The nerves are generally buried deep within muscle masses, and are thereby well protected except against penetrating wounds. There are, however, certain vulnerable sites, such as that of the radial nerve in the spiral groove where it may be damaged by a fractured humerus, the lateral popliteal nerve at the head of the fibula, and the ulna nerve behind the medial epicondyle of the humerus. Seddon (1943) defined three grades of injury, and Sunderland (1968) five. The following classification incorporates both:

1 Blockage of nerve conduction without loss of continuity of the axon (*neurapraxia*—Seddon). This is transient;

2 Damage to the axon with subsequent Wallerian degeneration, though

148

TABLE 6.1. Major types of condition causing peripheral nerve damage. The order is arbitrary

Trauma: direct
        entrapment
        familial pressure-sensitive neuropathy

Infection: diphtheria
        leprosy

General metabolic disease: diabetes mellitus
                acute intermittent porphyria
                uraemia
                hepatic failure
                thyroid disease
                hypoglycaemia

Metabolic diseases specifically affecting the nervous system

Old age

Vitamin deficiencies and malabsorption

Exogenous toxins

Acute idiopathic post-infectious polyneuropathy

Hereditary neuropathies: familial amyloidosis
              hereditary sensory neuropathy
              peroneal muscular atrophy
              Refsum's disease

Carcinoma

Ischaemia and collagen-vascular disease

Brachial plexus neuropathy

Radiation

Tropical diseases

Tumours of nerve

Chronic idiopathic neuropathy

Recurrent neuropathy

the connective tissue including the Schwann cell basement membrane remains intact (*axontmesis*—Seddon). Regeneration occurs at 1–2 mm/day and is usually effective unless the lesion is very proximal;

3   Damage to the axon and connective tissue, but preservation of the perineurium and fascicular architecture of the nerve. Regeneration is less complete than 2, but is still relatively effective;

4   Damage to the axon, connective tissue and perineurium, though the nerve remains macroscopically intact. Regeneration is poorly orientated and less effective;

5   Complete anatomical section of the nerve.

Types 3–4 are included in Seddon's term *neurotmesis*. The clinical problem is to decide not only upon the site of the lesion, but also upon the grade of injury, for the treatment of each group is different. This problem has been very fully discussed by Sunderland (1968). Grade 1 may be recognized by waiting for 5 or 6 days to see if recovery occurs, but all the remainder require regeneration which is a slow process. If anatomical continuity of the nerve is destroyed (grade 5), then regeneration is likely to be poor or absent. More effective regeneration can be achieved in grade 5 by nerve suture, reapproximating the nerve ends and allowing the regenerating nerves some chance of re-entering the Schwann cell tubes of the distal nerve. The decision whether to explore the nerve depends upon the likelihood that anatomical discontinuity has been produced. Nerve lesions associated with penetrating wounds are particularly likely to produce grade 5 damage. The decision also depends on whether the site is proximal or distal. If distal, such as a lesion of the ulnar nerve in the hand, the 30 days or so necessary for the appearance of the earliest signs of regeneration can be allowed to see whether this is going to occur. If no recovery can be seen by this time, the site of lesion may be explored to see whether anatomical discontinuity exists. On the other hand where the lesion is very proximal, such as in penetrating wounds of the buttock, the patient may have to wait 200 or more days before the first signs of recovery appear. Though suture of the nerve even years after injury *may* lead to useful recovery, and though regeneration from a proximal lesion *may* continue for several years, reinnervation after about 18 months is generally less effective. Thus where the lesion is likely to be associated with grade 5 injury, or where it is very proximal, exploration is generally indicated.

One situation in which this general rule does not apply is in nerve root avulsion. As described on page 257, distraction injuries may cause one or more nerve roots to be torn away from their attachment to the spinal cord. Surgical correction of this is considered impossible, and it is thus important to diagnose this proximal lesion in order to avoid an unnecessary exploration. The typical situation for nerve root avulsion is where a patient is thrown from a moving vehicle or falls from a height on to the tip of his shoulder. This leads to the shoulder and neck being pulled away from one another, and may avulse the cervical nerve roots or tear the brachial plexus. Avulsion may be detected by myelography in which the avulsed root sleeves can be clearly seen (fig. 9.1). If the roots are avulsed, then all the muscles innervated by those roots will show denervation changes, including fibrillation potentials, after about 5 days following the injury. The presence of fibrillation potentials in the spinalis muscles after this time shows that the lesion is more proximal than the brachial plexus, and probably consists of avulsion of the roots. Where root avulsion is present no recovery can be expected in the distribution of those roots.

A grade 2–5 lesion of the brachial plexus, like any other such lesion of a peripheral nerve distal to the posterior root ganglion, will cause the distal parts of the axons to degenerate. After about 5 days, the axon flare (page 74) and the sensory nerve action potential (page 88) will have disappeared in the anaesthetic area. The significance of the findings indicating a brachial plexus lesion depend on whether the roots are avulsed proximally. If not, then some recovery can occur despite the proximal site. Exploration to reveal grade 5 nerve damage and to allow the torn nerves to be sutured is therefore indicated.

The next question is 'when?'. Where extensive wounding has occurred, primary suture is less frequently successful and most surgeons prefer primary debridement of the wound and observation of the nerve, followed by secondary suture of the nerve 1–4 weeks later (Sunderland 1968, Ducker et al. 1969). In severe wounds, a gap may remain between the nerve ends which cannot be reduced by traction. A nerve graft may be required to bridge the gap. An autograft is the best, though this necessitates causing a lesion of another nerve. Heterografts are only moderately effective, though immunosuppression during the time the nerve axons are growing through the graft will produce a better result (Pollard et al. 1971).

During regeneration of axons down the nerve, patients are often aware of Tinel's sign (or symptom). Light percussion over the course of the nerve at the site of the advancing front of the axons will produce a tingling sensation referred to the area of innervation of that nerve. During the time when the denervated skin area is being reinnervated, sensation is distorted, and moderate stimuli may produce an unpleasant sensation (protopathic pain of Head). Only later does large fibre function become re-established with the return of the discrimination of light touch (epicritic sensation of Head). Where nerve regeneration cannot occur because of anatomical disruption of the nerve, the outgrowth of exuberant axons may produce a neuroma. Pressure upon this is often extremely painful particularly at amputation stumps. Excision, the injection of sclerosing fluids like phenol, and percussion with a vibrator may help relieve this condition.

One other condition of aberrant sensation which may follow injury is *causalgia* (Richards 1967, Abbots and Mitts 1970). Firstly clearly described by Weir Mitchell and colleagues in 1864 (see page 9), this is a severe intractable burning pain with trophic changes in the limb. The muscles atrophy, and the skin becomes thin, red and shiny. It is severely debilitating to the patient, and is greatly affected by psychological factors. Some individuals suffer severe psychiatric illnesses. The patient comes to protect the limb from any contact or change in temperature. Rarely seen other than with incomplete and proximal lesions of the median and sciatic nerves, it is commonest after missile wounds, but even then occurs only in about 5 per cent of cases. Causalgia may develop immediately or after a latent period following injury. The exact mechanism defies elucidation, but may be due to false peripheral synapses between the autonomic and motor fibres on the one hand and the sensory fibres on the other. Sympathectomy may be dramatically curative.

Entrapment or compression neuropathies

In addition to direct external compression, nerves may be compressed by a number of local factors including tumours and haematomata. These may all be grouped together as the *compression neuropathies*.

The nerve may also be compressed at many sites by anatomical structures within the body producing the so-called *entrapment neuropathies* (Kopell and Thompson 1963, Staal 1970). The commonest such condition is compression of the median nerve in the carpal tunnel which runs between the carpal bones and the flexor retinaculum and contains not only the median nerve but also the flexor tendons. The patient is usually a woman of middle age who recently has increased in weight, who uses her hands excessively or who has become pregnant. The exact cause of the condition is not clear, probably the combination of the anatomically narrower canal in the female, with fibrous thickening and oedema resulting from increased work, leading to excessive pressure within the canal. Myxoedema, acromegaly, amyloid infiltration, arthritis, and ganglion formation may predispose to the condition by narrowing the space available for the median nerve within the canal. The symptoms are of pains, numbness and paraesthesiae in the thumb, index and middle fingers, particularly at night. The hands are worse when hung down, and eased by being raised, and are worse after hard work. The signs include sensory impairment on the tips of the affected fingers, and weakness of the abductor pollicis brevis muscle with flattening of the thenar eminence. There is slowing of sensory and motor nerve conduction of the median nerve through the carpal tunnel, and electromyographic signs of denervation of the abductor pollicis brevis. Conservative therapy, including the application of night splints with the wrist in the mid-position, corticosteroid injections into the carpal tunnel and diuretics, may be effective in relieving symptoms. Failing this, surgical decompression, preferably by open division of the carpal ligament is indicated. It is normal for the nerve, at sites where it is exposed to pressure, to be slightly thickened with an increased amount of epi- and endo-neurial connective tissue. When compression occurs, however, there is narrowing of the nerve with pallor of the superficial blood vessels. Thomas and Fullerton (1963) found loss of the larger myelinated nerve fibres at the level of the compression in a patient with the carpal tunnel syndrome.

Nerve entrapment at many other sites is now recognized in man, the common feature being the presence of a firm structure such as bone, tendon or fascial layer against which the nerve may be compressed. A number of the commoner sites of entrapment are shown in table 6.2 with the motor and sensory symptoms and signs which result. If the nerve is sensory or mixed, pain results either locally or referred to the area of skin innervated by nerve, together with paraesthesiae and loss of superficial sensation. In entrapments of mixed or motor nerves, weakness and wasting occur relatively late. Pain may often be produced by pressing over the site of compression, and the symptoms are often precipitated by rendering the limb ischaemic for a few minutes.

A number of other nerve lesions have been described under this term by Kopell and Thompson (1963), including those of the superficial and deep peroneal, saphenous, sciatic, ilio-inguinal, and obturator nerves in the lower limb, and the radial, suprascapular, and dorsal scapular nerves in the upper limb. Several of these are occupational and result from repeated or unusual actions. They are considered in the next section. In all entrapments and compression neuropathies, the treatment is rest and the avoidance of the precipitating movement. Local infiltration of the site

TABLE 6.2 Commonest sites of nerve entrapment

Nerve	Site of entrapment	Symptoms and signs	
		Sensory	Motor
Median	Carpal tunnel at wrist	Pain, paraesthesiae, numbness thumb and 1st 2 fingers. Tender over carpal tunnel	Weakness and wasting abductor pollicis brevis
Median	Pronator teres muscle in forearm	Pain and tenderness over pronator teres. As for carpal tunnel	Weak pronation. As for carpal tunnel
Ulnar	Deep motor branch in palm	Nil	Weakness, wasting ulnar-innervated small muscles of hand
Ulnar	Loge de Guyon at wrist	Pain, paraesthesiae, numbness ulnar 2 fingers. Tender over compression site	As deep branch
Ulnar	Medial epicondyle at elbow	Pain, paraesthesiae, numbness ulnar border forearm and hand. Tenderness over compression site	Weak flexors of wrist and ulnar 2 fingers. As deep branch
Posterior tibial	Tarsal tunnel at ankle	Pain, paraesthesiae, numbness toes and sole of foot. Tender over compression site	Rare
Common peroneal (lateral popliteal)	Head of fibula at knee	Pain, paraesthesiae, numbness shin and dorsum of foot. Tender over fibular head	Weak dorsiflexion and eversion of foot
Lateral cutaneous of thigh	Inguinal ligament at anterior superior iliac spine	Pain, paraesthesiae, numbness lateral thigh	Nil
Digital of foot	Transverse intertarsal ligament	Pain, paraesthesiae, numbness inter-digital cleft	Nil

of compression with corticosteroids may bring relief. If these manoeuvres fail, surgical decompression of the nerve is indicated. In the case of the ulnar nerve, transposition into the antecubital region, or epicondylectomy is required.

Animal models of entrapments have been developed in recent years. These will allow further investigation of the aetiology, pathogenesis and treatment of this group of conditions. Aguayo *et al.* (1971) experimentally produced an entrapment by fitting a Silastic tube around the median popliteal nerve of young rabbits, and allowing growth to cause compression. The outer fibres of the nerve were more affected than the inner ones, and there was narrowing of axons, thinning of the myelin sheaths, segmental demyelination at the level of the compression and axonal swelling above. Distally a few fibres underwent axonal degeneration and regeneration. A natural animal model of pressure neuropathy was discovered by Fullerton and Gilliatt (1967a and b) in guinea pigs housed in cages with wire floors. The repeated trauma of the wire and compression of the ulnar, median and plantar nerves causes changes ranging from segmental demyelination at the level of compression to total Wallerian degeneration from that level distally.

Occupational neuropathies

Everyday activities produce innumerable minor traumata to nerves without significant long-term effects. If however an activity is repeated many thousands of times per day as it may be in the patient's occupation, damage may become apparent (Spaans 1970). The continued use of scissors may produce a digital neuropathy. Continuous kneeling may compress the sciatic nerve between the heel and the pelvis and the digital nerve over the hyperextended toes. Carrying a weight on the shoulders may damage the suprascapular nerve. The ballet dancer compressing the common peroneal nerve at its passage through the tibialis anterior muscle, the secretary injuring the same nerve by sitting cross-legged and the writer leaning on the ulnar nerve at the elbow are further examples of people developing occupational neuropathies.

Very frequent flexion and extension of the elbow may damage the ulnar nerve, and similar damage may result if this nerve is forced to take an abnormally long course or is distorted by local bony abnormalities. This occurs following some fractures of the humerus at the elbow, and the term *tardy ulnar nerve palsy* is given to this condition.

Familial pressure palsies

Rare individuals may have the tendency to develop palsies of the peripheral nerves following relatively minor episodes of nerve compression or ischaemia, and this tendency often runs in families. A proportion of these individuals have evidence of a widespread subclinical polyneuropathy, the nerve conduction velocity suggesting in some the presence of segmental demyelination (Earl *et al.* 1964). Behse *et al.* (1972) found bizarre abnormalities of the myelin sheaths, with grossly abnormal 'sausage-shaped' areas of thickening in the nerves of such patients.

Diphtheritic neuropathy

Diphtheria was once the scourge of many parts of the world, but immunization in early childhood and the frequent use of antibiotics have now made it a rare disease. Kinnier Wilson's textbook (1954) gives a full review. The responsible organism is *Corynebacterium diphtherii*, which usually causes an acute pharyngitis characterized by a grey membrane, but which can infect a skin wound. The dangerous complications are delayed and are due to a cardiotoxin and a neurotoxin. In experimental animals, the severity of the neuropathy is proportional to the dose of neurotoxin used. However, the amount of neurotoxin produced by the *Corynebacterium* varies with the virulence of the strain. In human infections it is therefore impossible to relate the severity of the infection to the severity of the delayed complications.

The major systemic nerve damage due to the neurotoxin is usually delayed for 30–50 days after the onset of pharyngitis, though in some patients local cranial nerve paralysis may develop 5–12 days after infection. This is usually relatively benign. The major paralysis often begins in the palate, but rapidly spreads to involve all the nerves, both motor and sensory. The patient may require tracheostomy and artificial respiration to prevent death from paralysis of bulbar and respiratory muscles.

Neither the reason for the delay nor the mode of action of the diphtheria toxin is known. It is rapidly fixed in the body; 1 hour after injection into experimental animals its effect can no longer be neutralized by an injection of massive doses of antitoxin. As discussed on page 137 *et seq.*, the toxin causes segmental demyelination, by damaging the Schwann cells of the peripheral nerves in a patchy fashion. There is breakdown of the myelin sheaths, but the axons remain intact unless the neuropathy is very severe.

This produces a marked slowing of nerve conduction leading to a complete conduction block and paralysis. However remyelination occurs quickly, and the paralysis recovers in 15–30 days unless death from neurological or cardiological complications supervenes.

Neuropathy of leprosy

This is probably the major cause of severe peripheral nerve disease in the world today. The chronic infection with *Mycobacterium leprae* insidiously damages the peripheral nervous system over many years. There is a predilection for the cutaneous nerves, the resultant severe anaesthesia causing neuropathic phenomena like painless injuries, chronic infections, Charcot joints, and mutilation. There may be loss of digits and facial structures, penetrating ulcers, and osteomyelitis.

Two polar forms of leprosy may be distinguished, *lepromatous* and *tuberculoid*, though *intermediate* forms are common. In the *lepromatous form*, hypertrophic skin lesions are frequent, and the nerves are teeming with *Mycobacterium leprae* in all elements of the nerve including the perineurium, Schwann cells and axons (fig. 6.1) (Job 1970). Initially there is little damage or cellular response. Later segmental demyelination and to a lesser extent axonal degeneration appear, with proliferation of Schwann cells and some fibrosis. The immunological response is humoral with a marked increase in serum immunoglobulins and enlargement of the lymph nodes, but the lepromin skin test is negative. The neuropathy is generally distal, symmetrical and predominantly sensory in type, though mononeuritis multiplex may be seen (Rosenberg and Lovelace 1968). The *Mycobacterium* may have a predilection for skin areas of lower temperature (Sabin 1969).

In the *tuberculoid form* of the neuropathy there is atrophy and depigmentation of the skin, and neuropathic phenomena are prominent. It is extremely difficult to find bacilli in the nerve, and the immunological response is cellular with a positive lepromin skin test. The pattern is usually of a mononeuritis multiplex. In striking contrast to lepromatous leprosy, in the tuberculoid form there is extensive infiltration with lymphocytes and macrophages, and marked proliferation of Schwann cells. Severe axonal loss from axonal degeneration predominates, with little segmental demyelination. There is a predilection for pressure sites with marked fibrosis, nodular thickening and tethering to underlying structures (Dastur 1955).

Thus the diagnosis in the lepromatous form may be confirmed by nerve biopsy, but in the tuberculoid form it must rest on a positive lepromin test.

Therapy with DDS and other sulphones has been available for a number of years and is known to be slowly effective in suppressing the disease. Even so, relapses can occur after many years of therapy. The recent success in growing *Mycobacterium leprae* in the mouse foot-pad (Rees and Waters 1971) has allowed the experimental investigation of the treatment of this difficult disease. Many other drugs have now been screened, and it has been shown that DDS is bacteriostatic, while rifampicin is rapidly bactericidal. When the disease is suppressed, it is possible to consider palliative

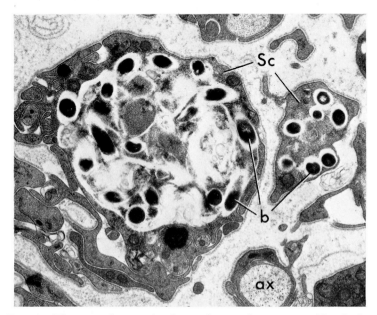

FIG. 6.1 Electron micrograph of a sural nerve from a case of borderline lepromatous leprosy. The Schwann cells (Sc) contain numerous leprosy bacilli (b). ax—axon. × 11,000. (Figure kindly provided by Dr R.H.M. King.) (*From* Bradley and Thomas 1970.)

procedures such as tendon transplants, and excision of fibrosed segments with heterologous nerve grafts (Antia *et al.* 1970).

Neuropathy of diabetes mellitus

Distal symmetrical predominantly sensory polyneuropathy

This is the commonest neuropathy associated with diabetes mellitus. Patients complain of numbness and paraesthesiae of the toes and feet, spreading to the legs. Later the fingers may be involved. The positive sensory phenomena of burning feet and tender calves are common. Loss of touch, pain and vibration sensation extend proximally in a glove and stocking distribution, and the distal reflexes become depressed. Neuropathic phenomena are common in severely affected cases. Relatively painless perforating ulcers of the feet are the most frequent, and are exacerbated by the impaired tissue metabolism and poor blood supply so common in these patients. The marked loss of joint position sense and Charcot joints combined with pupillary abnormalities which may result from recurrent attacks of uveitis or an autonomic neuropathy, present a picture similar to that of tabes dorsalis (*diabetic pseudotabes*).

The prevalence of the polyneuropathy is impossible to define for it depends on the intensity of the search. Patients complain of symptoms relatively infrequently unless they suffer from 'burning feet' or ulcers. Clinical examination reveals that a greater proportion of diabetics have an asymptomatic polyneuropathy, while electrophysiological and pathological studies show that subclinical damage to nerves is even more frequent. Perhaps about 5 per cent of diabetics have significant symptoms and signs of a distal predominantly sensory polyneuropathy (Bruyn and Garland 1970). It is generally believed that the neuropathy is less common in children though quite a high incidence of asymptomatic clinical and electrophysiological abnormalities are found in children (Lawrence and Locke 1963, Gamstorp *et al.* 1966).

There is a tendency for the prevalence and severity of a neuropathy to vary with the age at presentation and the degree of control of the diabetes, though the relationship is not precise (Rundles 1945). Gregersen (1967, 1968a and b) showed that the average motor and sensory nerve conduction velocities were decreased, and the vibration perception threshold raised in a large group of diabetic patients whether recently diagnosed or longstanding. The impairment is greater in those with symptomatic neuropathies, those with diabetes of longer duration, and those with poor control (Ward *et al.* 1971). Greenbaum (1964) showed that the neuropathy tended to begin around the time of diagnosis or at times of poor control of blood sugar levels. Interestingly in early diabetes there is a widespread sensory abnormality which also involves the threshold for taste and the critical fusion frequencies for sound and light (Chochinov *et al.* 1972).

However individual patients may vary from this prediction. Particularly in the older group, diabetes may be brought to light only when investigating a patient presenting with a peripheral neuropathy. Similarly in other patients the neuropathy advances despite adequate control of the blood sugar level and the absence of hypoglycaemic episodes which may themselves damage the peripheral nerves (see page 173). The explanation rests upon an understanding of the underlying biochemical defect in diabetes which probably causes impairment of the transport of glucose into cells long before hyperglycaemia and the classic symptoms of polyuria and polydipsia appear. The nerves may be undergoing damage during the whole of the 'pre-diabetic phase', and the underlying defect is not necessarily corrected by the administration of insulin. It is important to remember that the demonstration of impaired glucose tolerance does not prove that the neuropathy is due to the diabetes. The increased incidence of other diseases of the 'autoimmune' type like pernicious anaemia must be remembered.

The most marked and earliest pathological change is segmental demyelination; in the more severe form there is also loss of fibres due to axonal degeneration (Thomas and Lascelles 1966). Changes in the small endoneurial blood vessels are common in diabetes with progressively increasing medial and intimal hyperplasia, thickening of the basement membrane or capillaries, accumulation of PAS-positive material in the walls, and occlusion of some of the blood vessels. Many believe that the vascular changes are responsible for the neuropathy. However the lack of correlation between the neural degeneration and blood vessel changes has prompted many to conclude that the neuropathy is metabolic in origin (Greenbaum et al. 1964, Thomas and Lascelles 1966, Chopra et al. 1969). Neither the blood vessel nor the nerve fibre changes are restricted to diabetes, and a nerve biopsy could not be diagnostic of the condition.

In the nerve of patients with long-standing diabetic neuropathy 'onion-bulb' formation may be found (Ballin and Thomas 1968). Identical changes are now recognized in a wide variety of different diseases as emphasized elsewhere (see pages 141 et seq. and 188 et seq.). Onion bulbs simply indicate the presence of chronic repetitive segmental demyelination.

Proximal acute mononeuropathies

Patients with diabetes, especially those with a distal sensory polyneuropathy, frequently have weak and wasted quadriceps femoris muscles (Hirson et al. 1953). Goodman (1954) reviewed 17 cases of femoral neuropathy, finding 16 of them to be diabetic. This chronic predominantly motor femoral neuropathy is perhaps a tenth as common as the chronic mainly sensory distal symmetrical polyneuropathy, and is similarly often asymptomatic. Occasionally patients develop severe pain in the distribution of one femoral nerve, followed by wasting and weakness of the quadriceps muscle with loss of the knee jerk and sometimes a small area of superficial sensory loss on the front of the thigh. The pain may last 2 or 3 months, then gradually remit. The femoral nerve is the commonest to be involved, but others including the obturator and lateral popliteal nerves may also be affected. The control of the blood sugar level is often poor at the time of presentation, and with better control the condition improves. Casey and Harrison (1972) studied 12 patients 10 months to 12 years after the onset of the condition, and found that 11 had improved, and 7 had made a good functional recovery.

The history of the condition is interesting. Bruns (1890) first reported a proximal mononeuropathy in diabetes, recognizing the site of the lesion to lie in the peripheral nerve. Other reports appearing from time to time thereafter failed to diagnose the site of the lesion correctly (Bruyn and Garland 1970). Interest in the condition was reawakened by the description by Garland of 5 further cases (Garland and Taverner 1953, Garland 1955). He also originally mistook the site of the damage, terming the condition 'diabetic myelopathy' because 3 cases had extensor plantar responses, and 4 an increased concentration of protein in the C.S.F. Since then, electrophysiological studies have shown that the condition is due to a neuropathy (Chopra and Hurwitz 1968), and pathological studies have revealed degenerative changes in the lumbar plexus and other nerves (Lindén 1962). Raff et al. (1968) showed that there was ischaemic damage of the nerves in this condition. In serial sections of the femoral, obturator and posterior tibial nerves of a patient with this condition, they found numerous small infarcts, particularly of the small bridging fasciculi. Both axonal degeneration and segmental demyelination were found. Of more than 30 such infarcts, only 3 could be related to the occlusion of a nearby small endoneurial artery. In the remainder there was no local obstruction, though there was diffuse endothelial proliferation and narrowing of many arterioles and capillaries.

Autonomic neuropathy

Symptoms of autonomic neuropathy in diabetes other than impotence are relatively rare, though evidence of autonomic involvement is relatively common on investigation. Diabetic autonomic neuropathy is described on page 226.

Neuropathy of old age

Increasing age brings a mixed bag of joys and sorrows, the latter comprising the many ills to which the ageing body is liable. It is well known that from the seventh decade onwards vibration sensation, two-point discrimination, taste discrimination, and coordination become impaired, the ankle jerks become depressed and deafness and cataracts appear (Critchley 1931, Howell 1949). A decrease of the maximum conduction velocity occurs in motor and sensory nerves (Kaeser 1970). By the age of 80 years the decrease is about 10 per cent of the maximum velocity at the age of 30 years and is more in those with generalized deterioration including dementia.

Though degeneration of the nerves is prominent from the seventh decade onwards, it probably occurs progressively from early adult life. Dyck, et al. (1972) showed a progressive increase of pressure sensation threshold with age from the third decade. Campbell and McComas (1970) found that the estimated number of motor units in the extensor digitorum brevis muscle fell significantly beyond the age of 60. Jennekens et al. (1971) found that the extensor digitorum brevis muscle in fact shows changes of denervation and reinnervation progressively from the first decade. Harriman et al. (1970) found the complexity of the intramuscular terminal innervation and spherical axonal swellings to be more marked with increasing age.

Though the changes are earlier and greater distally, particularly in the lower limb, they also involve more proximal parts of the nervous system (Gardner 1940, Cottrell 1940). The nerves show degenerative changes of the vasa nervorum, increased fibrosis, and both segmental demyelination and axonal degeneration with regeneration (Vizoso 1950, Lascelles and Thomas 1966, Arnold and Harriman 1970). The non-myelinated nerve fibres are also involved in the process, showing progressive degeneration; complex plates of Remak cells develop (Ochoa and Mair 1969).

The problem with all degenerative conditions associated with age is to know whether they are due to ageing itself or to some other disease which is common in old age. This is almost a philosophical point, and it is probably more relevant to ask why some patients show degenerative changes at 45 years while others show none at the age of 80 years. This variability makes it very important to choose 'controls' carefully in any study of peripheral nerve function in a certain disease. It is necessary not only to match for age and sex, but also potentially for the degree of 'infirmity'. The neuropathy of old age certainly has many possible origins including ischaemia, entrapments, the cumulative effect of multiple traumata throughout life with a gradual decrease in the regenerative capacity, and an underlying cancer.

Neuropathies due to vitamin deficiencies

Peripheral nerve damage occurs in a number of vitamin deficiencies. Clinically the most important are the neuropathies of beriberi, pernicious anaemia and malabsorption. Leaving aside the deficiency of vitamin B_{12}, deficiencies of other vitamins usually occur in the setting of malnutrition and it is rare for deficiency of a single vitamin to occur clinically. Similarly in experimental work it has been difficult to prove the requirement of an individual vitamin for peripheral nerve function. For an extensive recent review of deficiency neuropathies the reader is referred to Erbslöh and Abel (1970).

Thiamine—vitamin B_1

The active form of this vitamin is thiamine pyrophosphate which is the coenzyme for at least three important enzymes of carbohydrate metabolism, pyruvate decarboxylase, α-ketoglutarate decarboxylase and transketolase. Deficiency causes an accumulation of pyruvate and lactate, with impairment of energy metabolism both in the neuron and Schwann cells. Though starvation alone in the presence of vitamin therapy may cause a peripheral neuropathy, the typical setting for thiamine deficiency was such as that occurring in the Japanese prisoner-of-war camps in the Second Word War. The diet consisted predominantly of polished rice, which contains carbohydrate with no vitamins because of the removal of the rice husks during polishing. The result was damage to the peripheral nerves (*dry beriberi*) and to the heart with congestive cardiac failure (*wet beriberi*). The incidence of symptomatic neuropathy depended upon the severity of deprivation, though most of the prisoners showed signs of a distal, symmetrical polyneuropathy. In 50 per cent this was mixed sensorimotor, in 30 per cent mainly sensory and 20 per cent mainly motor (Cruickshank 1952). A burning sensation in the feet, numbness of the feet, lower legs and occasionally fingers, and tender calves were the commonest sensory problems. A foot drop was the commonest motor problem. Optic neuritis occurred in some patients. Treatment with thiamine at a dose of more than 100 mg/day led to a slow recovery which often took more than 6 months. Those who had suffered prolonged and severe starvation made a lesser degree of recovery, the dysaesthetic phenomena being particularly resistant.

In experimental thiamine deficiency in rats, the maximum motor conduction velocity of the sciatic nerve was decreased by 50–60 per cent of normal suggesting a major degree of segmental demyelination (Erbslöh and Abel 1970). Earlier reports of the pathological changes in thiamine deficiency suggested the presence of segmental demyelination and Collins *et al.* (1964) showed that the earliest change was an increase in the normal irregularities of the myelin sheaths. Nevertheless it is clear that axonal degeneration predominates (Collins *et al.* 1964, Prineas 1970). This is in keeping with the slow recovery seen in the clinical situation which suggests axonal degeneration with recovery by axonal regrowth.

Vitamin B_{12}

The exact function of vitamin B_{12} is not clear. It is involved in the metabolism of methyl units, in nucleic acid metabolism, and probably in cell membrane synthesis. Deficiency is most commonly due to loss of intrinsic factor, which is produced by the gastric mucosa and required for the intestinal absorption of vitamin B_{12}. This deficiency is usually due to autoimmune damage of the gastric parietal cells by circulating antibodies. There is a familial tendency, and the disease usually presents in middle age. More rarely there is congenital absence of intrinsic factor, and the disease presents in the juvenile. Other causes of malabsorption of vitamin B_{12} include the blind loop syndromes, ileal resection, the fish tapeworm, and the dietary fads of vegans. The mechanism of damage of the peripheral nerves in vitamin B_{12} deficiency is not certain. Clinically the central nervous system changes predominate. Particularly there is progressive damage to the pyramidal tracts and posterior columns in the spinal cord. In addition many patients have symptoms of a polyneuropathy with paraesthesiae in the hands and feet and a mild glove and stocking impairment of the modalities of sensation conveyed by the larger fibres, together with loss of the ankle jerks.

There is slowing of the maximum motor and sensory conduction velocities in the distal parts of the peripheral nerves to about 80–90 per cent of normal, with no change in the proximal parts (Mayer 1965). The response to treatment with intramuscular vitamin B_{12} at a dose of 1000 µg/day is relatively quick, the paraesthesiae disappearing within a few days and the distal reflexes returning within 1–2 months. Similarly the distal nerve conduction velocity returns to normal within 1 month. However the spinal cord damage is much less responsive to therapy, and the prognosis is entirely dependent upon this. The physiological studies suggest that the neuropathy is a 'dying back' type of axonal degeneration, and this suggestion is supported by pathological studies in man, there being loss of the larger myelinated fibres in distal sensory nerves with the changes of axonal degeneration in teased single fibres (Greenfield and Carmichael 1935, McLeod et al. 1969). However in experimental vitamin B_{12} deficiency in monkeys segmental demyelination apparently predominates (Torres et al. 1971).

Other B group vitamins

Deficiency of pyridoxine (vitamin B_6), whose active derivative pyridoxal-5-phosphate is a coenzyme for many decarboxylases and transaminases, experimentally causes a peripheral neuropathy (Follis and Wingrobe 1945, Vilter et al. 1953). This is predominantly a distal, symmetrical sensory polyneuropathy, though central nervous system changes also occur. In the pig it is probably mainly an axonal degeneration, though single fibre studies have not been undertaken. Isoniazid produces an essentially identical neuropathy (see below page 166) by interfering with pyridoxine metabolism, probably forming the isonicotinyl hydrazone of pyridoxine (Aspinall 1964).

In pellagra, which is due mainly to nicotinic acid deficiency, a painful burning distal symmetrical sensory polyneuropathy may occur, though the central nervous system changes predominate. The burning feet syndrome may at times be due to riboflavin deficiency.

Malabsorption and other causes of vitamin deficiencies

A variety of neuropathic and myopathic syndromes have been reported with diseases causing malabsorption. A progressive symmetrical distal mixed polyneuropathy is the commonest, with sensory ataxia, paraesthesia and spontaneous pains (Cook and Smith 1966). Malabsorptions of all types may cause deficiencies particularly of the fat-soluble vitamins and folic acid. However supplementation with all known vitamins, the replacement of pancreatic enzymes, or the administration of a gluten-free diet where appropriate, will still not correct some of the neuropathies. Pathological changes are axonal and distal, though more studies are required of this interesting group of conditions (Cook et al. 1966).

Alcoholics frequently have a peripheral neuropathy similar in presentation to those with thiamine deficiency and have been shown to be deficient in thiamine, folic acid, pyridoxin, pantothenic acid and riboflavin (Fennelly *et al.* 1964). There is evidence of malabsorption of thiamine (Tomasulo *et al.* 1968). Their high caloric intake in the form of alcohol with deficiency of thiamine may be responsible for the nerve damage in many. Some, however, fail to improve with replacement of vitamins of the B group. The direct toxic effect of alcohol and the possible effect of liver damage must also be considered.

Epileptics frequently show signs of a peripheral neuropathy with areflexia, slight slowing of maximum motor and sensory conduction velocities, and denervation on electromyography (Horwitz *et al.* 1967). The serum folic acid is often low in these patients but usually replacement has no effect upon the neuropathy. The peripheral nerve damage is probably due to the chronic effects of the anticonvulsants, perhaps exacerbated by recurrent anoxic and traumatic episodes during the epileptic fits.

Neuropathies due to exogenous toxins

A wide range of chemical agents, including inorganic substances particularly metals, and organic chemicals, may cause damage to the peripheral nervous system. The short length of this section devoted to toxic neuropathies is no indication of their importance, but is simply due to the large number of such chemicals and the small amount which is known about the action of most of them (Cohen 1970, Le Quesne 1970).

Care is required before accepting all reports of neuropathies due to toxic substances, particularly those recording the uncommon reactions to drugs. The neuropathy may in fact be due to the underlying disease for which the drug was first given, or the association may be fortuitous. Moreover allergic immunological reactions to almost any agent can occur. The agent acts as a hapten, binds to protein, which then becomes an antibody against which the body reacts. Such reactions are usually no more common with one agent than another, the 'allergic predisposition' being more the character of the individual.

Other idiosyncratic reactions may indicate an underlying metabolic abnormality. Isoniazid intoxication occurs particularly in slow inactivators of the drug, in whom hepatic acetylation is slow with consequent high blood levels and the excretion of the major part of the drug unchanged in the urine (Evans *et al.* 1960, Evans 1963). This tendency is inherited as an autosomal recessive trait, heterozygotes showing intermediate rates of inactivation. Isoniazid neuropathy results from pyridoxine deficiency, the drug forming the isonicotinyl hydrazone of pyridoxine. It may be treated either by withdrawal of the drug or administration of pyridoxine in a dose of 10 mg/100 mg of isoniazid. The clinical picture is of a mixed sensori-motor distal neuropathy, sometimes with spontaneous burning pains. The maximum motor and sensory nerve conduction velocity are slightly slowed and the sensory nerve action potential is decreased in amplitude. The nerve shows axonal degeneration both of myelinated and unmyelinated nerve fibres (Cavanagh 1967, Hildebrand et al. 1968, Ochoa 1970).

Deficient detoxication due to hepatic disease or deficient excretion from renal failure may lead to excessive blood levels of potentially neurotoxic drugs. Nitrofurantoin neuropathy is an example of the latter. Clinical signs and symptoms of intoxication are uncommon unless the patient is in renal failure, though electrophysiological studies may reveal subclinical peripheral nerve damage (Toole et al. 1968). The peripheral neuropathy is a mixed sensorimotor distal neuropathy affecting both the hands and feet and often progressing rapidly. Axonal degeneration is the pathological change, and thus recovery on withdrawal of the drug is relatively slow.

Careful observation is often required, particularly of the effect of the withdrawal of the agent to establish in the first instance that a drug is potentially neurotoxic. Thalidomide was an example in point. The drug was first marketed in 1956, but not until 1960 was it first suggested that a sensory neuropathy with characteristic painful dysaesthesiae and nocturnal cramps might be due to the drug. Even then many patients still received the drug until the teratogenic effects became recognized and the drug was withdrawn. Electrophysiological and pathological studies indicate axonal degeneration in this neuropathy. Unfortunately many of the patients had been left with permanent and often disabling painful dysaethesiae (Fuller-ton and O'Sullivan 1968).

Often painstaking detective work is required to reveal the cause of a neuropathy in a patient. His place of work and any chemicals to which he has been exposed at home or at work must immediately be suspected. For instance acrylamide, a very potent peripheral nerve toxin, is used in many industries to make polyacrylamide as a water-proofer, flocculator or chemical grout. Absorption may occur through the skin or by inhalation of the powder. The monomer is readily water-soluble. The neuropathy affects the distal parts of the larger sensory and motor fibres, producing axonal degeneration. Its onset may be acute or insidious (Fullerton 1969). Recent work with rat poisons should suggest the possibility of thallium intoxication which causes an acute sensory motor polyneuropathy and alopecia. The pathological change is predominantly axonal degeneration (Bank et al.

1972). Suicidal or homicidal attempts must never be forgotten, and arsenic should be mentioned in this respect. This usually produces a mixed sensorimotor distal polyneuropathy, often with painful dysaesthesiae. Indigestion, skin pigmentation and hyperkeratosis are frequent accompaniments (Chhuttani *et al.* 1967). A number of other metals and metaloids are toxic to the peripheral nerves. Lead compounds cause a predominantly motor axonal neuropathy characteristically producing wrist- and foot-drop (Fullerton 1966). Gold compounds used in the treatment of rheumatoid arthritis may produce a distal sensorimotor neuropathy (Walsh 1970). Cytotoxic agents, particularly vincristine, used in the treatment of neoplastic conditions like leukaemia can produce distal sensorimotor polyneuropathies (Bradley *et al.* 1970).

Mass epidemics of paralysis due to peripheral and central nervous degeneration have resulted from contamination of food oils with agents containing organophosphates including triorthocresyl phosphate. These outbreaks have proved particularly difficult to diagnose since for an unknown reason there is a delay of 5–20 days between the ingestion and the first symptoms. There is a severe sensorimotor distal polyneuropathy with axonal degeneration of the largest fibres. Recovery is slow in the peripheral nervous system and minimal in the central nervous system (Cavanagh 1964). Endemic diseases such as the ataxic tropical neuropathies seen in East and West Africa may be due to cyanide released from foods like cassava containing cyanogens (see page 199).

Chronic alcoholism is a potent cause of peripheral nerve damage. Probably the excessive blood alcohol level itself is toxic, but the damage is increased by the commonly associated cirrhosis (page 172) and malnutrition (page 165). A mixed sensorimotor distal polyneuropathy is a common finding on examination, though this is asymptomatic in many cases. Foot-drop may develop and the sensory nerve damage may be so severe that acrodystrophic neuropathic phenomena like deep painless ulcers, Charcot joints and loss of digits occur (Bureau *et al.* 1957, Mota-Revatllat 1966). *Alcoholic acrodystrophic neuropathy* is particularly common in the South of France and Spain. The life-long chronic intake of 2 to 4 litres of wine every day with a normal diet is probably responsible for this particular neuropathy. Motor and sensory nerve conduction studies show mild slowing more marked in those with severe neuropathies, and of the order seen in axonal neuropathies (Mawdsley and Meyer 1965). Electromyographic signs of denervation are frequent. The pathological changes are of axonal degeneration (Walsh and McLeod 1970).

Poisons may affect many sites and are rarely entirely specific, though many have a predilection for certain parts of the peripheral nervous system. Botulinum toxin blocks the release of transmitter vesicles at the neuro-muscular junctions (Duchen 1970). Saxitoxin and tetrodotoxin block the depolarization of axonal and neuronal membranes (Evans 1969). Diph-theria toxin damages Schwann cells causing segmental demyelination with relative sparing of the axons. However, in most toxic neuropathies, the primary change is axonal degeneration. Frequently the pattern of degenera-tion is the 'dying-back' type affecting the distal parts of the large fibres (see page 136). The presence of a mild toxic neuropathy may predispose to the development of a second disease of the nerve such as entrapment (Hopkins and Morgan-Hughes 1969).

Drugs and other agents are usually screened for neurotoxic effects prior to release. Unfortunately there are considerable differences in the suscepti-bility of various species. For instance the rat is more resistant to lead, vin-cristine and triorthocresyl phosphate than are the guinea pig and many other animals.

The list of agents which may be responsible for peripheral nerve dam-age is legion. A few are shown in table 6.3. The importance of the recogni-tion of the toxic nature of a peripheral neuropathy cannot be too highly stressed for the poison may then be withdrawn and the patient allowed to recover. In addition, toxic neuropathies potentially offer biochemical keys for unlocking the treasury of knowledge of peripheral nerve biochemistry, though at present this offer remains largely unfulfilled.

Acute porphyric neuropathy

Acute nervous crises occur in porphyria, particularly of the acute inter-mittent type. They take the form of severe episodes of abdominal pain, psychiatric disorders, and peripheral neuropathies. The neuropathy is acute, severe and chiefly motor, leading to flaccid paralysis and loss of re-flexes (Ridley 1969). There is a proximal predominance, the upper limbs being involved more than the lower. The cranial nerves, trunk and respira-tory muscles and sphincters are often involved. In about a half there is some sensory involvement, which may be either proximal or distal and in-volving all modalities. The most classic picture is of a bathing trunk distri-bution of sensory loss, proximal paralysis and paradoxical preservation of the ankle jerks. Muscle wasting is rapid.

Pathological changes are predominantly of axonal degeneration, which

TABLE 6.3. Some of the causes of toxic neuropathies

METALS	Lead, arsenic (inorganic and organic), mercury (inorganic and organic), thallium, gold
INDUSTRIAL ORGANIC POISONS	*Solvents:* hexane, petrol, trichlorethylene, carbon tetrachloride, carbon disulphide, dimethylsulphoxide
	Insecticides and herbicides: dieldrin, aldrin, 2,4-D, DDT
	Others: TOCP, acrylamide, diethylthiocarbamate, p-bromophenylacetylurea
DRUGS	*Anticonvulsants:* phenytoin
	Chemotherapeutic: isoniazid, furans (nitrofurantoin, furaltadone), ethambutol, ethionamide, amphotericin B, sulphonamides, clioquinol, chloroquin
	Antimitotic: nitrogen mustards, ethoglucid, Vinca alkaloids (vincristine, vinblastine)
	Sedatives: thalidomide, glutethimide
	Others: imipramine, monoamine oxidase inhibitors, disulfiram, hydrallazine, stilbamidine, nitrofurazone, ergotamine
FOODS	Cyanogens (cassava, cycasin), alcohol, lathyrogens
BACTERIA AND VIRUSES	Diphtheria, [Guillain-Barré-Strohl syndrome]

in the motor nerves affects particularly the distal parts of the larger fibres in the intramuscular nerves, and in the sensory fibres affects predominantly the centrally directed axons of the dorsal roots (Cavanagh and Mellick 1965). In both instances there is therefore a 'dying-back' distribution in individual axons, though the longest fibres are not involved as in the more common type of 'dying back' neuropathy. It has been suggested that the effects fall particularly on those motor fibres supplying the largest motor units. This is unlikely to be the whole explanation of the proximal predominance since it takes no account of the proximal sensory loss. In some cases there may be an associated segmental demyelination (Thomas 1971).

If severe, respiratory and bulbar paralysis may endanger life, and tracheostomy and artificial respiration are often required. A few patients make a rapid recovery, though in most the recovery is relatively slow as might be expected with axonal regeneration. Sørensen and With (1971) reviewed 95 patients with acute intermittent porphyria, 41 of whom had had paralytic episodes. Of these 41, 17 had died, and 12 of the 24 survivors had residual paralyses after 3 years which in most cases remained permanent thereafter. Recovery was poorer in males.

Attacks of acute intermittent porphyria occur either spontaneously or precipitated by drugs. Alcohol in excess, barbiturates and sulphonamides are particularly responsible. There is a dominant mode of inheritance of the tendency, with incomplete penetrance (Pratt 1967). It has been shown that the attacks are associated with the induction of high levels of δ-amino-laevulic acid synthetase in the liver causing an increased excretion of δ-amino-laevulic acid and porphobilinogen in the urine (Cavanagh and Ridley 1967, Sweeney et al. 1970). The enzyme requires pyridoxal-5-phosphate as its coenzyme, and it has been suggested that the induction of this enzyme causes a deficiency of pyridoxine which produces the neuropathy. However, the picture of porphyric neuropathy differs from that of deficiency of pyridoxine, and there is no correlation between the pyridoxal-5-phosphate level and the neuropathy (Hamfelt and Wetterberg 1968). Meyer et al. (1972) doubted that δ-amino-laevulic acid synthetase induction causes the syndrome, and found a decrease of the red cell urobilinogen I-synthetase activity, though the part played by this in the neuropathy is not clear.

Metabolic neuropathies

Under this heading might be included diabetes mellitus and porphyria, which have already been considered, as well as the neuropathies of general medical diseases including hepatic, renal and thyroid disease, and hypoglycaemia (Henson and Urich 1970). In all, the incidence of symptomatic neuropathy is greatly exceeded by that of asymptomatic damage of the nerves producing either signs on examination or abnormalities of electrophysiological studies.

Uraemic neuropathy

With the longer survival of patients with uraemia as a result of peritoneal or haemodialysis, it has been recognized that many such patients develop a chronic distal symmetrical predominantly sensory polyneuropathy. It is usually not seen until the blood urea exceeds 250 mg/100 ml, and the creatinine clearance falls below 5 ml/min. However, the severity of the neuropathy is not entirely related to the degree of uraemia or electrolyte disturbance. The exact cause of the neuropathy is not clear, though there is some evidence of an inhibitor of transketolase in uraemics which is removed by dialysis but not overcome by thiamine administration (Sterzel et al. 1971). Dialysis may prevent the progression of the neuropathy and allow some recovery (Jebsen et al. 1967). However occasionally the neuropathy acutely appears or deteriorates following the institution of dialysis therapy. In these patients, dialysis may cause acute changes in osmotically active substances and loss of essential nutrients. The neuropathy usually remits following successful renal transplantation.

The symptoms, which are present in about 75 per cent of patients having chronic dialysis, include burning paraesthesiae, restless legs, hyperpathia and numbness spreading upwards from the feet, and only later involving the hands. Motor involvement is milder, though a foot-drop may result. There is mild slowing of the maximum motor and sensory nerve conduction velocities by about 5–10 per cent, with a decrease of the amplitude of the sensory nerve action potentials, the changes being suggestive of an axonal neuropathy. However pathological studies have shown definite segmental demyelination as well as signs of axonal degeneration, though as emphasized on page 119, segmental demyelination is easier to see than axonal degeneration in teased single fibre studies. There may be a relative loss of Schwann cells (Asbury et al. 1963). Segmental demyelination is marked in some fibres and little in others suggesting that an abnormality of the axon leads to secondary segmental demyelination (Jennekens et al. 1969, Dyck et al. 1971).

Hepatic neuropathy

The central nervous effects of chronic liver failure far outweigh the peripheral ones. Few patients with chronic liver failure have symptoms of the latter, though a fifth have signs of peripheral nerve damage usually with depression of reflexes distally. A fifth have slight slowing of the maximum conduction velocity in the main nerve trunks of the order of 10 per cent (Knill-Jones et al. 1972) and up to two-thirds have an increased peripheral latency of sensory and motor conduction and a decrease of the sensory nerve action potential (Seneviratne and Peiris 1970). The peripheral nerves of most patients show segmental demyelination with a lesser degree of loss of myelinated nerve fibres due to axonal degeneration. In patients with alcholic cirrhosis, the toxic effects of the alcohol and the effects of vitamin deficiencies cannot be excluded. However, damage can be found in primary biliary cirrhosis; Thomas and Walker (1965) reported three patients with cutaneous xanthomata, who had a mild distal symmetrical sensory polyneuropathy with xanthomatous infiltrations within the peripheral nerve causing loss of myelinated nerve fibres.

Neuropathies associated with thyroid disease

The carpal tunnel syndrome is relatively common in *myxoedema* due to infiltration of the tissue within the tunnel by myxoid material (Murray and Simpson 1958), and other entrapments may also occur. About 45 per cent of myxoedematous patients have sensory symptoms, and 10 per cent of these have signs of a mild distal symmetrical predominantly sensory polyneuropathy (Nickel and Frame 1958). In most there is slowing of the maximum sensory nerve conduction velocity by about 30 per cent, and a decrease of amplitude of the sensory nerve action potentials; in some there is slowing of the maximum motor nerve conduction velocity. Dyck and Lambert (1970) showed physiological and histological evidence of segmental demyelination and remyelination of myelinated nerve fibres with no change in unmyelinated nerve fibres in myxoedematous neuropathy. The symptoms and signs of the neuropathy largely recover with thyroid replacement.

In *thyrotoxicosis* a proximal myopathy is the main neuromuscular disorder. However electromyographic evidence of distal denervation has been reported in this condition, and some patients have mild symptoms and signs of sensory involvement suggesting the presence of a peripheral neuropathy (Ludin *et al.* 1969).

Hypoglycaemic neuropathy

The peripheral nervous system is by no means as sensitive to hypoglycaemia as the central nervous system, but cases of a distal symmetrical mixed polyneuropathy have been reported in patients with insulinomata (Danta 1969). Central nervous system symptoms predominate, but there may be initial sensory symptoms in the limbs and later a rapidly progressing distal motor neuropathy. Cases which have come to autopsy show degeneration of the perikarya within the spinal cord and dorsal root ganglia.

The part played by hypoglycaemic episodes in 'brittle' diabetics who develop a neuropathy has to be considered.

Neuropathies with other metabolic abnormalities

In a few relatively rare diseases of peripheral nerve, metabolic abnormalities have been described which may perhaps be the cause of the nerve disease. Several of these diseases affect the central nervous system more than the peripheral.

Tangier disease consists of the deposition of cholesterol esters throughout the reticuloendothelial system, particularly the tonsils, associated with a very low plasma cholesterol, and absent α-lipoproteins in the plasma. A progressive or recurrent sensorimotor neuropathy has been recorded in this disease, with loss both of myelin sheaths and axons (Kocen *et al.* 1967, Engel *et al.* 1967). The relationship between the biochemical abnormality and the neuropathy requires clarification.

Bassen-Kornzweig's disease involves neurological damage including ataxia from posterior column and spinocerebellar tract degeneration, pyramidal tract degeneration, atypical retinitis pigmentosa, areflexia and anterior horn cell degeneration. There is also malabsorption, particularly of fat. β-lipoproteins are absent from the plasma. The plasma cholesterol is very low. The red cell membrane is abnormal, leading to the formation of burr-cells (acanthocytes) (Farquhar and Ways 1966). The exact part played by the abetalipoproteinaemia is not certain.

The stigmata of *Fabry's disease* (*angiokeratoma corporis diffusum*) include characteristic skin lesions, corneal opacities, dilated conjunctival capillaries, and the abnormal deposition of lipids in many tissues. Atheromatous degeneration of the arteries leads to cerebral and myocardial infarction, and renal failure. Accumulation of lipid, which consists mainly of ceramide trihexosides, also occurs throughout many neurons. Spontaneous pains in the limbs are a frequent feature of the disease, without further evidence of a neuropathy, but lipid deposits in the perineurium and a moderate loss of myelinated nerve fibres may be found in peripheral nerves (Kocen and Thomas 1970). Ceramide trihexosidase is deficient in these patients, presumably leading to the formation of abnormal membranes, including myelin.

In *metachromatic leucodystrophy*, though central nervous white matter degeneration predominates, the peripheral nervous system is also involved. This leads to progressive areflexia and sometimes hypotonia supervening upon the picture of decorticate spasticity. Nerve conduction velocities are greatly slowed. Pathologically, the nerves show an increased amount of the normal irregularities of the myelin sheaths (fig. 6.2), and extensive segmental demyelination (fig. 6.3). There are numerous Schwann cell inclusions which stain metachromatically with basic dyes such as toluidine blue and cresylfast violet (see frontispiece). Under the electron microscope these

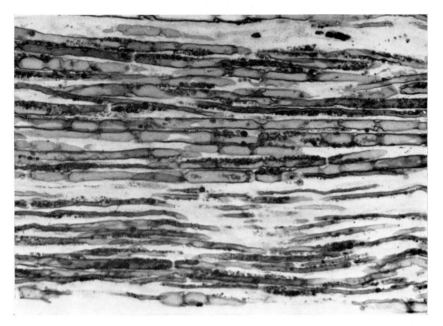

FIG. 6.2. Longitudinal section of a sural nerve biopsy from a child with metachromatic leucodystrophy, showing numerous coarsely granular inclusions and irregularities in the myelin sheaths. Weigert-Pal. × 250. (*From* Bradley and Thomas 1973.)

are seen as multilaminated bodies similar to myelin in the process of degradation (fig. 6.4). These consist of ceramide hexoside sulphates (sulphatides), and are believed to result from a deficiency of the lysosomal enzyme aryl sulphatase A which degrades sulphatide by removing the sulphate radical.

Globoid cell leucodystrophy in man and the dog is associated with segmental demyelination in the peripheral nerves, and the accumulation of cholesterol crystals and acid phosphatase activity in the Schwann cell cytoplasm. Foamy macrophages are found in the peripheral nerves, though

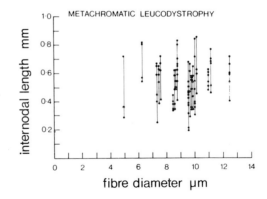

FIG. 6.3. Internodal length spectrum of single teased fibres from the sural nerve of a child with metachromatic leucodystrophy showing the pattern of segmental demyelination and remyelination.

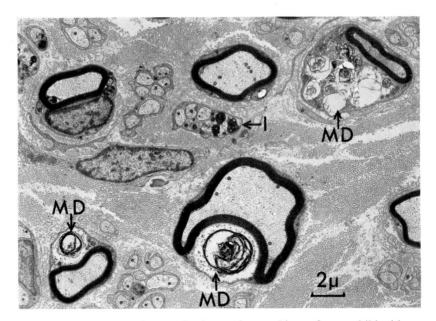

FIG. 6.4. Electron micrograph of a sural nerve biopsy from a child with metachromatic leucodystrophy showing several granules of metachromatic material (MD) in the Schwann cell cytoplasm of several myelinated nerve fibres. Abnormal granular inclusions (I) are also present in Remak cell cytoplasm.

large accumulations such as seen in the brain do not occur. Spongiform change may be seen in the peripheral nerves in *Canavan's disease*. Axon swellings may be seen in the peripheral nerves in cases of *neuroaxonal dystrophy*. However the changes in none of these conditions are as diagnostic as those in metachromatic leucodystrophy.

The accumulation of phytanic acid in *Refsum's disease* and of ceramide hexosides and ceramide hexoside sulphates in *hypertrophic neuropathy of the Dejerine-Sottas variety* is described on page 190. The occasional finding of aminoaciduria or of an abnormal pyruvate tolerance test (Hockaday *et al.* 1966) suggests the presence of an underlying biochemical defect awaiting to be discovered.

Acute idiopathic post-infectious polyneuropathy (Guillain-Barré-Strohl syndrome)

Clinical features

Landry (1859) described a group of patients with acute ascending paralysis which is now recognized probably to comprise both patients with post-infectious polyneuropathy and transverse myelitis. Guillain, Barré and Strohl (1916) collected a series of patients with polyradiculoneuritis, stressing the albumino-cytologic dissociation in the cerebrospinal fluid. Though many such patients have been described since, and much is known about the aetiology of the condition, the criteria for diagnosis still remain difficult to define. Though it is probable that there is one single disease entity here, a spectrum of symptoms is seen ranging from the acute with a relatively good prognosis to the subacute and chronic cases where continuing activity of the disease causes a worsening of the prognosis. In order to achieve a group with a relatively homogeneous clinical course and prognosis, many require rigid criteria to be satisfied before making the diagnosis. Emphasis is particularly given to the duration between the onset and peak of the weakness. Osler and Siddell (1960), in a list of twelve criteria, set 2 weeks as the limit for this interval. Prineas (1970a) allowed 3 weeks. Ravn (1967) accepted 46 days. Pleasure *et al.* (1968) set the limit at 2 months, while two of the cases of Asbury *et al.* (1969) worsened over 3 months. All such cases seemed essentially to be of the same disease, which illustrates the difficulty in defining acceptable diagnostic criteria.

Over 50 per cent of patients give a history of some preceding viral infection 2–4 weeks prior to the onset of the neuropathy. Over a quarter begin with paraesthesiae in the feet spreading proximally, and then involving the hands. Over a third have moderately severe pains, particularly in the back and limbs, which may cause diagnostic difficulties. Sensory loss is usually slight and may be absent in a third of patients, while motor involvement is the most striking feature. In a half of patients weakness is diffuse from the onset, while in the remainder it spreads up from the lower limbs to involve the upper limbs, the respiratory and then the bulbar muscles in the most severe cases. On an average the condition progresses for 1–2 weeks, and at its maximum tracheostomy and artificial respiration are required to support life in about 20–30 per cent of cases. In terms of a peripheral neuropathy, such a progress is *acute*.

The paresis is at its maximum for 1–4 weeks, those with milder weakness having paradoxically longer to wait before the onset of recovery. Thereafter there is gradual recovery, though it may take 3–6 months in some, and about 3–6 per cent of patients have relapses.

The cerebrospinal fluid protein concentration is raised in almost all patients at some time during the illness, though it may be normal in the first 7 days. The maximum rise is seen from the tenth to twentieth days, and the level may rise to 1800 mg/100 ml. The proportion of γ-globulin is raised in most cases. Papilloedema, which occurs in 5–10 per cent of cases, may be due to the increased protein concentration causing impairment of the absorption of cerebrospinal fluid (Morley and Reynolds 1966). Though Guillain *et al.* (1916) emphasized the albumino-cytologic dissociation, about a quarter of patients have a raised cell count in the C.S.F., though rarely to more than 40 cells/mm³. As described below, infiltration with lymphocytes and segmental demyelination predominate in the roots with lesser involvement of the peripheral nerves. Pathologically involved nerves show a decrease of maximum conduction velocity to 50 per cent of normal. However the standard nerve conduction studies undertaken early in the condition and in those cases where only the nerve roots are involved may show entirely normal maximum conduction velocities.

The overall prognosis for recovery is good considering the parlous state of some of the patients. It might be hoped that death would never result even in those requiring intermittent positive pressure ventilation, though most series still have a mortality rate of more than 10 per cent. About 18 per cent of patients followed for more than 3 years still have some residual permanent signs and symptoms, and these residua are commoner in children. Those more severely paralysed have a worse prognosis; of those on a respirator, 17 per cent remain severely disabled, and an additional 10 per cent have residual signs but lead a normal life (Hewer *et al.* 1968).

No other features of the disease have been found to aid in forecasting the outcome.

A less common variation of this condition affects predominantly the cranial nerves including the extraocular muscles, ataxia and areflexia being the sole indication of peripheral nerve involvement (Fisher 1956, Elizan *et al.* 1971) Autonomic involvement can also occur in the Guillain-Barré-Strohl syndrome, and may even occur without peripheral nerve involvement (see page 227).

Pathology

The primary pathological change in the Guillain-Barré-Strohl syndrome, and in its experimental counterpart, *experimental allergic neuritis* produced by immunizing an animal against peripheral nerve antigen by injecting peripheral nerve dispersed in Freund's adjuvant (Waksman and Adams 1955, Aström *et al.* 1968), is segmental demyelination. If the process is very severe, axonal degeneration occurs. Inflammatory cells, predominantly lymphocytes, infiltrate the perivascular spaces and interstitium, particularly in the nerve roots. Their presence may confirm the diagnosis of the Guillain-Barré-Strohl syndrome, though nerve biopsy is rarely required to make the diagnosis. In the tissues, infiltrating lymphocytes are believed to release a cytotoxic agent which damages the myelin and Schwann cells. Macrophages then make their appearance in the peripheral nerve. There is some argument whether macrophages play a major part in the breakdown of what may perhaps be normal myelin, as seems more likely for they may be seen infiltrating underneath the basement membrane and splitting off the myelin (Wisniewski *et al.* 1969, Carpenter 1972), or whether the major myelin breakdown occurs within Schwann cells without the direct intervention of macrophages.

Aetiology

Uncertainty still exists concerning the exact aetiology of this condition, though most agree that a preceding viral infection is important. The condition may, however, occur following other precipitants such as surgical operations. Some authors have found an increased incidence of antibodies to a wide range of viruses in the sera of these patients. In many cases of the Guillain-Barré-Strohl syndrome antibodies to nervous tissue (Melnick 1963), circulating myelinotoxins (Cook *et al.* 1971) and lymphocytes in the peripheral blood sensitive to peripheral nerve antigen (Cook *et al.* 1970, Currie and Knowles 1971) may be found. It has been suggested that those with a higher proportion of reactive lymphocytes in the peripheral blood at the onset of the disease have a worse prognosis. IgM, complement and lymphocytes are found in the peripheral nerves in the Guillain-Barré-Strohl syndrome.

The argument continues about whether the antibodies or the lymphocytes are the primary cause of the syndrome, and what attracts the antibodies and lymphocytes into the peripheral nerve. Perhaps the most plausible suggestion is that during the preceding illness a virus enters the Schwann cell, replicating there. Lymphocytes and antibodies reacting against this are thereby attracted into the nerve, where they damage the infected Schwann cells. The mechanism is similar therefore to that suggested for postviral encephalomyelitis by Webb and Gordon Smith (1966). The finding of similar pathological changes in a proven viral disease of chickens (Marek's disease) supports this suggestion (Wight 1969), though occasional cases arising during immunosuppressive therapy and following other precipitations show that this is not the complete explanation.

Treatment

If the autoimmune theory were true, it would be sensible to treat with immunosuppressive agents, including corticosteroids, adrenocorticotrophin and cytotoxic drugs. There is, however, argument about the effectiveness of these agents, Occasional cases show a dramatic response to corticosteroid therapy, but others show an equally dramatic relapse when the dosage is reduced and some become corticosteroid-dependent (Matthews *et al.* 1970).

The theoretical objection to such treatment is that when symptoms and signs have appeared, the lymphocytes are already in the tissue. The best time to administer immunosuppressive therapy would be *before* this, which is obviously impossible in the clinical situation. Large double-blind controlled trials are required to elucidate the matter. The author's practice is to give a short trial of about 1 week of corticosteroid treatment when the condition is deteriorating or severe. If no improvement appears, cytotoxic immunosuppressive therapy is added for the second week. If there is still no improvement, both treatments are withdrawn. The most important treatment is the general support, including tracheostomy and artificial respiration where required.

Recurrent polyneuropathy

Recurrent attacks of polyneuropathy may occur in the familial pressure-sensitive neuropathies, and a number of the hereditary neuropathies including acute intermittent porphyria. They may also be seen in the metabolic neuropathies when the underlying metabolic disease relapses. Idiopathic recurrent polyneuropathy is also a recognized syndrome. The first attack may be indistinguishable from acute idiopathic post-infectious polyneuropathy, or it may have a more subacute onset. The attacks may be frequent, and may be sufficiently severe to necessitate artificial respiration (Hewer *et al.* 1968). Permanent residua may develop following several attacks, or there may be complete recovery between each relapse. Segmental demyelination, sometimes with lymphocytic infiltration of the nerves, is the initial pathological change in most cases, and nerve hypertrophy with 'onion bulb' formation may develop (Austin 1958). A few cases may be due to a recurrent vasculitis, and axonal degeneration is more common in these.

Many of these patients respond well to corticosteroid therapy, either using prednisone or adrenocorticotrophin. However those patients who respond may show disastrous relapses with very small reductions in dosage. Personally observed cases, who have been almost totally quadriplegic, have been returned to almost normal peripheral nerve function with 80 IU of adrenocorticotrophin or 60 mg of prednisone daily. However the incautious reduction of dosage by as little as 10 per cent may produce a dramatic relapse. It is important that the dosage of corticosteroid therapy should be reduced extremely slowly in these cases. When the patient is found to have a steroid-sensitive recurrent polyneuropathy, the author's practice is to maintain the dose of corticosteroid required to suppress the condition for 2–3 months. The dosage is then reduced by 5 mg of prednisone of 5 IU of adrenocorticotrophin every month, until the dose eventually reaches zero or a relapse occurs necessitating a return to a higher dose level. At lower doses, the reduction must be by an even smaller amount. In this way corticosteroid therapy was eventually withdrawn in three out of five personally observed patients, leaving them with relatively normal peripheral nerve function; one was left with severe residual damage, and one died when his neuropathy eventually became unresponsive to corticosteroid therapy. Immunosuppressive therapy is worthy of trial in this group of patients.

Hereditary neuropathies

Hereditary diseases of the peripheral nerve make up only a small part of the whole group of peripheral neuropathies. Acute intermittent porphyria, which has an autosomal dominant form of inheritance, has already been mentioned (page 169). A number of other inherited conditions in which central nervous degeneration predominates have also been mentioned already. These include metachromatic leucodystrophy, Bassen-Kornzweig's disease, Tangier disease, globoid cell leucodystrophy and neuroaxonal dystrophy (pages 174–175) which have an autosomal recessive mode of inheritance, and Fabry's disease (page 175) which has a sex-linked recessive mode of inheritance. Friedreich's ataxia should be added to this list; usually inheritance is of an autosomal recessive type, and the peripheral nerves show axonal degeneration (McLeod 1971). A number of other diseases of peripheral nerve may be inherited including amyloidosis, hereditary sensory radicular neuropathy, peroneal muscular atrophy, hypertrophic neuropathy and Refsum's disease.

Amyloidosis

Three main types of familial amyloidosis with different clinical patterns have been described. All have a dominant mode of inheritance.

Andrade type

This condition is endemic in the part of northern Portugal around Oporto (Andrade 1952). It also occurs in Portuguese descendants in other parts of the world, and in those with no Portuguese blood. The disease begins between 25–35 years of age, and leads to death within 7–15 years. It presents with sensory symptoms in the lower limbs, which include painful dysaesthesiae and spontaneous shooting pains. Pain and temperature sensation and autonomic function are preferentially lost (*viz* unmyelinated and small myelinated fibres are particularly involved), leading to trophic ulceration of the feet. The autonomic involvement produces diarrhoea, sphincter impairment, impotence in the male, decreased gastrointestinal motility, postural hypotension, and disordered cardiac conduction. Death may be due to inanition, or to chronic renal failure due to chronic pyelonephritis or amyloid infiltration of the kidneys.

The maximum motor and sensory nerve conduction velocities may be normal or only decreased by about 10 per cent, though there is a progressive fall in the sensory nerve action potential amplitude until total failure of peripheral nerve conduction. Dyck and Lambert (1969) showed that the loss of the C potential in the sural nerve *in vitro* corresponded to the loss of unmyelinated nerve fibres seen pathologically.

Amyloid is present both in the adventitia and media of small arterioles, and in masses free within the endoneurium (see frontispiece). It is also found in the kidneys, skin blood vessels and rectal submucosa. It shows the characteristic staining reactions with Congo red and thioflavin T, and is composed of characteristic non-branching fibrils of 7–10 nm diameter (Coimbra and Andrade 1971). The nerve fibres may be compressed by the endoneurial deposits. The most striking feature in the cases of Dyck and Lambert (1969) was the loss of unmyelinated nerve fibres corresponding closely to the loss of pain and temperature sensation and of the C potential. Axonal degeneration of the myelinated nerve fibres also occurs.

Rukavina type

A large kinship of Swiss origin with amyloid polyneuropathy was described from Indiana by Rukavina et al. (1956), and subsequently a further un-related kinship of German origin has been reported from Maryland (Mahloudi et al. 1969). This condition is much more benign than the Andrade type, males however being more severely affected than females. It presents usually at about the age of 45 with a bilateral carpal tunnel syndrome (page 152 et seq.). At this stage surgical decompression can be curative of the local symptoms, and amyloid is found infiltrating the flexor retinaculum causing the compression.

Later in the disease there develops a progressive distal symmetrical polyneuropathy affecting particularly the larger myelinated fibres, and the legs more than the arms. This often remains mild, and some patients live to the eighties with little disability. Vitreous opacities are common, requiring surgical evacuation of the vitreous. Autonomic and renal involvement occur only late in this type of amyloidosis. Electrophysiological studies show a minimal decrease of the maximum motor nerve conduction velocity in the nerve trunks, though the terminal motor and sensory latencies are increased.

Van Allen type

Van Allen et al. (1969) reported a large kinship in Iowa originating from the British Isles, who presented with a painful distal symmetrical sensori-motor polyneuropathy starting in the lower limbs at about the age of 30–35 years. The carpal tunnel syndrome was not seen, nor was there significant autonomic disturbance. However a progressive nephropathy and peptic ulceration were prominent features. Progressive renal failure caused death within 15 or 20 years, by which time there was significant loss of all modalities of sensation distally in the arms and legs, with amyotrophy. The C.S.F. protein concentration was raised in most cases. Amyloid was present within the nerve roots, the posterior root ganglia, and the sympathetic nerves and ganglia. Again the blood vessel walls and interstitium were particularly affected.

It seems impossible to ascribe all the changes occurring in the Andrade and Van Allen types to the direct effects of the amyloid within the peripheral nerve itself. Amyloid in the walls of many blood vessels may produce infarction of peripheral nerve (Asbury 1970). However, neither the compressive effect of amyloid masses within the perineurium, nor the ischaemia resulting from vascular infiltration, would seem sufficient to explain the particular loss of unmyelinated fibres seen in the Andrade type of disease. The infiltration of the posterior root and autonomic ganglia with amyloid leading to total replacement of many of the neurons is probably the cause of the unmyelinated and later myelinated nerve fibre degeneration and loss (Appenzeller 1970). In all, unfortunately only palliative symptomatic therapy is available.

Congenital and hereditary sensory neuropathies

A number of disease entities in which there is a hereditary or congenital sensory neuropathy have now been recognized. These include congenital non-progressive sensory neuropathy, hereditary progressive sensory neuropathy, and hereditary sensory radicular neuropathy, all of which are described below. All are associated with a marked impairment of all modalities of sensation distally in the limbs, the loss of pain and temperature sensation resulting in repeated injuries, infections, distal mutilation and arthropathic joints. The tendon reflexes are abolished, but motor involvement is minimal or absent. The terms, Morvan's syndrome and acrodystrophic neuropathy have been applied to these conditions, which have often been misdiagnosed in the past as syringomyelia. Other diseases which may produce a similar clinical picture include diabetic sensory polyneuropathy (see page 158 *et seq.*), alcoholic acrodystrophic neuropathy (see page 168), the sensory neuropathy of carcinoma (see pages 191–192), and tabes dorsalis (see page 264).

In addition there are three conditions recognized in which there is congenital absence of pain sensation over the whole body. In the first, *congenital insensivitiy to pain*, from birth there is absence of the normal appreciation and reaction to pain unassociated with other neurological deficits (Jewesbury 1970). These patients have otherwise normal sensation, and are usually able to discriminate accurately between hot and cold, and sometimes between a sharp and a blunt pin. There is however no reaction to pain of any variety, and such patients have been exhibited in fairgrounds as 'The Human Pin Cushion'. Repeated episodes of painless injury and infection produce progressive mutilation with ulceration and neuropathic joints. The sensory nerves in the skin are normal, and full autopsy examination has so far failed to reveal any underlying abnormality of the nervous system (Baxter and Olszewski 1960). The anatomical site and pathophysiology of this disease is therefore unknown, though a cortical localization has been suggested. Acquired cortical lesions, particularly of the supramarginal gyrus of the dominant parietal lobe, may produce a state termed by Schilder (1931), pain asymbolia, in which there is no lack of sensation and no analgesia in the common sense, but the psychic reaction to pain is absent. Osuntokun *et al.* (1968) described two half-sibs who had congenital pain asymbolia with auditory imperception. In these children there was no appreciation of pain nor of the significance of the spoken word despite normal intelligence.

A different condition is *congenital insensivity to pain with anhidrosis* (Vassella *et al.* 1968). These patients may have recurrent episodes of unexplained fever. Swanson *et al.* (1965) found at autopsy in one case the absence of the small primary sensory neurons and axons of the posterior root ganglia, the posterior roots and Lissauer's tract. No anatomical cause of the anhidrosis could be discovered.

The third of this group of conditions is *familial dysautonomia (Riley-Day syndrome*; see page 225), in which in addition to the total absence from birth of pain sensation over the whole of the body, there is also emotional lability, absent lacrimation, postural hypotension, absent fungiform papillae on the tongue and hyperhidrosis (Riley *et al.* 1949). Other neurological features including nystagmus, poor muscle tone and coordination, and areflexia are often present. The patients are usually of Jewish descent. The anatomical basis of the disease is the absence of unmyelinated nerve fibres in the peripheral and autonomic nerves (Aguayo *et al.* 1971). In view of this abnormality of the peripheral nerves and the areflexia, familial dysautonomia should be classified as a peripheral neuropathy and not as one of the syndromes of congenital insensitivity to pain.

Congenital non-progressive sensory neuropathy

A number of cases have been described in which from birth there is evidence of a distal polyneuropathy in the limbs, involving all modalities of sensation (Ogden *et al.* 1959, Winkelmann *et al.* 1962, Murray 1973). The characteristic feature is the impairment of all modalities of sensation distally in the limbs, the face and trunk usually being spared. The tendon and axon reflexes are lost, but a motor deficit is rarely present. Pain sensation is affected less than that of touch and position, but distally in the limbs pain sensation is totally absent producing the mutilating changes described above. This mutilation becomes progressively worse during life, but repeated clinical investigation shows no change in the degree of sensory loss. The nerves show a striking almost total loss of myelinated nerve fibres with relative preservation of the unmyelinated nerve fibres, and no evidence of active degeneration.

Progressive sensory neuropathy

These cases are very similar to the non-progressive sensory neuropathy described above, except that the onset is usually in the early years of life, and there is a definite clinical progression (Johnson and Spalding 1964, Schoene *et al.* 1970). The familial pattern of cases is compatible with an autosomal recessive mode of inheritance. The clinical and pathological features are indistinguishable from those of the non-progressive congenital sensory neuropathy, and separation of the two conditions rests upon repeated clinical examinations.

Fig. 6.5 shows a sural nerve biopsy from a patient with a progressive sensory neuropathy beginning in childhood. There are no myelinated, and very few unmyelinated nerve fibres remaining. There is no family history of a similar condition. This patient illustrates that the clear-cut demarcation described in this section is not always possible. This 15-year-old boy developed distal ulceration and neuropathic joints from the first few years of life, and had signs of a distal sensory neuropathy involving all modalities in the limbs. There was however in addition the total absence of reaction to all forms of pain over the whole of the body which had probably also been present from the earliest years of life. The pattern suggests that there was congenital damage to the unmyelinated and small myelinated nerve fibres of the whole body, the process later spreading to involve the larger myelinated fibres distally in the limbs.

Hereditary sensory radicular neuropathy

Under this title Denny-Brown (1951) described the pathological changes in a condition reported previously by many authors without pathological confirmation. It was first described in 1852 by Nélaton. The disease generally has an autosomal dominant mode of inheritance, and presents with painless penetrating ulcers and mutilation of the feet and later hands from the second to fourth decades, though a childhood onset may occur in a few families

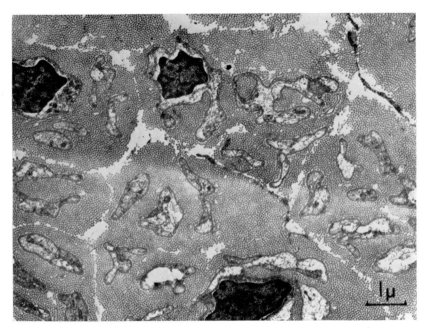

FIG. 6.5. Electron micrograph of a sural nerve biopsy from a patient with progressive sensory neuropathy beginning in childhood showing total loss of myelinated and almost total loss of unmyelinated nerve fibres. Only atrophic Schwann cell processes and collagen remain.

(Heller and Robb 1955). Thévenard (1942) termed the condition 'l'acropathie ulcéro-mutilante familiale'. The patients have a marked loss of pain and temperature sensation distally, other modalities of sensation later becoming involved. The tendon reflexes distally are lost, though proximally they may be preserved. Lightning-like pains in the limbs may occur. Early in the condition the maximum motor and sensory conduction velocities are normal, though there may be a slight decrease in the amplitude of the nerve action potential, and an increased terminal latency. Though signs of motor involvement are usually absent, electromyography may show signs of slight denervation distally. The condition progresses gradually, death resulting from uncontrolled infection or from secondary amyloidosis due to repeated infections.

The primary pathological change is shrinkage and loss of the small neurons of the posterior root ganglia and of the small myelinated and unmyelinated fibres in the peripheral nerves (Denny-Brown 1951, Turkington and Stiefel 1965, Wallace 1970). It is presumed that the primary site of the disease is in the posterior root ganglion small neurons. Later there is quite extensive damage to the larger neurons and fibres. Denny-Brown's finding of amyloid in the posterior root ganglia has been absent in other cases, and may have been simply due to secondary amyloidosis. A number of other neurological features have been reported in some families with this condition, including peroneal muscular atrophy, nerve deafness, optic atrophy and central nervous involvement.

Charcot-Marie-Tooth disease and hypertrophic neuropathy

The history of peroneal muscular atrophy goes back to the descriptions by Charcot and Marie (1886) and Tooth (1886) who described families with progressive distal wasting and weakness producing a 'stork-leg' appearance, motor involvement later spreading to the hands with relatively little involvement of the sensory nerves. That of hypertrophic neuropathy goes back to the original description by Dejerine and Sottas (1893) of a brother and sister presenting in their teens with a relatively rapidly progressive distal sensorimotor neuropathy, in whom the peripheral nerves were hypertrophied with 'onion-bulb' formation. It is only in recent times that the relationship between these diseases and a number of other conditions with a similar clinical and pathological picture has been elucidated. This has mainly been the result of the work of Dyck and Lambert (1968a and b) who surveyed a large number of individuals from families with this condition, and made the following separations.

Charcot-Marie-Tooth disease of the hypertrophic type with dominant inheritance

This group include kinship similar to those of Charcot and Marie (1886), Tooth (1886) and Roussy and Lévy (1926). The earliest sign is usually pes cavus, and some gait disturbance often appears by the second decade due to progressive atrophy of the anterior and posterial tibial groups of muscles. A progressive foot-drop develops, and later there is difficulty in manipulating the fingers. Sensory impairment appears late and is less severe than the motor deficit, involving especially the large fibre modalities. A number of relatives may have no symptoms though there is very marked slowing of nerve conduction (Bradley and Aguayo 1969). The condition is very slowly progressive, and many are still walking with aids 30 years after the onset. The maximum motor and sensory nerve conduction velocities are of the order seen in demyelinating neuropathies, namely 5–20 m/s, and the nerve shows extensive segmental demyelination, and hypertrophy with 'onion-bulb' formation.

Charcot-Marie-Tooth disease of the hypertrophic type, sporadic, dominant with poor expression, or recessive inheritance

These cases are identical to those above, but with a different family pattern.

Hypertrophic neuropathy of the Dejerine-Sottas type

The onset is usually within the first few years of life, with delayed walking. The condition progresses slowly so that the patient becomes wheelchair-bound from 20–30 years of age. There is a progressive symmetrical glove and stocking loss of sensation involving predominantly the larger fibres. The electrophysiological and pathological changes are essentially similar to those described in the dominantly inherited group above, though the remaining myelin sheaths tend to be thinner.

Neuronal type of Charcot-Marie-Tooth disease with a dominant inheritance

The clinical pattern is similar to the first type, but the onset is in middle age, there is less hand and more leg involvement, and no enlargement of the peripheral nerves. The maximum motor nerve conduction velocity in the ulnar and median nerves is normal, and sensory loss is mild compared with motor impairment. Sensory nerve biopsies show very slight loss of the larger myelinated nerve fibres and no segmental demyelination or hypertrophic change. The site of the lesion may be in the motor axons or anterior horn cells, with very little involvement of the posterior root ganglion neurons.

Progressive spinal muscular atrophy of the Charcot-Marie-Tooth type

These are sporadic cases with onset in the second and third decades of life. Onset in the first decade has occurred in some personally observed cases. There is distal symmetrical weakness of the lower limbs subsequently spreading to the hands and forearms. Wasting is severe and extends to the mid-thigh and forearm. There is no sensory abnormality clinically or electrophysiologically. The maximum motor nerve conduction velocity is normal, and the nerves are not hypertrophied.

Peroneal muscular atrophy may also occur with other diseases in which there is central nervous degeneration. In Dyck and Lambert's series, the first type was most frequent at about 70 per cent, and the second type the next most common at about 10 per cent. At present there is no knowledge of the aetiology of the condition, though Dyck *et al.* (1970) found evidence of an abnormal metabolism of ceramide hexosides and ceramide hexoside sulphates in hypertrophic neuropathy of the Dejerine-Sottas type.

Refsum's disease (heredopathia atactica polyneuritiformi)

This condition, which is probably inherited in an autosomal recessive manner, was first described by Refsum (1946). The symptoms first appear in the first and second decades of life, with the development of a chronic progressive symmetrical distal sensorimotor polyneuropathy which may show relapses and remissions. Extensive hypertrophy of the peripheral nerves with onion-bulb formation is characteristic (Cammermeyer 1956). There is cerebellar dysfunction with ataxia and nystagmus, and retinitis pigmentosa which is described as 'atypical' because it lacks the classical 'bone corpuscle' pigment cells. The C.S.F. protein concentration is raised, and there are often nerve deafness, ichthyosis, cardiac and pupillary abnormalities. The condition is rare, only about fifty such cases having been described in the literature, but is of interest because of a knowledge in part of the underlying biochemistry of the condition and treatment thereof. There is an increased amount of one of the free fatty acids, namely phytanic acid (3,7,11,15-tetramethyl-hexadecanoic acid) in the blood and many tissues of the body (Klenk and Kahlke 1963), derived from phytols in the diet, the exclusion of which produces a considerable improvement in the patients (Steinberg *et al.* 1970).

Hypertrophic neuropathy may occur in many other conditions including diabetes (see page 160), relapsing polyneuropathy (Austin 1958), acromegaly (Stewart 1966), and multifocal enlargement of peripheral nerves (Adams *et al.* 1965, Simpson and Fowler 1966).

Carcinomatous neuropathy

Neoplastic conditions may have direct effects upon peripheral nerves, either by direct compression or infiltration, or by compression by haematoma or interstitial haemorrhage in those conditions with bleeding diatheses. There may also be a remote effect of the neoplasm without the intervention of one of these mechanisms. The generalized wasting occurring in patients with cancer has been known since time immemorial, and for more than 40 years it has been recognized that cancer can produce degeneration of the nervous system by its remote effect without direct invasion. It is now recognized that almost any cancer can cause neuropathy, but that it is especially common with carcinoma of the bronchus, ovary, breast and stomach, with reticuloses such as leukaemia and Hodgkin's disease, and with dysproteinaemic syndromes, such as multiple myelomatosis and Waldenström's macroglobulinaemia. Certain tumours tend to produce certain types of neuropathy. The central and peripheral nervous systems as well as the neuromuscular junction and the muscle may be affected. Though some doubt the existence of carcinomatous neuropathy (Wilner and Brody 1968), and others have suggested that it is largely due to malnutrition (Hildebrand and Coërs 1967), it is generally acknowledged that there is an increased incidence of these syndromes with carcinoma. In fact Newman and Gugino (1964) followed up 8 patients, who were more than 65 years of age, with an unexplained neuropathy, and found that all developed carcinoma within 18 months. The number of patients was small, and there was no control series, but this report does suggest that cancer is an important cause of chronic progressive polyneuropathy in old age.

The incidence of carcinomatous polyneuropathy is difficult to define since it depends on how intensive is the search. Croft and Wilkinson (1965) found 'neuromyopathy' in 16 per cent of patients with carcinoma of the lung, though they included those with simple areflexia which might have been due to ageing. Trojaborg *et al.* (1969) found clinical signs of a peripheral neuropathy in only 5 per cent of patients with carcinoma of the lung, and Hildebrand and Coërs (1967) found such signs in only 4 per cent of a group of patients with various carcinomata. From 2–5 per cent of patients with reticulosis have signs of peripheral neuropathy (Hutchinson *et al.*

1958; Currie and Henson 1971). Electrophysiological evidence of peripheral nerve damage was present in 32 per cent of Trojaborg's series. Histological abnormalities of the terminal motor innervation were present in 41 per cent of Hildebrand and Coërs' series, particularly in patients with cachexia. The commonest electrophysiological abnormalities are signs of denervation on electromyography with a slight increase in the terminal latency of motor conduction, though with normal sensory and motor nerve conduction velocities in the main nerve trunks.

The commonest peripheral nerve disease due to carcinoma is a mixed sensorimotor distal symmetrical polyneuropathy which makes up more than 80 per cent of such cases (Croft *et al.* 1967). In some this is an insignificant part of their terminal carcinomatous illness, but in others it may be severe and the presenting complaint. It may occasionally be relapsing and remitting. A pure sensory neuropathy may occur in cancer patients due to degeneration of the neurons of the posterior root ganglia, with perivascular lymphocytic infiltration in the ganglia (Denny-Brown 1948). A form of motor neuron disease has also been reported in association with carcinoma (Brain *et al.* 1965), though it is uncertain whether this is more than a chance association. The critical criterion of cure of the carcinomatous syndrome following total removal of the carcinoma has been shown in few if any patients.

There is some uncertainty about the underlying pathology in the mixed sensorimotor neuropathies of carcinoma. Croft *et al.* (1967) found changes suggestive of segmental demyelination in 10 cases, which were confirmed by teasing single nerve fibres in two. Henson and Urich (1970) found both axonal degeneration and segmental demyelination, the latter predominating. However, Webster *et al.* (1967) in a patient with carcinoma of the bronchus, and Walsh (1971) in 5 patients with multiple myeloma found only axonal degeneration. The aetiology of the condition is uncertain. Lymphocytic infiltration in the posterior root ganglia and peripheral nerves raises the possibility of an autoimmune process. Another possibility is the action of a faculative virus allowed to infiltrate the nerves as a result of the carcinomatous process. Occasionally patients with carcinomatous neuropathy may improve with corticosteroid therapy.

Ischaemic neuropathies and collagen-vascular diseases

Though the peripheral nerves have an extensive plexus of blood vessels (see page 38), occlusion of several major feeding vessels or of many smaller vasa nervorum can cause a neuropathy. This is usually acute, mixed sensorimotor in type, and in the distribution of a mononeuritis multiplex.

Neuropathy in arteriosclerosis

Large artery disease causes symptoms which relate much more to the ischaemic muscles (intermittent claudication) or gangrene of the whole limb, but in a survey of 32 patients with symptomatic arterial disease, two-thirds had paraesthesiae (Eames and Lange 1967). Nearly 90 per cent had sensory abnormalities on examination, usually patchy, asymmetric and distal in the lower limbs. About half had depressed ankle jerks, and half weakness of one or both legs. A third had muscle wasting which was often asymmetrical. Pathological examination showed often severe loss of myelinated fibres with both Wallerian degeneration and segmental demyelination (Eames and Lange 1967, Chopra and Hurwitz 1967). These changes probably result both from poor perfusion due to the major artery disease, and from secondary changes of the endoneurial vessels, with increased perivascular connective tissue, osmiophilic inclusions in the endothelial cell cytoplasm, endothelial proliferation, and occasionally complete occlusion by fibrin. It is uncertain whether these changes are due to coexistent hypertension or microembolization from proximal atheroma.

An acute asymmetric mononeuropathy may occur in subacute bacterial endocarditis due to embolization of the major feeding vessels (Jones and Siekert 1968). The proximal ischaemic mononeuropathy of diabetes has already been described (page 160), and the part played by ischaemia in the distal symmetrical polyneuropathy of diabetes has been discussed (page 158). Ischaemia due to amyloid infiltration of the walls of the blood vessels may play a part in amyloid neuropathy (page 182).

Collagen-vascular disease

Most collagen-vascular diseases can damage the nerves by ischaemia. The incidence of peripheral nerve involvement is highest in polyarteritis nodosa, where up to 20–30 per cent of patients have a neuropathy (Lovshin and Kernohan 1948, Bleehan et al. 1963). The picture is usually of a mononeuritis multiplex with acute lesions of individual nerves, though later it may blend into a progressive distal symmetrical sensorimotor polyneuropathy. Individual infarcts of the nerve are often painful. A combined sural

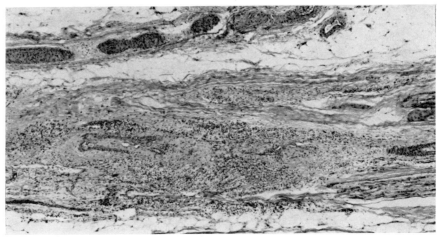

Fig. 6.6a

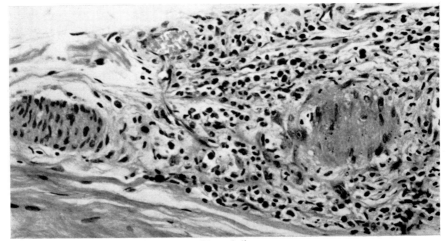

Fig. 6.6b

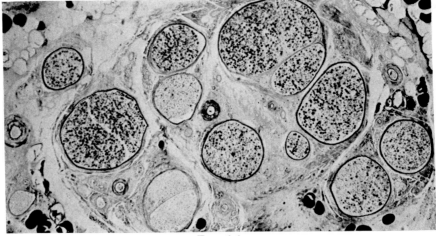

Fig. 6.6c

nerve and gastrocnemius muscle biopsy is often a useful diagnostic procedure in this disease for it will often reveal a damaged small artery. The vessel is occluded with typical inflammatory necrosis of the wall, and the surrounding collection of mixed inflammatory cells containing polymorphs, lymphocytes and eosinophils (fig. 6.6). The nerve shows axonal degeneration secondary to the ischaemic damage. The treatment of polyarteritis nodosa with corticosteroids alone is not as effective as might be wished, and combination with cytotoxic immunosuppressive agents is probably justified.

The incidence of involvement of the peripheral nervous system in systemic lupus erythematosus varies from 3–13 per cent (Dubois 1966, Johnson and Richardson 1968), central nervous system involvement being somewhat more frequent. Again there is usually an acute mononeuritis multiplex, though some start with a distal symmetrical sensorimotor polyneuropathy. Occasionally a Guillain-Barré-like picture may occur. A peripheral neuropathy can occur in giant cell arteritis (Warrell et al. 1968), scleroderma (Richter 1954, Kibler and Rose 1960), dermatomyositis (McEntee and Mancall 1965) and Wegener's granulomatosis (Stern 1970).

Rheumatoid neuropathy

Several types of clinically symptomatic peripheral neuropathies have been described in rheumatoid arthritis. They are best classified into four types (modified from Pallis and Scott 1965).

1 Lesions of major nerves of upper and lower limbs
These make up about 40 per cent of this group of conditions. They are mainly due to compression of the nerve within a fascial sheath or bony canal by an effusion within a joint, swelling of the joint capsule, osteophytes or displacement of a bone. Lesions of the lateral popliteal nerve at the

---

FIG. 6.6 Polyarteritis nodosa. *a* Longitudinal section of a small artery in a sural nerve biopsy showing occlusion, recanalization and a periarterial inflammatory focus. H. & E. × 30. *b* High power view of another vessel showing hyaline degeneration of the vessel wall and a periarterial collection of inflammatory cells of mixed type. H. & E. × 200. *c* Transverse section of a sural nerve biopsy showing total loss of myelinated nerve fibres from some fascicles and a patchy loss from others. Weigert-Pal. × 30. (*From* Bradley and Thomas 1974. Pathology of peripheral nerve disease. Chap. 7 in *Disorders of Voluntary Muscle*, ed. Walton J. N. Churchill-Livingstone, Edinburgh. In press.

fibular head and of the median nerve in the carpal tunnel are the commonest, with all the features of an entrapment neuropathy (see page 152). Local injection of corticosteroids or surgical decompression may be required to relieve the pressure. Occasionally such lesions of the major nerves may be due to an underlying arteritis.

2 *Digital neuropathy* (about 20 per cent)

This is due to occlusion of the individual digital arteries producing sensory loss on one side of one finger. The condition is usually not severe.

3 *Distal symmetrical sensory polyneuropathy of lower limbs* (about 30 per cent)

This condition is insidious in onset, with paraesthesiae and numbness and loss of pain and vibration sense up to the ankles. The ankle jerks may be absent.

4 *Distal symmetrical mixed sensorimotor polyneuropathy of upper and lower extremities*

This is the smallest group at less than 10 per cent of the whole group, but is the most severe and has the poorest prognosis. It often presents initially as a mononeuritis multiplex before progressing to a distal symmetrical sensorimotor polyneuropathy. The course is relatively rapid over a few months, and most patients die within 2 years from a widespread vasculitis.

All forms of neuropathy are commonest in seropositive cases with nodules (Hart 1966), and this is particularly true of type 4 (Chamberlain and Bruckner 1970). There is evidence that corticosteroid therapy of rheumatoid arthritis predisposes to the development of a peripheral neuropathy, though the mechanism is not clear (Ferguson and Slocumb 1961).

Electrophysiological investigations may help elucidate the condition in patients with rheumatoid arthritis. In type 1, nerve conduction will show a focal delay at the point of compression. Many patients with type 3 neuropathy have maximum sensory conduction velocities reduced to about 50 per cent of normal, that is to the level expected of segmental demyelination. In type 4 neuropathy there is little or no slowing prior to the development of total conduction block, together with severe electromyographic evidence of denervation, the whole picture suggesting axonal degeneration.

Pathological studies have generally shown a diffuse vasculitis with occlusion of the vasa nervorum, more marked in the type 4 than the type 3 cases. The infarcts are particularly in the upper arm and mid-thigh levels, involving the centre of the fasciculi, suggesting that these are watershed zones (Dyck *et al.* 1972). The nerves may show segmental demyelination, though Wallerian degeneration predominates, particularly in the more severe cases (Haslock *et al.* 1970, Weller *et al.* 1970). The correct way of treating rheumatoid neuropathy is still under investigation. In the type 3 sensory polyneuropathy, it is best to avoid corticosteroid therapy as far as possible. In the type 4 neuropathy, cytotoxic immunosuppressive agents are worthy of trial because of the poor prognosis. D-penicillamine may also be of value (Golding 1973).

Dysglobulinaemic neuropathies

Cryoglobulins may occur in the plasma in a number of conditions, including chronic infections and collagen-vascular diseases. Macroglobulins may occur in these disorders and in lymphoproliferative disorders. Both may be associated with peripheral nerve disease, which may either be a mononeuritis multiplex or a distal symmetrical mixed polyneuropathy (Dayan and Lewis 1966, Logothetis *et al.* 1968). Axonal degeneration and loss is the predominant pathological change. Probably in these patients, hyperviscosity of the plasma leads to underperfusion of the capillaries, and ischaemic damage.

Brachial plexus neuropathy (neuralgic amyotrophy)

This is an interesting disorder, the pathological basis of which still awaits clarification. The typical history is of a patient who develops an extremely severe pain in one shoulder and arm which may last for 1 day to 3 months, though the average is about a week. During this time, or as the pain remits signs of nerve damage appear. These are predominantly motor, though some sensory symptoms and signs may occur. The affected muscles rapidly become paralysed and atrophied. The distribution of the motor and sensory involvement may indicate a lesion of one cord of the brachial plexus, or of a single cervical nerve root, or of one peripheral nerve, commonly the long thoracic nerve. Quite frequently the pattern is mixed, though the muscles around the shoulder joint are especially involved (Turner and Parsonage 1957, McGee and Dejong 1960, Gathier and Bruyn 1970a).

The power occasionally recovers within a month, but in most cases it takes 6 months to 2 years to do so. The rate of recovery is roughly proportional to the distance of the affected muscle from the brachial plexus. In most cases, the long thoracic, or circumflex nerve lesions have recovered by about a year, while the anterior and posterior interosseous nerve lesions often take 18 months to 3 years to recover. Most cases however eventually make a relatively full recovery.

The duration of recovery suggests that in a few cases the predominant lesion is focal segmental demyelination or distal axonal degeneration, while in most there is a proximal site of axonal degeneration. The loss of axonal reflexes in the anaesthetic area in patients with neuralgic amyotrophy supports the suggestion of axonal degeneration. Electrophysiological studies show marked denervation changes in affected muscles with an increase in conduction time from the supraclavicular fossa to the affected muscle (Kraft 1969). This would be compatible either with segmental demyelination or terminal axonal degeneration. The cases reported by Weikers and Mattson (1969) had diffuse slowing of up to 25 per cent in the maximum conduction velocity in the median, ulnar and lateral popliteal nerves, and increased terminal latencies, suggesting a more widespread disease. The only pathological study so far available showed axonal degeneration (Tsairis et al. 1972).

The condition is at least four times as common in males as in females, and the right side appears preferentially to be involved. A wide range of precipitating factors have been incriminated including infections, trauma, surgical operations and immunization. A very similar syndrome may occur in serum sickness, though nerves other than those around the shoulder are more often involved in the latter condition (Allen 1931, Gathier and Bruyn 1970b). Recurrences of neuralgic amyotrophy may occasionally be seen, and rarely cranial nerve or other distant nerve lesions may also occur. Adequate analgaesia is the most important element of the treatment. Corticosteroid or adrenocorticotrophin therapy has been used in the acute condition without striking benefit.

Radiation neuropathy

The peripheral nerves are relatively resistant to x-radiation damage, but *may* be damaged if they are included in the field of deep x-ray therapy (Innes and Carsten 1961, Stoll and Andrews 1966, Haymaker 1969). The commonest radiation damage of peripheral nerves is where the brachial plexus is injured as a result of x-ray therapy for carcinoma of the breast, though the lumbosacral plexus may also be damaged by x-ray therapy of the pelvic areas. A dose of more than 5000 rads is liable to cause a progressive syndrome of paraesthesiae, muscle weakness and atrophy. Occasionally, as in radiation myelopathy, a sudden onset suggests a vascular occlusion secondary to endarteritis. The progressive syndrome probably also has a vascular basis, radiation damage to parenchymatous elements *per se* being less important. An interval of 3 months to 3 years following radiotherapy is usual. Once excessive irradiation has occurred no treatment is known to prevent the neuropathy developing. Immediate and late anterior horn cell degeneration following electrocution injuries may also be mentioned in this context (Panse 1970).

Tropical neuropathies

Peripheral nerve disease is particularly common in the tropical developing countries. The most important, *leprosy* (page 157), and the neuropathies due to *vitamin deficiencies* (page 163) have already been described. A neuropathy similar to that occurring in non-tropical malabsorption syndromes (page 165) may develop in *tropical sprue*. Certain foods such as cassava containing cyanogens may cause chronic cyanide intoxication if improperly cooked. The cyanide damages the peripheral nerves perhaps by its effect upon vitamin B_{12} metabolism (Osuntokun 1968). This *tropical ataxic neuropathy* has been described from many parts of Africa and the West Indies. The initial symptoms are of paraesthesiae and numbness in the legs, and lead on to a distal symmetrical predominantly sensory polyneuropathy, though motor involvement also occurs. Ataxia is a major feature, probably due to posterior column degeneration. Nerve deafness and optic atrophy are frequent accompaniments. The motor nerve conduction velocity is reduced in these patients by 30 per cent. Further studies are required to elucidate the pathological changes occurring in the nerves. Cycasin in starch prepared from the Cycads in Guam produces an ataxic neuropathy in animals, and may perhaps play a part in the amyotrophic lateral sclerosis-Parkinsonism-dementia complex which is endemic in Guam (Hirono and Shibuya 1967).

African *trypanosomiasis* (*T. gambiense* or *rhodesiense*) frequently produces an ataxic gait with loss of deep sensation and reflexes, and often signs of cortico-spinal tract damage. The posterior root ganglia show marked inflammatory infiltration, which is also present in the peripheral nerves. A vasculitis is often seen and there is probably both axonal degeneration and

segmental demyelination (Janssen *et al.* 1956). The South American try-
panosome (*T. cruzi*) specifically damages not only the heart but also the
autonomic ganglion cells of the viscera, producing megacolon and megaoesophagus (see page 228). The anterior horn cells may also be attacked. In
many other diseases which characteristically occur in warm climates such
as malaria, schistosomiasis, sickle cell anaemia and lathyrism, the major
neurological complications are of the central nervous system, though peripheral lesions may also occur.

Tumours of nerve

The major tumour of nerve results from neoplastic but benign overgrowth
of the Schwann cells and fibroblasts. It is extremely rare for a primary
overgrowth of axons to produce a tumour. A traumatic neuroma is the result of disorganized outgrowth of axons from a sectioned nerve, but it cannot be described as neoplastic.

The proportion of fibroblastic and Schwann cell proliferation differs
considerably from tumour to tumour and the histological appearance may
thus vary greatly. This has led to a long controversy about the origin and
title of the various tumours. Neurinoma, neurofibroma, Schwannoma and
neurilemmoma are only a few of the names which have been used (Russell
and Rubinstein 1963, Kramer 1970).

The tumours are sometimes single or may be multiple in the dominantly
inherited disease, *multiple neurofibromatosis* or von Recklinghausen's
disease. This interesting disease is associated with many other developmental and neoplastic changes of the central nervous system, bone and skin.
The latter include multiple café-au-lait spots, and sessile and pedunculated
skin lesions. Von Recklinghausen's neurofibromata may be focal on nerve
trunks, or diffusely aggregated into plexiform neuromata, particularly on
the cutaneous nerves (fig. 6.7). The tumour may cause no symptoms if it
enlarges slowly giving the axons time to accommodate to distortion. More
usually compression of nerve occurs, producing pain and loss of function in
the distribution of the nerve. This is particularly the case where the tumour
arises within the vertebral canal or intervertebral foramen, when its site of
origin is usually the posterior nerve root. Enlargement of the intervertebral
foramen may occur in these cases, and a dumb-bell extension within and
outside the canal is not uncommon. Pain in a radicular distribution is
characteristic.

Rarely do these tumours undergo malignant degeneration to a sarcoma, and such sarcomata are rarely seen outside von Recklinghausen's disease.

Chronic idiopathic polyneuropathy

The aetiology of the conditions outlined so far in this chapter are to a greater or lesser extent known. However in a proportion of patients with peripheral nerve disease no aetiology can be discovered despite intensive investigation. Most of such patients have a chronic progressive sensorimotor distal polyneuropathy. Some of these patients may eventually prove to have an underlying carcinoma, but in many this is not so.

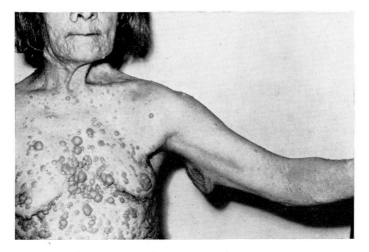

FIG. 6.7 A patient with multiple neurofibromatosis showing numerous pedunculated skin lesions, and a plexiform neuroma on the left arm.

The absolute frequency of this condition is difficult to define. In a general hospital in the United Kingdom, about 40 per cent of the patients with peripheral nerve disease fall into the 'idiopathic' group (Prineas 1970). Because the more easily diagnosed conditions are filtered off prior to referral, the proportion of idiopathic cases rises to 50–70 per cent in specialized neurological units (Elkington 1952, Matthews 1952, Rose 1960, Bradley 1967 unpublished data).

A number of these patients may show a response to corticosteroid therapy, and it is always worth considering this. However as pointed out above (page 181), this sometimes results in the development of profound relapses upon withdrawal of the corticosteroid therapy, and the development of a steroid-dependent state. It is important therefore to decide whether the patient's symptoms and incapacity warrant this potential risk.

REFERENCES

Traumatic nerve lesions

ABBOTS K.H. and MITTS M.G. (1970) Reflex neurovascular syndromes. In *Handbook of Clinical Neurology*, vol. 8, ed. Vinken P.J. and Bruyn G.W., pp. 321–356. North-Holland, Amsterdam.

AGUAYO A., NAIR C.P.V. and MIDGLEY R. (1971) Experimental progressive compressive neuropathy in the rabbit. Histological and electrophysiological studies. *Arch. Neurol. (Chic.)* **24**, 358–364.

BEHSE F., BUCHTHAL F., CARLSEN F. and KNAPPEIS G.G. (1972) Hereditary neuropathy with liability to pressure palsies. Electrophysiological and histopathological aspects. *Brain* **95**, 777–794.

DUCKER T.B., KEMPE, L.G. and HAYES G.J. (1969) The metabolic background for peripheral nerve surgery. *J. Neurosurg.* **30**, 270–280.

EARL C.J., FULLERTON P.M., WAKEFIELD G.S and SCHUTTA H.S. (1964) Hereditary neuropathy, with liability to pressure palsies. *Quart. J. Med.* **33**, 481–498.

FULLERTON P.M. and GILLIATT R.W. (1967a) Pressure neuropathy in the hind foot of the guinea pig. *J. Neurol. Neurosurg. Psychiat.* **30**, 18–25.

FULLERTON P.M. and GILLIATT R.W. (1967b) Median and ulnar nerve neuropathy in the guinea pig. *J. Neurol. Neurosurg. Psychiat.* **30**, 393–402.

KOPELL H.P. and THOMPSON W.A.L. (1963) *Peripheral Entrapment Neuropathies.* Williams and Wilkins, Baltimore.

POLLARD J.D., GUY R.S. and McLEOD J.G. (1971) Peripheral nerve grafting. *Proc. IInd. Int. Congr. Muscle Dis.*, Perth, W. Australia.

RICHARDS R.L. (1967) Causalgia. A centennial review. *Arch. Neurol. (Chic.)* **16**, 339–350.

SEDDON H.J. (1943) Three types of nerve injury. *Brain* **66**, 237–288.

SPAANS F. (1970) Occupational nerve lesions. In *Handbook of Clinical Neurology*, vol. 7, ed. Vinken P.J. and Bruyn G.W., pp. 326–343. North-Holland, Amsterdam.

STAAL A. (1970) The entrapment neuropathies. In *Handbook of Clinical Neurology*, vol. 7, ed. Vinken P.J. and Bruyn G.W., pp. 285–325. North-Holland, Amsterdam.

SUNDERLAND S. (1968) *Nerve and Nerve Injuries.* Livingstone, Edinburgh.

THOMAS P.K. and FULLERTON P.M. (1963) Nerve fibre size in the carpal tunnel syndrome. *J. Neurol. Neurosurg. Psychiatr.* **26**, 520–527.

Diphtheritic neuropathy

WILSON S.K.A. (1954) *Neurology*, 2nd edn., Bruce A.N., pp. 738–747. Butterworth, London.

Neuropathy of leprosy

ANTIA N.H., PANDYA S.S. and DASTUR D.K. (1970) Nerves in the arm in leprosy.
I: Clinical, electrodiagnostic and operative aspects. *Int. J. Leprosy* **38**, 12–29.

DASTUR D.K. (1955) Cutaneous nerves in leprosy: the relation between histopathology and cutaneous sensibility. *Brain* **78**, 615–633.

JOB C.K. (1970) *Mycobacterium leprae* in nerve lesions in lepromatous leprosy.
Arch. Path. (Chic.) **89**, 195–207.

REES R.J.W. and WATERS M.F.R. (1971) Recent trends in leprosy research. *Brit.
med. Bull.* **28**, 16–21.

ROSENBERG R.N. and LOVELACE R.E. (1968) Mononeuritis multiplex in lepromatous leprosy. *Arch. Neurol. (Chic.)* **19**, 310–314.

SABIN T.D. (1969) Temperature-linked sensory loss. A unique pattern in leprosy.
Arch. Neurol. (Chic.) **20**, 257–262.

Neuropathy of diabetes mellitus

BALLIN R.H.M. and THOMAS P.K. (1968) Hypertrophic changes in diabetic
neuropathy. *Acta neuropath. (Berl.)* **11**, 93–102.

BRUNS L. (1890) Über neuritische Lähmungen beim Diabetes mellitus. *Berl. Klin.
Wschr,* **27**, 509–515.

BRUYN G.W. and GARLAND H. (1970) Neuropathies of endocrine origin. In *Handbook of Clinical Neurology*, vol. 8, ed. Vinken P.J. and Bruyn G.W., pp. 29–71.
North-Holland, Amsterdam.

CASEY E.B. and HARRISON M.J.G. (1972) Diabetic amyotrophy: a follow-up study.
Brit. med. J. **1**, 656–659.

CHOCHINOV R.H., ULLYOT L.E. and MOORHOUSE J.A. (1972) Sensory thresholds
in patients with juvenile diabetes and their close relatives. *New Engl. J. Med.*
286, 1233–1237.

CHOPRA J.S. and HURWITZ L.J. (1968) Femoral nerve conduction in diabetes and
chronic occlusive vascular disease. *J. Neurol. Neurosurg. Psychiat.* **31**, 28–33.

CHOPRA J.S. and HURWITZ L.J. and MONTGOMERY D.A.D. (1969) The pathogenesis of sural nerve changes in diabetes mellitus. *Brain* **92**, 391–418.

GAMSTORP I., SHELBURNE S.A.JR., ENGELSON G., REDONDO D. and TRAISMAN H.S.
(1966) Peripheral neuropathy in juvenile diabetes. *Diabetes* **15**, 411–418.

GARLAND H. (1955) Diabetic amyotrophy. *Brit. med. J.* **2**, 1287–1290.

GARLAND H. and TAVERNER D. (1953) Diabetic myelopathy. *Brit. med. J.* **1**, 1405–
1408.

GOODMAN J.J. (1954) Femoral neuropathy in relation to diabetes mellitus. *Diabetes*
3, 266–271.

GREENBAUM D. (1964) Observations on the homogeneous nature and pathogenesis
of diabetic neuropathy. *Brain* **87**, 215–232.

GREENBAUM D., RICHARDSON P.C., SALMON M.V. and URICH H. (1964) Pathological observations on six cases of diabetic neuropathy. *Brain* **87**, 201–214.

GREGERSEN G. (1967) Diabetic neuropathy: influence of age, sex, metabolic control,
and duration of diabetes on motor conduction velocity. *Neurol. (Minneap.)* **17**,
972–980.

GREGERSEN G. (1968a) Latency time, maximal amplitude and electromyography in diabetic patients. *Acta med. Scand.* **183**, 55–60.

GREGERSEN G. (1968b) Vibratory perception threshold and motor conduction velocity in diabetics and non-diabetics. *Acta med. Scand.* **183**, 61–65.

HIRSON C., FEINMANN E. L. and WADE H. J. (1953) Diabetic neuropathy. *Brit. med. J.* **1**, 1408–1412.

LAWRENCE D. G. and LOCKE S. (1963) Neuropathy in children with diabetes mellitus. *Brit. med. J.* **1**, 784–485.

LINDÉN L. (1962) Amyotrophia diabetica. *Svenska Läk.-Tidn.* **59**, 3368–3373.

RAFF M. C., SANGALANG V. and ASBURY A. K. (1968) Ischaemic mononeuropathy multiplex associated with diabetes mellitus. *Arch. Neurol. (Chic.)* **18**, 487–499.

RUNDLES R. W. (1945) Diabetic neuropathy: a general review with a report of 125 cases. *Medicine (Balt.)* **24**, 111–160.

THOMAS P. K. and LASCELLES R. G. (1966) The pathology of diabetic neuropathy. *Quart. J. Med.* **35**, 489–509.

WARD J. D., FISHER D. J., BARNES C. G., JESSOP J. D. and BAKER R. W. R. (1971) Improvement in nerve conduction following treatment in newly diagnosed diabetics. *Lancet* **1**, 428–430.

Neuropathy of old age

ARNOLD N. and HARRIMAN D. G. F. (1970) The incidence of abnormality in control human peripheral nerves studied by single axon dissection. *J. Neurol. Neurosurg. Psychiat.* **33**, 55–61.

CAMPBELL M. J. and McCOMAS A. J. (1970) The effects of ageing on muscle function. *5th Symp. Current Res. in Musc. Dyst.*

COTTRELL L. (1940) Histological variations with age in apparently normal nerve trunks. *Arch. Neurol. Psychiat. (Chic.)* **43**, 1138–1150.

CRITCHLEY M. (1931) The neurology of old age. *Lancet* **1**, 1119–1127, 1221–1230, 1331–1336.

DYCK P. J., SCHULTZ P. W. and O'BRIEN P. C. (1972) Quantitation of touch-pressure sensation. *Arch. Neurol. (Chic.)* **26**, 465–473.

GARDNER E. D. (1940) Decrease in human neurones with age. *Anat. Rec.* **77**, 529–536.

HARRIMAN D. G. F., TAVERNER D. and WOOLF A. L. (1970) Ekbom's syndrome and burning paraesthesiae. A biopsy study by vital staining and electron microscopy of the intramuscular innervation, with a note on the age changes in motor nerve endings in distal muscles. *Brain* **93**, 393–406.

HOWELL T. H. (1949) Senile deterioration of the central nervous system. A clinical study. *Brit. med. J.* **1**, 56–58.

JENNEKENS F. G. I., TOMLINSON B. E. and WALTON J. N. (1971) Data on the distribution of fibre types in five human limb muscles. An autopsy study. *J. neurol. Sci.* **14**, 245–257.

KAESER H. E. (1970) Nerve conduction velocity measurements. In *Handbook of Clinical Neurology*, vol. 7, ed. Vinken P. J. and Bruyn G. W., pp. 116–196. North-Holland, Amsterdam.

LASCELLES R. G. and THOMAS P. K. (1966) Changes due to age in internodal length in the sural nerve in man. *J. Neurol. Neurosurg. Psychiat.* **29**, 40–44.

OCHOA J. and MAIR W. G. P. (1969) The normal sural nerve in man. II. Changes in the axons and Schwann cells due to ageing. *Acta neuropath. (Berl.)* **13**, 217–239.

VIZOSO A. D. (1950) The relationship between internodal length and growth in human nerves. *J. Anat. (Lond.)* **84**, 342–353.

Neuropathies due to vitamin deficiencies

ASPINALL D. L. (1964) Multiple deficiency state associated with isoniazid therapy. *Brit. med. J.* **2**, 1177–1178.

COLLINS G. H., WEBSTER H. de F. and VICTOR M. (1964) The ultrastructure of myelin and axonal alterations in sciatic nerves of thiamine deficient and chronically starved rats. *Acta neuropath. (Berl.)* **3**, 511–521.

COOKE W. T. and SMITH W. T. (1966) Neurological disorders associated with adult coeliac disease. *Brain* **89**, 683–722.

COOKE W. T., JOHNSON A. G. and WOOLF A. L. (1966) Vital staining and electron microscopy of the intramuscular nerve endings in the neuropathy of adult coeliac disease. *Brain* **89**, 663–682.

CRUICKSHANK E. K. (1952) Dietary neuropathies. *Vitam. and Horm.* **10**, 1–45.

ERBSLÖH F. and ABEL M. (1970) Deficiency neuropathies. In *Handbook of Clinical Neurology*, vol. 7, ed. Vinken P. J. and Bruyn G. W., North-Holland, Amsterdam.

FOLLIS R. H. JR. and WINTROBE M. M. (1945) A comparison of the effects of pyridoxine and pantothenic acid deficiency on nervous tissue of swine. *J. exp. Med.* **81**, 539–552.

FENNELLY J., FRANK O., BAKER H. and LEEVY C. M. (1864) Peripheral neuropathy of the alcoholic. Aetiologic role of aneurin and other B-complex vitamins. *Brit. med. J.* **2**, 1290–1292.

GREENFIELD J. G. and CARMICHAEL F. A. (1935) The peripheral nerves in cases of subacute combined degeneration of the cord. *Brain* **58**, 483–491.

HORWITZ S. J., KLIPSTEIN F. A. and LOVELACE R. E. (1967) Folic acid and neuropathy in epilepsy. *Lancet* **2**, 1305–1306.

MAYER R. F. (1965) Peripheral nerve function in vitamin B_{12} deficiency. *Arch. Neurol. (Chic.)* **13**, 355–362.

McLEOD J. G., WALSH J. C. and LITTLE J. M. (1969) Sural nerve biopsy. *Med. J. Austral.* **2**, 1092–1096.

PRINEAS J. (1970) Peripheral nerve changes in thiamine deficient rats. *Arch. Neurol. (Chic.)* **23**, 541–548.

TOMASULO P. A., KATER R. M. H. and IBER F. L. (1968) Impairment of thiamine resorption in alcoholism. *Amer. J. clin. Nutr.* **21**, 1340–1344.

TORRES I., SMITH W. T. and OXNARD C. E (1971) Peripheral neuropathy associated with vitamin-B_{12} deficiency in captive monkeys. *J. Path.* **105**, 125–146.

VILTER R. W., MÜLLER J. F., GLAZER H. S., JARROLD T., ABRAHAM J., THOMPSON C. and HAWKINS V. R. (1953) The effect of vitamin B_6 deficiency by desoxypyridoxine in human beings. *J. Lab. clin. Med.* **42**, 335–357.

Neuropathies due to exogenous toxins

BANK W. J., PLEASURE D. E., SUZUKI K., NIGRO M. and KATZ R. (1972) Thallium poisoning. *Arch. Neurol. (Chic.)* **26**, 456–464.

BRADLEY W. G., LASSMAN L. P., PEARCE G. W. and WALTON J. N. (1970) The neuromyopathy of vincristine in man. Clinical, electrophysiological and pathological studies. *J. neurol. Sci.* **10**, 107–131.

BUREAU Y., BARRIÈRE H., KERNEIS J.-P. and DE FERRON A. (1957) Acropathies ulcero-multinantes pseudosyringomyeliques non-familiales des membres inferieurs. *Presse med* **65**, 2127–2132.

CAVANAGH J. B. (1964) Peripheral nerve changes in orthocresyl phosphate poisoning in the cat. *J. Path. Bact.* **87**, 365–383.

CAVANAGH J. B. (1967) Pattern of change in peripheral nerves produced by isoniazid intoxication in rats. *J. Neurol. Neurosurg. Psychiat.* **30**, 26–33.

CHHUTTANI P. N., CHAWLA L. S. and SHARMA T. D. (1967) Arsenical neuropathy. *Neurol. (Minneap.)* **17**, 269–274.

COHEN M. M. (1970) Toxic neuropathy. In *Handbook of Clinical Neurology*, Vol. 7, ed. Vinken P. J. and Bruyn G. W., pp. 510–526, North-Holland, Amsterdam.

DUCHEN L. W. (1970) Changes in motor innervation and cholinesterase localization induced by botulinum toxin in skeletal muscle of the mouse: differences between fast and slow muscles. *J. Neurol. Neurosurg. Psychiat.* **33**, 40–54.

EVANS D. A. P. (1963) Pharmacogenetics. *Amer. J. Med.* **34**, 639–662.

EVANS M. H. (1969) Mechanism of saxitoxin and tetrodotoxin poisoning. *Brit. med. Bull.* **25**, 263–267.

EVANS D. A. P., MANLEY K. A. and McKUSICK V. A. (1960) Genetic control of isoniazid metabolism in man. *Brit. med. J.*, **2**, 485–491.

FULLERTON P. M. (1966) Chronic peripheral neuropathy produced by lead poisoning in guinea pigs. *J. Neuropath. exptl. Neurol.* **25**, 214–236.

FULLERTON P. M. (1969) Electrophysiological and histological observations on peripheral nerves in acrylamide poisoning in man. *J. Neurol. Neurosurg. Psychiat.* **32**, 186–192.

FULLERTON P. M. and O'SULLIVAN D. J. (1968) Thalidomide neuropathy. A clinical, electrophysiological and histological follow-up study. *J. Neurol. Neurosurg. Psychiat.* **31**, 543–551.

HILDEBRAND J., JOFFROY A. and COËRS C. (1968) Myoneural changes in experimental isoniazid neuropathy. Electrophysiological and histological study. *Arch. Neurol. (Chic.)* **19**, 60–70.

HOPKINS A. P. and MORGAN-HUGHES J. A. (1969) Effect of local pressure in diphtheritic neuropathy. *J. Neurol. Neurosurg. Psychiat.* **32**, 614–623.

LE QUESNE P. M. (1979) Iatrogenic neuropathies. In *Handbook of Clinical Neurology*, ed. Vinken P. J. and Bruyn G. W., pp. 527–551. North-Holland, Amsterdam.

MAWDSLEY C. and MAYER R. F. (1965) Nerve conduction in alcoholic polyneuropathy. *Brain* **88**, 335–356.

MOTA-REVETLLAT J. (1966) Acropatia ulceromutilante: enfermedad de Thevenard. Forme esporadica. *Med. Clin. (Barcelona)* **47**, 322–328.

OCHOA J. (1970) Isoniazid neuropathy in man. Quantitative electron microscopic study. *Brain* **93**, 831–850.

TOOLE J. F., GERGEN J. A., HAYES D. M. and FELTS J. H. (1968) Neural effects of nitrofurantoin. *Arch. Neurol.* **18**, 680–687.

WALSH J. C. (1970) Gold neuropathy. *Neurol. (Minneap.)* **20**, 455–458.

WALSH J. C. and McLEOD J. G. (1970) Alcoholic neuropathy. An electrophysiological and histological study. *J. neurol. Sci.* **10**, 457–469.

Acute porphyric neuropathy

CAVANAGH J. B. and MELLICK R. S. (1965) On the nature of the peripheral nerve lesions associated with acute intermittent porphyria. *J. Neurol. Neurosurg. Psychiat.* **28**, 320–327.

CAVANAGH J. B. and RIDLEY A. R. (1967) The nature of the neuropathy complicating acute intermittent porphyria. *Lancet* **2**, 1023–1024.

HAMFELT A. and WETTERBERG L. (1968) Neuropathy in porphyria. *Lancet* **1**, 50.

MEYER U. A., STRAND, L. J., DOSS M., REES A. C. and MARVER H. S. (1972) Acute intermittent porphyria: demonstration of a genetic defect in porphobilinogen metabolism. *New Engl. J. Med.* **286**, 1227–1282.

PRATT R. T. C. (1967) *The Genetics of Neurological Disorders.* Oxford University Press, London.

RIDLEY A. (1969) The neuropathy of acute intermittent porphyria. *Quart. J. Med.* **38**, 307–333.

SØRENSEN A. W. S. and WITH T. K. (1971) Persistent pareses with porphyric attacks. *Acta med. Scand.* **190**, 219–222.

SWEENEY V. P., PATHAK M. A. and ASBURY A. K. (1970) Acute intermittent porphyria: increased ALA-synthetase activity during an acute attack. *Brain* **93**, 369–380.

THOMAS P. K. (1971) Morphological basis for alterations in nerve conduction in peripheral neuropathies. *Proc. roy. Soc. Med.* **64**, 295–298.

Metabolic neuropathies

ASBURY A. K., VICTOR M. and ADAMS R. D. (1963) Uraemic polyneuropathy. *Arch. Neurol. (Chic.)* **8**, 413–428.

DANTA G. (1969) Hypoglycaemic peripheral neuropathy. *Arch. neurol.* **21**, 121–132.

DYCK P. J., JOHNSON W. J., LAMBERT E. H. and O'BRIEN P. C. (1971) Segmental demyelination secondary to axonal degeneration in uremic neuropathy. *Proc. Mayo Clin.* **46**, 400–431.

DYCK P. J. and LAMBERT E. H. (1970) Polyneuropathy associated with hypothyroidism. *J. Neuropath. exp. Neurol.* **29**, 631–658.

ENGEL W. K., DORMAN J. D., LEVY R. I. and FREDRICKSON D. S. (1967) Neuropathy in Tangier disease. *Arch. Neurol. (Chic.)* **17**, 1–9.

FARQUHAR J. W. and WAYS P. (1966) Abetalipoproteinemia. In *Metabolic Basis of Inherited Diseases*, 2nd edn., ed. Stanbury J. B., Wyngaarden J. B. and Fredrickson D. S, pp. 509–522. McGraw-Hill, New York.

Henson R.A. and Urich H. (1970a) Metabolic neuropathies. In *Handbook of Clinical Neurology*, vol. 8, ed. Vinken P.J. and Bruyn G.W., p. 1–28. North-Holland, Amsterdam.

Hockaday T.D.R., Hockaday J.M. and Rushworth G. (1966) Motor neuropathy associated with abnormal pyruvate metabolism unaffected by thiamine. *J. Neurol. Neurosurg. Psychiat.* **29**, 119–128.

Jebsen R.H., Tenckhoff H. and Honet J.C. (1967) Natural history of uraemic polyneuropathy and effects on dialysis. *New Engl. J. Med.* **277**, 327–333.

Jennekens F.G.I., van Spijk D. van der Most and Dorhout Mees E.J. (1969) Nerve fibre degeneration in uraemic polyneuropathy. *Proc. Europ. Dial. Trans. Ass.* **6**, 191–197.

Knill-Jones R.P., Goodwill C.J., Dayan A.D. and Williams R. (1972) Peripheral neuropathy in chronic liver disease: clinical, electrodiagnostic and nerve biopsy findings. *J. Neurol. Neurosurg. Psychiat.* **35**, 22–30.

Kocen R.S. and Thomas P.K. (1970) Peripheral nerve involvement in Fabry's disease. *Arch. Neurol. (Chic.)* **22**, 81–88.

Kocen R.S., Lloyd J.K., Lascelles P.T., Fosbrooke A.S. and Williams D. (1967) Familial-lipoprotein deficiency (Tangier disease) with neurological abnormalities. *Lancet* **1**, 1341–1345.

Ludin H.P., Speiss H. and Koenig M.P. (1969) Neuromuscular dysfunction associated with thyrotoxicosis. *Europ. Neurol.* **2**, 269–278.

Murray I.P.C. and Simpson J.A. (1958) Acroparaesthesia in myxoedema: a clinical and electromyographic study. *Lancet* **1**, 1360–1363.

Nickel S.N. and Frame B. (1968) Neurologic manifestations of myxoedema. *Neurol. (Minneap.)* **18**, 511–517.

Seneviratne K.N. and Peiris O.A. (1970) Peripheral nerve function in chronic liver disease. *J. Neurol. Neurosurg. Psychiatr.* **33**, 609–614.

Sterzel R.B., Semar M., Lonergan E.T., Treser G. and Lange K. (1971) Relationship of nerve tissue transketolase to neuropathy of chronic uraemia. *Jl Clin. Invest.* **50**, 2295–2304.

Thomas P.K. and Walker J.G. (1965) Xanthomatous neuropathy in primary biliary cirrhosis. *Brain* **88**, 1079–1088.

Acute idiopathic post-infectious polyneuropathy

Asbury A.K., Arnason B.G. and Adams R.D. (1969) The inflammatory lesion in ideopathic polyneuritis. Its role in pathogenesis. *Medicine (Balt.)* **48**, 173–215.

Aström K.E., Webster H.deF. and Arnason B.G. (1968) The initial lesion in experimental allergic neuritis. A phase and electron microscopic study. *J. exp. Med.* **128**, 469–496.

Austin J.H. (1968) Recurrent polyneuropathies and their corticosteroid treatment. *Brain* **81**, 157–192.

Carpenter S. (1972) An ultrastructural study of an acute fatal case of the Guillain-Barré syndrome. *J. neurol. Sci.* **15**, 125–140.

Cook S.D., Dowling P.C., Murray M.R. and Whitaker J.N. (1971) Circulating demyelinating factors in acute ideopathic polyneuritis. *Arch. Neurol. (Chic.)* **24**, 136–144.

COOK S.D., DOWLING P.C. and WHITAKER J.N. (1970) The Guillain-Barré syndrome. Relationship of circulating immunocytes and disease activity. *Arch. Neurol. (Chic.)* **22**, 470–474.

CURRIE S. and KNOWLES M. (1971) Lymphocyte transformation in the Guillain-Barré syndrome. *Brain* **94**, 109–116.

ELIZAN T.S., SPIRE J.P., ANDIMAN R.M., BAUGHMAN F.A. and LLOYD-SMITH D.L. (1971) Syndrome of acute ideopathic ophthalmoplegia with ataxia and areflexia. *Neurol. (Minneap.)* **21**, 281–292.

FISHER C.M. (1956) An unusual variant of acute ideopathic polyneuritis (syndrome of ophthalmoplegia, ataxia and areflexia). *New Engl. J. Med.* **255**, 57–65.

GUILLAIN G., BARRÉ J. and STROHL H. (1916) Sur un syndrome de radiculonévrite avec hyperalbuminose du liquide cephalo-rachidien sans reaction cellulaire. *Bull. Mem. Soc. Med., Hop. Paris* **40**, 1462–1470.

HEWER R.L., HILTON P.J., CRAMPTON-SMITH A. and SPALDING J.M.K. (1968) Acute polyneuritis requiring artificial respiration. *Quart. J. Med.* **37**, 479–491.

LANDRY, O. (1869) Note sur la paralysie ascendante aigue. *Gaz. Hebd. Med. Chirurg.* **6**, 472–474, 486–488.

MATTHEWS W.B., HOWELL D.A. and HUGHES R.C. (1970) Relapsing corticosteroid-dependent polyneuritis. *J. Neurol. Neurosurg. Psychiat.* **33**, 330–337.

MELNICK S.C. (1963) 38 cases of the Guillain-Barré syndrome: an immunological study. *Brit. med. J.* **1**, 368–373.

MORLEY J.B. and REYNOLDS E.H. (1966) Papilloedema and the Landry-Guillain-Barré syndrome. *Brain* **89**, 205–222.

OSLER L.D. and SIDELL A.D. (1960) The Guillain-Barré syndrome. The need for exact diagnostic criteria. *New Engl. J. Med.* **262**, 964–969.

PLEASURE D.E., LOVELACE R.E. and DUVOISIN R.C. (1968) Prognosis of acute polyradiculoneuritis. *Neurol. (Minneap.)* **18**, 1143–1148.

PRINEAS J. (1970a) Polyneuropathies of undetermined cause. *Acta neurol. Scand.* Suppl. 44, 1–72.

RAVN H. (1967) The Landry-Guillain-Barré syndrome. *Acta. neurol. Scand.* Suppl. 30, 1–64.

THOMAS P.K., LASCELLES R.G., HALLPIKE J.F. and HEWSER R.L. (1969) Recurrent and chronic relapsing Guillain-Barré polyneuritis. *Brain* **92**, 589–606.

WAKSMAN B.H. and ADAMS R.D. (1955) Allergic neuritis: an experimental disease of rabbits induced by the injection of peripheral nervous tissue and adjuvants. *J. exp. Med.* **102**, 213–236.

WEBB H.E. and GORDON-SMITH C.E. (1966) Relation of immune responses to development of central nervous system lesions in virus infections of man. *Brit. med. J.* **2**, 1179–1181.

WISNIEWSKI H., TERRY R.D., WHITAKER J.N., COOK S.D. and DOWLING P.C. (1969) The Landry-Guillain-Barré syndrome. A primary demyelinating disease. *Arch. Neurol. (Chic.)* **21**, 269–276.

WIGHT P.A.L. (1969) The ultrastructure of sciatic nerves affected by fowl paralysis (Marek's disease). *J. comp. Path.* **79**, 563–570.

Hereditary neuropathies

ADAMS R.D., ASBURY A.K. and MICHELSEN J.J. (1965) Multifocal pseudohypertrophic neuropathy. *Trans. Amer. Neurol. Ass.* **90**, 30–32.

AGUAYO A.J., NAIR C.P.V. and BRAY G.M. (1971) Peripheral nerve abnormalities in the Riley-Day syndrome. *Arch. Neurol. (Chic.)* **24**, 106–116.

ANDRADE C. (1952) A peculiar form of peripheral nouropathy. Familial atypical generalised amyloidosis with special involvement of the peripheral nerves. *Brain* **75**, 408–427.

APPENZELLER O. (1970) *The Autonomic Nervous System.* North-Holland, Amsterdam.

ASBURY A.K. (1970) Ischemic disorders of peripheral nerve. In *Handbook of Clinical Neurology*, vol. 8, ed. Vinken P.J. and Bruyn G.W., pp. 154–164. North-Holland, Amsterdam.

AUSTIN J.H. (1958) Recurrent polyneuropathies and their corticosteroid treatment. *Brain* **81**, 157–192.

BAXTER D.W. and OLSZEWSKI J. (1960) Congenital universal insensitivity to pain. *Brain* **83**, 381–393.

BRADLEY W.G. and AGUAYO A. (1969) Hereditary chronic neuropathy. Electrophysiological and pathological studies in an affected family. *J. neurol. Sci.* **9**, 131–154.

CAMMERMEYER J. (1956) Neuropathological changes in hereditary neuropathies: manifestations of the syndrome of heredopathia atactica polyneuritiformis in the presence of interstitial hypertrophic polyneuropathy. *J. Neuropath. exp. Neurol.* **15**, 340–361.

CHARCOT J.M. and MARIE P. (1886) Sur une forme particulière d'atrophie musculaire progressive souvent familial débutant par les pieds et les jambes et atteignant plus tard les mains. *Rev. Med. (Paris)* **6**, 97–138.

COIMBRA A. and ANDRADE C. (1971) Familial amyloid polyneuropathy. An electron-microscopic study of the peripheral nerve in five cases. *Brain* **94**, 199–206.

DEJERINE J. and SOTTAS J. (1893) Sur la névrite interstitielle, hypertrophique et progressive de l'enfance. *C.R. Soc. Biol.* **45**, 63–96.

DENNY-BROWN D. (1951) Hereditary sensory radicular neuropathy. *J. Neurol. Neurosurg. Psychiat.* **14**, 237–252.

DYCK P.J. and LAMBERT E.H. (1968a) Lower motor and primary sensory neuron diseases with peroneal muscular atrophy. I. Neurologic, genetic and electrophysiological findings in hereditary polyneuropathies. *Arch. Neurol. (Chic.)* **18**, 603–618.

DYCK P.J. and LAMBERT E.H. (1968b) II. Neurologic, genetic and electrophysiologic findings in various neuronal degenerations. *Arch. Neurol. (Chic.)* **18**, 619–625.

DYCK P.J. and LAMBERT E.H. (1969) Dissociated sensation in amyloidosis. Compound action potential, quantitative histologic and teased fiber, and electron microscopic studies of sural nerve biopsies. *Arch. Neurol. (Chic.)* **20**, 490–507.

DYCK P.J., ELLEFSON R.D., LAIS A.C., SMITH R.C., TAYLOR W.F. and VAN DYKE R.A. (1970) Histologic and lipid studies of sural nerves in inherited hypertrophic neuropathy: preliminary report of a lipid abnormality in nerve and liver in Dejerine-Sottas diease. *Proc. Mayo Clin.* **45**, 286–327.

HELLER I.H. and ROBB P. (1955) Hereditary sensory neuropathy. *Neurol. (Minneap.)* **5**, 15–29.

JEWESBURY E.C.O. (1970) Congenital indifference to pain. In *Handbook of Clinical Neurology*, vol. 8, ed. Vinken P.J. and Bruyn G.W., pp. 187–204. North-Holland, Amsterdam.

JOHNSON R.H. and SPALDING J.M.K. (1964) Progressive sensory neuropathy in children. *J. Neurol. Neurosurg. Psychiat.* **27**, 125–130.

KLENK E. and KAHLKE W. (1963) Über das Vorkommen der 3, 7, 11, 15-tetra-methyl-Hexadecansaüre in den Cholisterinestern und anderen Lipoidfraktionen der Organe bein einem Krankheitsfall unbekannter Genese (Verdacht auf Heredopathia atactica polyneuritiformis [Refsum-Syndrom]). *Hoppe-Seylers Z. Physiol. Chem.* **333**, 133–139.

McLEOD J.G. (1971) An electrophysiological and pathological study of peripheral nerves in Friedreich's ataxia. *J. neurol. Sci.* **12**, 333–349.

MAHLOUDJI M., TEASDALL R.D., ADAMKIEWICZ J.J., HARTMANN, W.H., LAMBIRD P.A. and McKUSICK V.A. (1969) The genetic amyloidoses, with particular reference to hereditary neuropathic amyloidosis, Type II (Indiana or Rukavina type). *Medicine (Balt.)* **48**, 1–37.

MURRAY T.J. (1973) Congenital sensory neuropathy. *Brain* **96**, 387–394.

NÉLATON (1852) Affection singulière des os du pied. *Gaz. Hôp. Paris* **4**, 13–20.

OGDEN T.E., ROBERT F. and CARMICHAEL E.A. (1959) Some sensory syndromes in children: indifference to pain and sensory neuropathy. *J. Neurol. Neurosurg. Psychiat.* **22**, 267–276.

OSUNTOKUN B.O., ODEKU E.L. and LUZZATO L. (1968) Congenital pain asymbolia and auditory imperception. *J. Neurol. Neurosurg. Psychiat.* **31**, 291–296.

REFSUM S. (1946) Heredopathia atactica polyneuritiformis: familial syndrome not hitherto described. *Acta psychiat. Scand.* Suppl. 38.

RILEY C.M, DAY R.L., GREELEY D. McL. and LANGFORD W.S. (1949) Central autonomic dysfunction with defective lacrimation: report of five cases. *Pediatrics* **3**, 468–478.

ROUSSY G. and LÉVY G. (1926) Sept cas d'une maladie familiale particulière: Trouble de la marche, pied bots et aréfléxie tendineuse généralisée, avec accessoirement, légère maladresse des mains. *Rev. Neurol.* **1**, 427–450.

RUKAVINA J.G., BLOCK W.D., JACKSON C.E., FALLS H.F., CAREY J.H. and CURTIS A.C. (1956) Primary systemic amyloidosis: a review and an experimental, genetic and clinical study of 29 cases with particular emphasis on the familial form. *Medicine (Balt.)* **35**, 239–334.

SCHILDER P. (1931) Cortical bedingte Steigerung von Schmertzreaktionen. *Z. ges. Neurol. Psychiat.* **132**, 367–370.

SCHOENE W.C., ASBURY A.K., ÅSTRÖM K.E. and MASTERS R. (1970) Hereditary sensory neuropathy. A clinical and ultrastructural study. *J. neurol. Sci.* **11**, 463–487.

SIMPSON D.A and FOWLER M. (1966) Two cases of localized hypertrophic neurofibrosis. *J. Neurol. Neurosurg. Psychiat.* **29**, 80–84.

STEINBERG D., MIZE C.E., HERNDON J.H., JR., FALES H.M., ENGEL W.K. and
    VROOM F.Q. (1970) Phytanic acid in patients with Refsum's syndrome and re-
    sponse to dietary treatment. *Arch. int. Med.* **125**, 75–87.
STEWART B.M. (1966) Hypertrophic neuropathy of acromegaly. *Arch. Neurol.*
    (*Chic.*) **14**, 107–110.
SWANSON A.G., BUCHAN G.C. and ALVORD E.C.JR. (1965) Anatomic changes in
    congenital insensitivity to pain: absence of small primary sensory neurons in
    ganglia, roots and Lissauer's tract. *Arch. Neurol.* (*Chic.*) **12**, 12–18.
THÉVENARD A. (1942) L'acropathie ulcéro-mutilante familiale. *Rev. neurol.* **74**,
    193–212.
TOOTH H.H. (1886) *The Peroneal Type of Progressive Muscular Atrophy.* Thesis,
    University of London. H.K. Lewis, London.
TURKINGTON R.W. and STIEFEL J.W. (1965) Sensory radicular neuropathy. *Arch.
    Neurol.* (*Chic.*) **12**, 19–24.
VASSELLA F., EMRICH H.M., KRAUS-RUPPERT R., AUFDERMANN F. and TÖNZ O.
    (1968) Congenital sensory neuropathy with anhidrosis. *Arch. Dis. Childh.* **43**,
    124–130.
WALLACE D.C. (1970) Hereditary sensory radicular neuropathy. A familial study.
    Mervyn Archdale Med. Monographs, vol. 8. Australian Medical Association,
    Sydney.
WINKELMANN R.K., LAMBERT E.H. and HAYLES S.B. (1962) Congenital absence
    of pain. Report of a case and experimental studies. *Arch. Derm.* **85**, 325–331.

Carcinomatous neuropathy

BRAIN W.R., CROFT P.B. and WILKINSON M. (1965) Motor neurone disease as a
    manifestation of neoplasm. *Brain* **88**, 479–500.
CROFT P.B. and WILKINSON M. (1965) The incidence of carcinomatous neuromyo-
    pathy in patients with various types of carcinoma. *Brain* **88**, 427–434.
CROFT P.B., URICH H. and WILKINSON M. (1967) Peripheral neuropathy of sen-
    sorimotor type associated with malignant disease. *Brain* **90**, 31–66.
CURRIE S. and HENSON R.A. (1971) Neurological syndromes in the reticuloses.
    Brain **94**, 307–320.
DENNY-BROWN D. (1948) Primary sensory neuropathy with muscular changes
    associated with carcinoma. *J. Neurol. Neurosurg. Psychiat.* **11**, 73–87.
HENSON R.A. and URICH H. (1970) Peripheral neuropathy associated with malig-
    nant disease. In *Handbook of Clinical Neurology*, vol. 8, ed. Vinken P.J. and
    Bruyn G.W., pp. 131–148. North-Holland, Amsterdam.
HILDEBRAND J. and COËRS C. (1967) Neuromuscular function in patients with
    malignant tumours. *Brain* **90**, 67–83.
HUTCHINSON E.C., LEONARD B.J., MAUDSLEY C. and YATES P.O. (1958) Neuro-
    logical complications of the reticuloses. *Brain* **81**, 75–92.
NEWMAN M.K. and GUGINO R.J. (1964) Neuropathies and myopathies associated
    with occult malignancies. *J. Amer. med. Ass.* **190**, 575–577.
TROJABORG W., FRANTZEN E. and ANDERSEN I. (1969) Peripheral neuropathy and
    myopathy associated with carcinoma of the lung. *Brain* **92**, 71–82.

WALSH J.C. (1971) The neuropathy of multiple myeloma. An electrophysiological and histological study. *Arch. Neurol.* **25**, 404–414.

WEBSTER H. DE F., SCHRÖDER J.M., ASBURY A.K. and ADAMS R.D. (1967) The role of Schwann cells in the formation of 'onion bulbs' found in chronic neuropathies. *J. Neuropath. exp. Neurol.* **26**, 276–299.

WILNER E.C and BRODY J.A. (1968) An evaluation of the remote effects of cancer on the nervous system. *Neurol. (Minneap.)* **18**, 1120–1124.

Ischaemic neuropathies and collagen-vascular diseases

BLEEHAN S.S., LOVELACE R.E. and COTTON R.E. Mononeuritis multiplex in periarteritis nodosa. *Quart. J. Med.* **127**, 193–209.

CHAMBERLAIN M.A. and BRUCKNER F.E. (1970) Rheumatoid neuropathy. Clinical and electrophysiological features. *Ann. rheum. Dis.* **29**, 609–616.

CHOPRA J.S. and HURWITZ L.J. (1967) Internodal length of sural nerve fibres in chronic occlusive vascular disease. *J. Neurol. Neurosurg. Psychiat.* **30**, 207–214.

DAYAN A.D. and LEWIS P.D. (1966) Demyelinating neuropathy in macroglobulinaemia. *Neurol. (Minneap.)* **16**, 1141–1144.

DUBOIS E.L. (ed.) (1966) *Lupus Erythematosus.* McGraw-Hill, New York.

DYCK P.J., CONN D.L. and OKAZAKI H. (1972) Necrotizing angiopathic neuropathy. Three-dimensional morphology of fiber degeneration related to sites of occluded vessels. *Proc. Mayo Clin.* **47**, 461–475.

EAMES R.A. and LANGE L.S. (1967) Clinical and pathological study of ischaemic neuropathy. *J. Neurol. Neurosurg. Psychiat.* **30**, 215–226.

FERGUSON R.H. and SLOCUMB C.H. (1961) Peripheral neuropathy in rheumatoid arthritis. *Bull. Rheum. Dis.* **11**, 251–254.

GOLDING D.N. (1973) D-penicillamine in rheumatoid arthritis. *Brit. J. hosp. Med.* **9**, 805–813.

HART F.D. (1966) Complicated rheumatoid disease. *Brit. med. J.* **2**, 131–135.

HASLOCK D.I., WRIGHT V. and HARRIMAN D.G.F. (1970) Neuromuscular disorders in rheumatoid arthritis. A motor-point biopsy study. *Quart. J. Med.* **39**, 335–358.

JOHNSON R.T. and RICHARDSON E.P. (1968) The neurological manifestations of systemic lupus erythematosus. *Medicine (Balt.)* **47**, 333–369.

KIBLER R.F. and ROSE F.C. (1960) Peripheral neuropathy in the 'collagen diseases'. A case of scleroderma neuropathy. *Brit. med. J.* **1**, 1781–1784.

LOGOTHETIS J., KENNEDY W.R., ELLINGTON A. and WILLIAMS R.C. (1968) Cryoglobulinaemic neuropathy. Incidence and clinical characteristics. *Arch. Neurol. (Chic)* **19**, 389–397.

LOVSHIN L.L. and KERNOHAN J.W. (1948) Peripheral neuritis in periarteritis nodosa. *Arch. int. Med.* **82**, 321–338.

McENTEE W.J. and MANCALL E.L. (1965) Neuromyositis: a reappraisal. *Neurol. (Minneap.)* **15**, 69–75.

PALLIS C.A. and SCOTT J.T. (1965) Peripheral neuropathy in rheumatoid arthritis. *Brit. med. J.* **1**, 1141–1147.

RICHTER R.B. (1954) Peripheral neuropathy and connective tissue disease. *J. Neuropath. exp. Neurol.* **13**, 168–180.

STERN G. (1972) The peripheral nerves in Wegener's granulomatosis. In *Handbook of Clinical Neurology*, vol. 8, ed. Vinken P.J. and Bruyn G.W., pp. 112–117. North-Holland, Amsterdam.

WARRELL D.A., GODFREY S. and OLSEN E.G.J. (1968) Giant-cell arteritis with peripheral neuropathy. *Lancet* **1**, 1010–1013.

WELLER R.O., BRUCKNER F.E. and CHAMBERLAIN M.A. (1970) Rheumatoid neuropathy: a histological and electrophysiological study. *J. Neurol. Neurosurg. Psychiat.* **33**, 592–604.

Brachial plexus neuropathy

ALLEN I.M. (1931) Neurological complications of serum treatment with report of a case. *Lancet* **2**, 1128–1131.

GATHIER J.C. and BRUYN G.W. (1970a) Neuralgic amyotrophy. In *Handbook of Clinical Neurology*, vol. 8, ed. Vinken P.J. and Bruyn G.W., pp. 77–85. North-Holland, Amsterdam.

GATHIER J.C. and BRUYN G.W. (1970b) The serogenic peripheral neuropathies. In *Handbook of Clinical Neurology*, vol. 8, ed. Vinken P.J., and Bruyn G.W. pp. 95–111. North-Holland, Amsterdam.

KRAFT G.H. (1969) Multiple distal neuritis of the shoulder girdle. An electromyographic clarification of 'paralytic brachial neuritis'. *Electroenceph. J.* **27**, 722.

MAGEE K.R. and DEJONG R.N. (1960) Paralytic brachial neuritis. *J. Amer. Med. Ass.* **174**, 1258–1263.

TSAIRIS P., DYCK P.J. and MULDER D.W. (1972) Natural history of brachial plexus neuropathy. Report of 99 cases. *Arch. Neurol. (Chic.)* **27**, 109–117.

TURNER T.W.A. and PARSONAGE M.J. (1957) Neuralgic amyotrophy (paralytic brachial neuritis) with specific reference to prognosis. *Lancet* **2**, 209–212.

WEIKERS N.J. and MATTSON R.H. (1969) Acute paralytic brachial neuritis. A clinical and electrodiagnostic study. *Neurol. (Minneap.)* **19**, 1153–1158.

Radiation neuropathy

HAYMAKER W. (1969) The effect of ionizing radiation on the nervous system. In *The Structure and Function of Nervous Tissue*, vol. III, ed. Bourne G.H., pp. 441–518. Academic Press, New York.

INNES J.R.M. and CARSTEN A. (1961) Delayed effects of localized x-irradiation on the nervous system of experimental rats and monkeys. In *Fundamental Aspects of Radiosensitivity. Brookhaven Sympos. in Biol.* **14**, pp. 200–203. Brookhaven National Lab., New York.

PANSE F. (1970) Electrical lesions of the nervous system. In *Handbook of Clinical Neurology*, vol. 7, ed. Vinken P.J. and Bruyn G.W., pp. 344–387. North-Holland, Amsterdam.

STOLL B.A. and ANDREWS J.T. (1966) Radiation-induced peripheral neuropathy. *Brit. med. J.* **2**, 834–838.

Tropical neuropathies

HIRONO I. and SHIBUYA C. (1967) Induction of a neurological disorder by cycasin in mice. *Nature* **216**, 1311–1312.

JANSSEN P., VAN BOGAERT L. and HAYMAKER W. (1956) Pathology of the peripheral nervous system in African trypanosomiasis. *J. Neuropath. exp. Neurol.* **15**, 269–287.

OSUNTOKUN B.O. (1968) An ataxic neuropathy in Nigeria. A clinical, biochemical and electrophysiological study. *Brain* **91**, 215–248.

Tumours of nerve

KRAMER W. (1970) Tumours of nerves. In *Handbook of Clinical Neurology*, vol. 8, ed. Vinken P.J. and Bruyn G.W, pp. 412–512. North-Holland, Amsterdam.

RUSSELL D.S. and RUBINSTEIN L.J. (1963) *Pathology of Tumours of the Nervous System*, 2nd edn. Arnold, London.

Chronic idiopathic polyneuropathy

ELKINGTON J.ST.C. (1952) Recent work on the peripheral neuropathies. *Proc. roy. Soc. Med.* **45**, 661–664.

MATTHEWS W.B. (1952) Cryptogenic polyneuritis. *Proc. roy. Soc. Med.* **45**, 667–669.

PRINEAS J. (1970) Polyneuropathies of undetermined cause. *Acta neurol. Scand.* Suppl. **44**, 1–72.

7

Diseases of the Autonomic Nervous System

Consideration of diseases of the autonomic nervous system has been separated from that of other diseases of the peripheral nerve because of the very different anatomy and physiology of this system. A great number of autonomic nerve fibres run in the peripheral nerves, and autonomic dysfunction occurs along with motor and sensory dysfunction in diseases of the peripheral nerve. In addition there are a number of diseases more specifically involving autonomic nerves which must be described.

ANATOMY

The anatomy of the efferent parts of the autonomic nervous system is represented in figs. 7.1 and 7.2. This system has two different components, the *sympathetic* and *parasympathetic*. The *central* regulation of both is sited in the hypothalamus and to a lesser extent in the reticular formation of the brainstem. From these, central sympathetic and parasympathetic fibres descend through the brainstem to the spinal cord, where they synapse upon the appropriate *preganglionic neurons*. In the *sympathetic nervous system* these lie in the intermediolateral grey column of T1 to L2 levels of the spinal cord. Preganglionic axons, which are myelinated, leave the spinal cord in the anterior roots from whence they pass in the white rami to the various sympathetic ganglia, most of which lie in the paravertebral sympathetic chain. There they synapse upon *postganglionic neurons* whose axons are unmyelinated, and either join the peripheral nerves via the grey rami or run to the structures which they innervate in the various autonomic nerve plexuses including the carotid and splanchnic plexuses.

The arrangement of the *parasympathetic nervous system* is different. The preganglionic neurons lie in the brainstem related to the III, VII, IX and X cranial nerves, and in the S2–S4 segments of the spinal cord. The

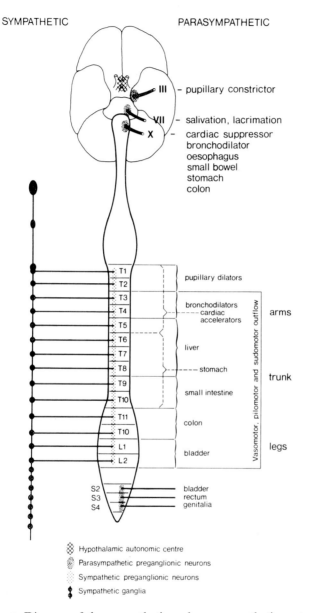

FIG. 7.1. Diagram of the sympathetic and parasympathetic centres and their areas of supply.

axons pass directly to the appropriate viscera in the cranial and sacral nerves. There they synapse upon postganglionic neurons which lie in relation to the smooth muscle and glands which they innervate.

The afferent impulses from the structures receiving autonomic nerve supply travel to the central nervous system in either the appropriate autonomic or spinal nerve.

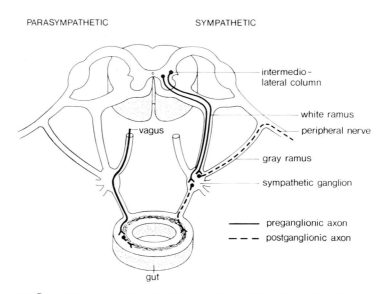

PARASYMPATHETIC   SYMPATHETIC

intermedio-lateral column

white ramus
peripheral nerve

vagus

gray ramus

sympathetic ganglion

———— preganglionic axon
— — — postganglionic axon

gut

FIG. 7.2. Diagram of the dual innervation of the viscera by the parasympathetic and sympathetic nervous systems.

PHYSIOLOGY

Transmitter substances

The transmitter substance released by preganglionic neurons of both the sympathetic and parasympathetic nervous system is acetylcholine:

$$CH_3-N^+-CH_2-CH_2-O-CH_3$$

with CH_3, CH_3, CH_3 groups and OH^-

Acetylcholine is also the transmitter of the postganglionic parasympathetic axons. Nor-adrenaline is the transmitter of the postganglionic sympathetic axons, though a small proportion of adrenaline is also released. Adrenaline is the major compound released from the adrenal medulla on sympathetic nerve stimulation.

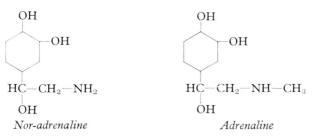

Nor-adrenaline   Adrenaline

Acetylcholine is also the synaptic transmitter of one part of the post-ganglionic sympathetic nervous system, namely the fibres innervating the piloerector muscles and the sweat glands of the skin.

Activation of the parasympathetic nervous system induces pupillary constriction, salivation, lacrimation, bronchoconstriction, slowing of the heart rate, and increased activity of the muscles in the walls of the hollow viscera including the stomach, bowel and bladder. Smooth muscle sphincters such as the pylorus are inhibited. Conversely activation of the sympathetic nervous system produces pupillary dilatation, inhibition of salivation, acceleration of the heart rate, decreased activity of the smooth muscle of the hollow viscera and stimulation of the smooth muscle sphincters, as well as cutaneous vasoconstriction, piloerection and sweating.

Tests of autonomic nervous function

Both systems in the normal state exhibit tone, that is there is a continuous slow rate of action potentials in autonomic nerves. This is capable of being recorded in man (Delius *et al.* 1972, Hagbarth *et al.* 1972). More usually the function of the autonomic nervous system is assessed by applying a series of tests. The object of these is to demonstrate either normal function, or define the site of dysfunction in this system. With lesions of the central autonomic pathways, reflex autonomic control of, for instance, the blood pressure and heart rate may remain intact, though alterations of this reflex control by central nervous influences such as stress become impossible. The abolition of the normal reflex control of autonomic nervous function may be due to lesions of the afferent or efferent part of the autonomic reflex arc. The latter can be recognized by demonstration of denervation supersensitivity, that is excessive sensitivity of the denervated structures to the normal transmitter substance. However not all denervated structures show this phenomenon, and sweating is one such exception. The tests may be grouped under the various fields of control exerted by the autonomic nervous system.

Control of arterioles and blood pressure

Postural control of blood pressure

When a normal individual is rapidly tilted from the horizontal position to the erect, though gravity tends to draw the blood towards the feet, there is immediate compensatory reflex vasoconstriction in the lower limbs and splanchnic territory. The blood pressure thus falls insignificantly. If there is an abnormality either of the afferent or efferent side of this baroreceptor reflex, then a marked fall in blood pressure occurs (*postural hypotension*), which may lead to syncope.

Cold pressor and stress tests

The sudden exposure of a part of the body to cold, for instance by dipping one foot in water at 5°C, normally induces vasoconstriction throughout the body. This may be measured either by a rise of blood pressure recorded by an intra-arterial catheter, or by hand plethysmography. In the latter, the vasoconstriction of the arterioles of the skin is demonstrated by the decreased rate of rise of volume of the hand upon venous occlusion. The stress of mental arithmetic induces a similar change. These tests require both the central and peripheral autonomic pathways to be intact.

Valsalva manoeuvre

If a normal subject blows against a fixed resistance of 20–40 mm Hg for 10 seconds or more, the increased intrathoracic pressure impairs venous return leading to a decrease in the systemic blood pressure. The baroreceptor reflex thereby induces vasoconstriction and an increase in the heart rate by increasing sympathetic outflow. When the subject stops blowing, the venous return is re-established and the stroke volume of the heart returns to normal. However the heart is pumping into a peripheral circulation which is still constricted, and there is therefore an overshoot of blood pressure (see fig. 7.3), with consequent slowing of the heart rate. A lesion of the afferent or efferent part of the reflex arc will block these responses so that there is simple hypotension during the manoeuvre with neither reflex tachycardia nor overshoot with bradycardia. The Valsalva manoeuvre tests not only the control of the arterioles, but also the reflex control of the heart rate.

Nor-adrenaline infusion test

The intravenous infusion of nor-adrenaline at a rate of 2–5 μg/min produces a very small rise of blood pressure in normal individuals whose baro-receptor control compensates for the increased vasoconstriction by a decreased sympathetic discharge rate to the blood vessels. Where there is a

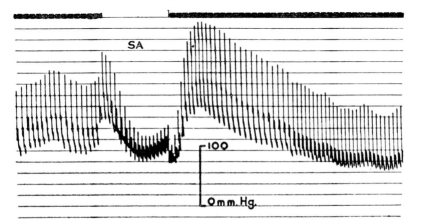

FIG. 7.3. Continuous record of the blood pressure in the brachial artery of a man during the performance of the Valsalva manoeuvre at the break in time signal (upper black line). (*From* Howard, Leathart, Dornhorst and Sharpey-Schafer 1951. *Brit med. J.* **2**, 382.)

postganglionic sympathetic lesion, the smooth muscles of the blood vessels become supersensitive to nor-adrenaline, and therefore the systolic and mean blood pressures rise by perhaps 20–50 mm Hg. This supersensitivity can only be due to a lesion of postganglionic sympathetic function.

Control of heart rate

Carotid sinus reflex

Massage of the carotid sinus in a normal individual stimulates the baro-receptors to produce an increased discharge rate in the autonomic afferent fibres. This leads to an increase in vagal discharge with consequent slowing of the heart rate. A lesion either of the afferent or efferent side of the reflex arc will abolish this response. This test should not be undertaken lightly since it may cause cardiac arrest in unusually sensitive individuals.

Intravenous atropine test

In a resting man, the heart rate is under the continuous control of the vagus nerve. This tonic activity may be demonstrated by blocking its effect with atropine, producing a rise in heart rate. An intravenous injection of 2 mg of atropine given over 3 to 4 minutes will increase the heart rate of a normal individual from 70 beats per minute to 100 beats per minute.

Control of skin temperature

In the normal state there is continuous tonic activity in the sympathetic nerves to the blood vessels of the skin. Therefore a preganglionic or an acute postganglionic lesion will normally induce vasodilatation, the skin becoming flushed and hot. Denervation supersensitivity may develop in a chronic postganglionic lesion, the skin becoming blue and cold due to excessive vasoconstriction. The temperature of one part of the body may be compared with that of another to demonstrate such temperature changes.

Control of sweating

Thermal sweating is under the control of the sympathetic nervous system, though it is cholinergic. A rise of central body temperature by more than a fraction of a degree normally produces increased sweating which may be demonstrated by sprinkling the body with quinizarin powder, or by applying starch-iodide paper. Absence of thermal sweating may be due to a lesion anywhere from the central sympathetic pathways to the postganglionic sympathetic axons. Sweating can also be induced by electrophoresing acetylcholine into the skin (MacMillan and Spalding 1969). A positive response to this test in the absence of thermal sweating indicates that the lesion is preganglionic. For some reason denervation supersensitivity is not a feature of the sweat glands in this test, though hyperhidrosis may occur in certain peripheral lesions of the sympathetic nerves including familial dysautonomia.

Control of visceral motor function

Hollow viscera

The hollow viscera like the bladder and rectum are under the control of the autonomic nervous system, though their smooth muscle also shows autonomous activity. The coordinated contracture of the smooth muscle, as in peristalsis or micturition, requires participation of the autonomic nervous system, and in particular of the parasympathetic part. The autonomic innervation of the bladder is also under central autonomic control, a lesion of which leads to imperfect emptying of the bladder (Bors and Comarr 1971). Pressure changes within the viscera may be recorded, but the interpretation of the changes is complicated by the mutually antagonistic effects of the sympathetic and parasympathetic nerves, and their opposite effects upon the sphincters.

Pupillary responses

The normal pupil shows reflex constriction to light and accommodation, and reflex dilatation in response to pinching the skin of the neck. These responses may be abolished by lesions of the afferent or efferent parts of the reflex. In addition the pupil offers the possibility of direct pharmacological assessment of the state of the autonomic nervous system. Instillation of 1 per cent atropine will block cholinergic transmission of the parasympathetic nerves causing dilatation of the pupil. The instillation of 2 per cent cocaine stimulates the adrenergic receptors thereby producing dilatation of the pupil. The instillation of 2·5 per cent methacholine (Mecholyl) into the conjunctival sac of normal individuals produces no response, but where there is a lesion of the preganglionic parasympathetic system with denervation supersensitivity, there is marked pupilloconstriction. On the other hand where there is a postganglionic lesion of the sympathetic nerves, 2 per cent cocaine does not cause the normal pupillary dilatation. The probable reason is that cocaine normally stimulates the release of catecholamines or potentiates their effects, neither of which occur in the absence of sympathetic nerve terminals.

PHARMACOLOGY

Ganglion-blocking drugs

The preganglionic neurons of both the sympathetic and parasympathetic nervous system release acetylcholine, the receptors on the postganglionic neurons being nicotinic in type. In both systems these receptors are completely blocked by such ganglion-blocking agents as hexamethonium, mecamylamine, pempidine and trimetaphan. The result is the inhibition of all normal functions of the autonomic nervous system, the patient becoming constipated and impotent, having urinary retention, postural hypotension, tachycardia, a dry mouth and hot dry skin, and being unable to focus his eyes or stand bright sunlight.

Drugs acting upon postganglionic transmission

Sympathetic nervous system

The action of adrenaline and nor-adrenaline may be divided into *α-effects* such as vasoconstriction of the skin and viscera and inhibition of smooth muscle, and the *β-effects* such as vasodilatation in skeletal muscle, dilatation of the bronchi, mobilization of hepatic glucose, and an increase in the heart rate. Agents like isoprenaline have very marked direct β-effects, while nor-adrenaline has marked direct α-effects. Other sympathomimetic drugs such as ephedrine, cocaine, and amphetamine stimulate structures innervated by postganglionic sympathetic neurons by releasing catecholamines stored in those nerve endings. Reserpine abolishes postganglionic sympathetic nerve activity by depleting those postganglionic nerve endings of transmitter catecholamines. Two classes of agent have been developed which separately block by competitive inhibition the two types of action of catecholamines, the α-blockers, which include phenoxybenzamine and phentolamine, and the β-blockers, which include propranalol and practalol. Monoamine oxidase inhibitors like phenelzine prevent the metabolism of catecholamines, and, though they have little effect upon the action of catecholamines released at postganglionic sympathetic nerve endings, they greatly potentiate the effect of circulating directly-acting sympathomimetic drugs.

Parasympathetic nerves

Acetylcholine and a number of cholimimetic drugs like carbachol, methacholine and pilocarpine act directly upon cholinergic receptors of structures innervated by parasympathetic postganglionic neurons. Atropine competitively blocks their effect. Agents like neostigmine and physostigmine inhibit acetylcholinesterase.

The organophosphorus compounds like diisopropyl fluorophosphate are very long acting anticholinesterases. All such anticholinesterases allow the accumulation of acetylcholine at the neuroeffector synaptic junction, and thus potentiate the effect of the parasympathetic nervous system.

For further details of the pharmacology of the autonomic nervous system the reader is referred to Goodman and Gillman (1970).

DISEASES OF THE AUTONOMIC NERVOUS SYSTEM

Central nervous diseases including idiopathic orthostatic hypotension (Shy-Drager syndrome)

Central nervous lesions, including those of the hypothalamus, mid-brain, central reticular formation and spinal cord, may damage the central control of the autonomic nervous system. Examples include the hyperpyrexia associated with some hypothalamic and pontine lesions, and the marked postural hypotension and loss of control of bladder function in cases of paraplegia. Postural hypotension is also a feature of the condition termed idiopathic orthostatic hypotension (Shy and Drager 1960, Bannister 1971), and may be seen in patients with Parkinson's disease, particularly during L-dopa therapy. In the former, there are often signs of degeneration of other systems within the central nervous system, including bulbar palsy and cerebellar ataxia. Degeneration and loss of the preganglionic sympathetic neurons lying in the intermediolateral columns of the spinal cord are responsible for loss of postural control of blood pressure. Some of these patients later develop features of Parkinson's disease, while patients with Parkinson's disease may have degeneration of the intermediolateral columns. Treatment with fludrocortisone to increase the blood volume, and where necessary with lower-body pressure suits, may prevent hypotensive episodes. In many patients the course of the disease is progressively downhill.

Familial dysautonomia (Riley-Day syndrome)

This is a rare disease, but of interest in relation to the autonomic nervous system. It occurs mainly in families of Jewish extraction, and is inherited in an autosomal recessive mode. The characteristic clinical features, present from birth, are emotional lability, absence of tears, insensitivity to pain, postural hypotension, absence of fungiform papillae on the tongue, and episodic hyperhidrosis, hyperpyrexia, hypertension, vomiting, and attacks of epilepsy. The tendon and corneal reflexes may be absent. There is decreased excretion of vanillyl mandelic acid (VMA) suggesting loss of adrenal secretion, while increased sensitivity to intravenous nor-adrenaline and to 2·5 per cent methacholine instilled into the conjunctival sac suggest loss of postganglionic sympathetic and parasympathetic neuron activity. Pathological studies have revealed absence of small neurons in the sympathetic and posterior root ganglia (Pearson et al. 1971), and absent unmyelinated nerve fibres with a decrease in the number of large myelinated nerve fibres in the peripheral sensory nerves (Aguayo et al. 1971). It seems likely that almost all the features of the disease are the result of congenital absence of these small neurons and their axons from the sensory and autonomic nervous system. The way in which this absence may come about has been suggested by experimental studies to be mentioned below (page 228).

Diabetic autonomic neuropathy

The autonomic nervous system is the part of the peripheral nervous system least commonly damaged by diabetes mellitus. Impotence in the male is probably the most frequent symptom, followed by diabetic diarrhoea. There is marked loss of potency in about 50 per cent of diabetic males (Martin 1953, Ellenberg 1971). Retrograde ejaculation may occur due to lack of relaxation of the external sphincter during orgasm. The bladder is frequently involved in diabetic autonomic neuropathy producing an increased residual volume and decreased detrusor muscle activity. It rarely leads to retention with overflow, though it predisposes to urinary infections.

Severe diabetic diarrhoea is relatively uncommon, though investigations demonstrate that gastrointestinal function is quite commonly abnormal (Rundles 1945, Bruyn and Garland 1970). The diarrhoea is usually postprandial or nocturnal, profuse, watery, explosive and distressing (Malins and Mayne 1969). Inexplicably treatment with small doses of tetracycline will often abolish diabetic diarrhoea. Similar explosive, nocturnal diarrhoea may also occur in other autonomic neuropathies including those of amyloidosis, and rheumatoid arthritis. Though impaired cardiovascular reflexes are found in 20 per cent of diabetics (Sharpey-Shaffer and Taylor 1960, Moorhouse et al. 1966), symptomatic postural hypotension is uncommon. Some patients exhibit peripheral red, shiny, atrophic skin with decreased sweating, while others have cold, white limbs with hyperhidrosis. The latter may perhaps be due to postganglionic degeneration with denervation supersensitivity (Pickering 1960).

The pathological basis of the autonomic dysfunction in diabetes probably rests in the degeneration of the neurons of the autonomic ganglia and their processes (Appenzeller and Richardson 1966, Hensley and Soergel 1968). Careful control of the diabetes is the only way of reversing the process at present.

Acute idiopathic postinfectious polyneuropathy

Autonomic involvement is not uncommon in the Guillain-Barré-Strohl syndrome (Appenzeller and Marshall 1963, Birchfield and Shaw 1964). Orthostatic hypotension on tipping patients on respirators is common, but spontaneous episodes of hypotension, hypertension and cardiac dysrhythmia may also occur (Davies and Dingle 1972). These may perhaps result from partial blockage of the cardiovascular reflexes on the afferent and efferent side, and from the high circulating levels of catecholamines together with denervation supersensitivity of the blood vessels and heart. A pure autonomic neuropathy has been described developing acutely after an upper respiratory tract infection and showing spontaneous though incomplete recovery over the next two years (Thomashefsky et al. 1972). An experimental model was developed by Appenzeller et al. (1965). In an analogous fashion to the production of experimental allergic neuritis, they immunized rabbits with sympathetic ganglia and Freund's adjuvant, and showed a lack of the normal reflex vasodilatation to heat 6–8 days after the injection. A similar autoimmune process damaging the autonomic nervous system may explain the human cases mentioned above.

Hereditary primary amyloidosis

Autonomic involvement is a striking feature of the hereditary amyloidosis of the Andrade type and may occur late in the Rukavina type (see page 182). Explosive nocturnal and postprandial diarrhoea, impotence, sphincter impairment, decreased gastrointestinal motility, postural hypotension and disordered cardiac conduction are frequently observed. This autonomic involvement is often responsible for the death of patients either by inanition from diarrhoea or by chronic pyelonephritis from urinary retention and infection. Sympathetic ganglia may be heavily infiltrated with amyloid, which may totally replace many of the neurons, resulting in loss of post-ganglionic sympathetic nerve fibres (Appenzeller 1970). Treatment at present is purely symptomatic.

South American trypanosomiasis (Chagas' disease)

Trypanosoma cruzi produces damage both to the heart and the autonomic ganglia either by releasing a toxin or perhaps by the direct effect of the try-panosomes on the autonomic nerve cells. The result is degeneration and loss of the ganglion cells and axons of the myenteric plexus with some inflammatory response (Smith 1967a). Gross autonomic paralysis with dilatation particularly of the oesophagus and colon results. Treatment of the disease in the early stages may prevent the development of megaoesophagus and megacolon.

Hirschsprung's disease resulting from congenital absence of myenteric ganglion cells in a segment of the colon and rectum may also be mentioned in this context. An acquired idiopathic degeneration of the myenteric plexus may cause chronic intestinal obstruction (Dyer *et al.* 1969).

Toxic damage to autonomic function

Chronic alcoholics may occasionally have evidence of loss of circulatory reflexes with postural hypotension. The sympathetic ganglia show abnormalities including giant sympathetic neurons, very similar to those seen in diabetic autonomic neuropathy (Appenzeller and Richardson 1966). Treatment with cytotoxic agents including vincristine may produce damage to the autonomic nervous system and thus constipation and intestinal obstruction (Smith 1967b, Bradley *et al.* 1970). Thallium intoxication may cause tachycardia, hypertension, increased salivation and fever, though the basis is not clear (Bank *et al.* 1972). Botulinum E intoxication may present with acute autonomic dysfunction, the toxin probably preventing the release of acetylcholine at the parasympathetic nerve endings on smooth muscle (Koenig *et al.* 1964). Treatment of mice and rats in the first weeks of life with antibody to nerve growth factor (an agent which stimulates the growth of neurons of the sympathetic nervous system in newborn animals) will produce a morphological state very similar to that occurring in familial dysautonomia (see page 225) (Levi-Montalcini and Angeletti 1966, Aguayo *et al.* 1972). Treatment of adult animals with 6-hydroxy-dopamine produces degeneration of the postganglionic sympathetic nerve endings

(Malmfors and Sachs 1968). Both these experimental tools offer ways of further investigating the autonomic nervous system.

Involvement of autonomic fibres in diseases of peripheral nerves

Many lesions of the peripheral nerves causing denervation of an area of skin are associated with trophic changes in the skin, which becomes thin, red, dry and shiny. In other patients the skin becomes cold, vasoconstricted with hyperhidrosis. The cause of these two responses is not certain, though the former may perhaps result from loss of postganglionic sympathetic control of the blood vessels, while the latter may be an example of denervation supersensitivity. Causalgia, which is a severe spontaneous pain occurring after partial lesions of the major nerve trunks has been ascribed to abnormal functional synapses between sympathetic and sensory fibres at the site of injury (see page 152).

REFERENCES

AGUAYO A. J., MARTIN J. B. and BRAY G. M. (1972) Effects of nerve growth factor antiserin on peripheral unmyelinated nerve fibres. *Acta neuropath. (Berl.)* **20**, 288–298.

AGUAYO A. J., NAIR C. P. V. and BRAY G. M. (1-71) Peripheral nerve abnormalities in the Riley-Day syndrome. *Arch Neurol. (Chic.)* **24**, 106–116.

APPENZELLER O. (1970) *The Autonomic Nervous System*. North-Holland Publishing Co., Amsterdam.

APPENZELLER O., ARNASON B. G. and ADAMS R. D. (1965) Experimental autonomic neuropathy: an immunologically induced disorder of reflex vasomotor function. *J. Neurol. Neurosurg. Psychiat.* **28**, 510–515.

APPENZELLER O. and MARSHALL J. (1963) Vasomotor disturbance in Landry-Guillain-Barré syndrome. *Arch. Neurol. (Chic.)* **9**, 368–372.

APPENZELLER O. and RICHARDSON E. P. (1966) The sympathetic chain in patients with diabetes and alcoholic polyneuropathy. *Neurol. (Minneap.)* **16**, 1205–1209.

BANK W. J., PLEASURE D. E., SUZUKI K., NIGRO M. and KATZ R. (1972) Thallium poisoning. *Arch. Neurol. (Chic.)* **26**, 456–464.

BANNISTER R. (1971) Degeneration of the autonomic nervous system. *Lancet* **2**, 175–179.

BIRCHFIELD R. J. and SHAW C. M. (1964) Postural hypotension in the Guillain-Barré syndrome. *Arch. Neurol. (Chic.)* **10**, 149–157.

BORS E. and COMARR A. E. (1971) *Neurological Urology. Physiology of micturition, its neurological disorders and sequelae*. Skarger, Basel.

BRADLEY W. G., LASSMAN L. P., PEARCE G. W. and WALTON J. N. (1970) The neuro-myopathy of vincristine in man. Clinical, electrophysiological and pathological studies. *J. neurol. Sci.* **10**, 107–131.

BRUYN G. W. and GARLAND H. (1970) Neuropathies of endocrine origin. In *Handbook of Clinical Neurology*, vol. 8, ed. Vinken P. J. and Bruyn G. W., pp. 29–71. North-Holland, Amsterdam.

DAVIES A. G. and DINGLE H. R. (1972) Observations on cardiovascular and neuro-endocrine disturbances in the Guillain-Barré syndrome. *J. Neurol. Neurosurg. Psychiat.* **35**, 176–179.

DELIUS W., HAGBARTH K.-E., HONGELL A. and WALLIN B. G. (1972) General characteristics of sympathetic activity in human muscle nerves. *Acta physiol. Scand.* **84**, 65–81.

DYER N. H., DAWSON A. M., SMITH B. F. and TODD I. P. (1969) Obstruction of bowel due to lesions of the myenteric plexus. *Brit. med. J.* **1**, 686–689.

ELLENBERG M. (1971) Impotence in diabetes: the neurologic factor. *Ann. intern. Med.* **75**, 213–219.

GOODMAN L. S. and GILMAN A. (1970) *The Pharmacological Basis of Therapeutics*, 4th edn. Macmillan, London.

HAGBARTH K.-E., HALLIN R. G., HONGELL A., TOREBJÖRK H. E. and WALLIN B. G. (1972) General characteristics of sympathetic activity in human skin nerves. *Acta physiol. Scand.* **84**, 164–176.

HENSLEY G. T. and SOERGEL K. H. (1968) Neuropathologic findings in diabetic diarrhoea. *Arch. Path.* **85**, 587–597.

KOENIG M. G., SPICKARD A., CARDELLA M. A. and ROGERS D. E. (1964) Clinical and laboratory observations on Type E botulism in man. *Medicine (Balt.)* **43**, 517–545.

LEVI-MONTALCINI R. and ANGELETTI P. U. (1966) Immunosympathectomy. *Pharmacol. Rev.* **18**, 619–628.

MALINS J. M. and MAYNE N. (1969) Diabetic diarrhoea. *Diabetes* **18**, 858–866.

MALMFORS T. and SACHS C. (1968) Degeneration of adrenergic nerves produced by 6-hydroxy-dopamine. *Europe. J. Pharmacol.* **3**, 89–92.

MARTIN M. M. (1953) Diabetic neuropathy. A clinical study of 150 cases. *Brain* **76**, 594–624.

McMILLAN A. L. and SPALDING J. M. K. (1969) Human sweating response to electrophoresed acetylcholine. *J. Neurol. Neurosurg. Psychiat.* **32**, 155–160.

MOORHOUSE J. A., CARTER S. A. and DOUPE J. (1966) Vascular responses in diabetic peripheral neuropathy. *Brit. med. J.* **1**, 883–888.

PEARSON J., BUDZILOVICH G. and FINEGOLD M. J. (1971) Sensory, motor and autonomic dysfunction: The nervous system in familial dysautonomia. *Neurol. (Minneap.)* **21**, 486–493.

PICKERING G. W. (1969) The anatomical and functional aspects of the neurological lesions of diabetes. *Proc. roy. Soc. Med.* **53**, 142–143.

RUNDLES R. W. (1945) Diabetic neuropathy: a general review with a report of 125 cases. *Medicine (Balt.)* **24**, 111–160.

SHARPEY-SHAFER E. P. and TAYLOR P. J. (1960) Absent circulatory reflexes in diabetic neuritis. *Lancet* **1**, 559–561.

SHY G.M. and DRAGER G.A. (1960) A neurological syndrome associated with orthostatic hypotension. *Arch. Neurol. (Chic.)* **2**, 511–527.

SMITH B. (1967a) The myenteric plexus in Chagas' disease. *J. Path. Bact.* **94**, 462–463.

SMITH B. (1967b) The myenteric plexus in drug-induced neuropathy. *J. Neurol. Neurosurg. Psychiat.* **30**, 506–510.

THOMASHEFSKY A.J., HORWITZ S.J. and FEINGOLD M.H. (1972) Acute autonomic neuropathy. *Neurol. (Minneap.)* **22**, 251–255.

8

Diseases of the Perikaryon

The separation of diseases primarily damaging the nerve cell body (*perikaryon*, or more accurately *cyton*) from those primarily damaging the peripheral *axon* is often very difficult. The very close inter-relationship of the perikaryon and axon, by which degeneration of one rapidly produces changes in the other, adds to this difficulty, a fact discussed on pages 135–136. The clinical pointer to a disease of the anterior horn cell is the presence of fasciculations (see page 76), though these are sometimes seen in diseases of other parts of the neuromuscular apparatus. Electrophysiological indications of denervation, including fibrillation potentials and a reduced interference pattern may occur equally in anterior horn cell or peripheral nerve disorders, but giant amplitude polyphasic muscle action potentials and a great enlargement in the motor unit territory is more common with anterior horn cell disease than with peripheral motor neuropathies (see page 104).

The recognition of posterior root ganglion disease is even more difficult. The clinical signs of a radicular distribution of sensory change occurs equally in posterior root or posterior root ganglion lesions. Electrophysiological signs of loss of sensory nerve action potentials and of H reflexes, and loss of the axon flare occur equally in disease of the posterior root ganglion or peripheral nerve. Pathological changes are again not critically diagnostic. Loss of motor or sensory nerve fibres and the changes of denervation and reinnervation on muscle biopsy which are described in chapter 4, may occur equally with perikaryal or peripheral nerve damage. In an individual patient, it is necessary to collect all the evidence, clinical, physiological and pathological, before attempting to decide the site of origin of the disease. Even then only at autopsy may the true state of affairs be revealed.

Despite these problems the group of disorders to be described in this chapter are accepted as arising from disease of the perikarya.

DISEASES OF ANTERIOR HORN CELLS

Virus diseases

Acute anterior poliomyelitis

This disease, until recently the scourge particularly of developed countries, has almost disappeared in immunized populations following the introduction of effective vaccines (Paul 1971). It is due to one of the enteroviruses, of which three distinct strains have been recognized. Type 1 (Brunhilde) is the commonest, and like type 3 (Leon) causes severe paralytic disease; type 2 (Lansing) is pathogenic for rodents, but may cause a milder disease in man. Infection is transmitted by faecal contamination of hands or food, the latter either as a result of faulty sanitation, inadequate hygiene, or carriage of the virus by house-flies.

In poorer countries, prior to the development of effective immunization, the incidence of paralytic poliomyelitis was lower than in developed countries. This was probably due to the fact that infection was acquired in early infancy in such poor countries at a time when the child was still partly protected by antibodies received from the mother; in more developed countries exposure occurred in epidemics when the full paralytic effect of the virus might become manifested (Paul et al. 1952).

From studies of the development of antibodies against the prevalent virus strain in such epidemics, it is known that more than 100 cases become infected with the virus for every case who develops symptoms (Melnick and Ledinko 1953). Of those who developed symptoms, only 30 to 60 per cent developed paralysis. The remainder had a non-paralytic illness, such as diarrhoea or pyrexia. It was possible to isolate the responsible virus from both symptomatic and asymptomatic cases. Pharyngeal secretions contained the virus in the first few days of symptoms, while virus could be isolated from the faeces for 3 or more weeks. This, combined with the fact that nasal instillation of virus induced the disease in monkeys, led to the belief that the virus entered the nervous system via the olfactory nerves. Only when a transient viraemia was demonstrated in the pre-paralytic phase, was it realized that infection of the nervous system occurred via the blood stream (Horstmann et al. 1954). For those interested in the historical developments of ideas of the aetiology and pathogenesis of poliomyelitis, Paul (1971) provides a full account. Russell (1956), van Bogaert (1958) and Bodian

(1959) have reviewed the clinical and pathological aspects of this now very well-understood disease.

Clinical

The full illness shows two phases. The '*minor illness*' consists of fever, malaise, headache and some gastrointestinal disturbance which may last for 1 or 2 days. This phase is associated with the viraemia (Horstmann *et al.* 1954), and is followed by a temporary improvement for 2–5 days during which the patient may be perfectly well, before the development of the '*major illness*', with fever and severe headache, pain in the back and limbs, neck stiffness and at times delirium. The cerebrospinal fluid white cell count may reach 250 per mm^3, the cells being both polymorphs and lymphoctyes early in the illness, and only lymphocytes later. The protein concentration rises in the second week to about 200 mg/100 ml. In 30–60 per cent of cases developing the 'major illness', paralysis occurs heralded by widespread fasciculation, and may be asymmetric and focal. Paralysis appears from the first to the fifth day of the 'major illness', and progresses for 1–3 days. In mild cases improvement may appear within a week, but in a few severe cases the first signs of recovery may not be seen for a month. Physical exertion taken during the early phase of the 'major illness' leads to a gross increase in the severity of paralysis. Paralysis is accompanied by rapid wasting of the involved muscles which show classical denervation atrophy. The bulbar and respiratory muscles are frequently involved, and without special treatment the patient will die. The disease is almost entirely restricted to the lower motor neuron, but rarely the inflammatory reaction and oedema resulting from widespread neuronal involvement may lead to more diffuse damage of the spinal cord with some signs of sensory disturbance. Recovery of function may begin within 1–3 weeks after the peak of paralysis and continue for several years. Recovery is partly due to restoration of function of neurons which are not irreversibly damaged, and partly due to the reinnervation of denervated muscle fibres by surviving motor neurons.

Pathology

The primary change is of damage to the neurons with nuclear pyknosis, cytolysis and neuronophagia. Less severely damaged neurons show chromatolysis. Infiltration of grey matter with microglial cells, and proliferation of astrocytes is prominent. Engorgement of blood vessels is widespread and there are often haemorrhages in the surrounding grey matter and perivascular inflammatory cell infiltrates. The anterior roots and peripheral nerves show consequent axonal degeneration and loss, and the skeletal muscle undergoes profound denervation atrophy. When some degree of recovery occurs, marked enlargement of the motor units within the muscles develops due to branching of the motor nerve fibres.

In man, an inflammatory reaction remains in the spinal cord for several weeks. In man and the monkey Bodian (1948) showed that up to a third of the motor neurons in a nucleus may be destroyed without there being detectable weakness. In severe cases of paralysis, more than two-thirds of the cells may be lost.

Treatment

The important form of treatment is prophylaxis, for once the disease is established, only symptomatic therapy is possible. Two major classes of vaccine have been developed (Paul 1971). Those derived from killed virus (Salk and British vaccines) which require to be injected have largely been replaced by oral live attenuated virus (Sabin vaccine). The latter has the advantage of convenience of administration, together with the theoretical advantage of the specific intestinal mucosal cell immunity. There is no evidence of reversion of the attenuated virus to the wild type, nor of significant passage from person to person. All children should receive this vaccine in early childhood as a part of their routine immunization. Treatment of the established case involves isolation, symptomatic analgesics and treatment of the fever, and passive movements of the affected limbs. Where there are respiratory and bulbar symptoms, artificial respiration and tracheostomy are required. There is still a small population of individuals in the world living with the help of respirators following previous outbreaks of polio.

Rabies

Rabies is an endemic disease of carnivores, particularly dogs, wolves and vampire bats. The virus resides in the salivary glands, is transmitted by biting, and in man may produce a fatal encephalomyelitis. There is evidence that the virus reaches the nervous system by retrograde passage along the axons from the site of the bite to the spinal cord and thence to the brain, since the incubation period for the development of the encephalitis is longer the further from the brain the bite happens to be.

Clinical

The interval between the bite and the appearance of the symptoms varies from 25–70 days, depending on the proximity to the head. Local changes at the bite give no indication of whether rabies virus has been innoculated or not, and during the latent period there are no symptoms. In the typical disease, the first generalized symptom is depression and sleeplessness, followed by the development of painful pharyngeal spasms. These rapidly spread to involve all muscles of swallowing and respiration, and later the whole skeletal musculature. They are induced by any sound, and particularly by drinking and later by even the thought of water, which is why the disease is called 'hydrophobia'. Death is usually from dehydration, pneumonia or exhaustion. In a few cases, the changes are confined to the spinal cord with consequent lower motoneuron paralysis.

Pathology

The damage is widespread throughout the central nervous system (Sükrü-Aksel 1958), and also involves the posterior root and sympathetic ganglia and peripheral nerves (Tangchai and Vejjajiva 1971). Endothelial damage, necrosis of the nervous tissue, and extensive inflammatory cell infiltration occur. Neurons throughout the central nervous system develop characteristic Negri bodies, eosinophilic round inclusions 5–10 μm in diameter containing basophilic granules. There is also extensive neuronophagia and glial proliferation. In the spinal cord the anterior and posterior grey horns are equally affected.

Investigations

In the countries where the disease is endemic, every effort should be made to catch the animal that has bitten a person, to observe whether it develops signs of rabies, and to examine the central nervous system for evidence of the virus.

Treatment

In most cases, despite symptomatic measures, rabies proves fatal. A rare case may however survive (Hattwick et al. 1972). Immunization with a vaccine prepared from the nervous system of rabbits innoculated with rabies has been available for many years, but unfortunately the presence of the foreign brain protein gives a relatively high incidence of allergic encephalomyelitis in patients receiving this. A vaccine derived from virus grown on duck embryos has proved to be neither effective nor totally free of the risk of encephalomyelitis, and current efforts are being devoted to produce a vaccine by growing the virus in tissue culture (*Lancet* 1972). Moreover, unless immunization is undertaken very early in the incubation period it is ineffective.

As a result of the control of wild life populations and the eradication of infected animals, the disease has become rare in Western Europe. Great Britain had eliminated the disease by strict quarantine regulations governing the importation of any potentially infected animal.

Herpes zoster

Shingles is primarily a disease of the posterior root ganglion caused by the zoster-varicella virus, and is described below (page 245 *et seq.*). In many cases, however, the disease spreads to the spinal cord with inflammation mainly of the posterior and anterior horns and some degree of destruction of the anterior horn cells with consequent lower motoneuron paralysis (*British Medical Journal* 1970). The inflammation may in fact involve the cord several segments from the level of the affected posterior root ganglion. In the abdominal wall this may cause an area of paradoxical movements of the muscles. Long tract damage may sometimes be severe (Gordon and Tucker 1945). Clinical signs of such cord damage are however not common. The spinal cord lesions are usually permanent, though some reinnervation of the paralysed muscles may occur from the adjacent myotomes.

'Degenerative diseases'

Motor neuron disease (amyotrophic lateral sclerosis; progressive muscular atrophy; progressive bulbar palsy)

Grouped under the term *motor neuron disease* are several different syndromes with varying degrees of upper motor neuron damage and lower motor neuron denervation of muscles innervated by the spinal cord and medulla. The course in all is progressively downhill. The pathological changes are very similar in almost all groups, though occasional unusual features have been reported. The different clinical pattern may eventually be found to be related to differences in aetiology, but at present it is clearer to consider them as a single disease group the aetiology of which is at present unknown (Norris and Kurland 1969).

Clinical

This is a disease of late middle life, the onset of symptoms usually being about the age of fifty, though patients may be seen from the age of twenty to ninety (Vejjajiva, Foster and Miller 1967). Males are affected about twice as commonly as females. The pattern of symptoms and signs depends upon the clinical type of the disease. In progressive muscular atrophy, weakness and wasting are usually seen first in the small muscles of the hands, later spreading to more proximal muscles in the arms and legs. The wasting may however begin in other muscle groups, and in progressive bulbar palsy the tongue and palate are the earliest involved. Fasciculation is common in the early stages, often preceding significant wasting. In amyotrophic lateral sclerosis, the wasting and weakness of muscles is accompanied by progressive degeneration of the corticospinal tract producing upper motor neuron signs beginning in the legs. These include spasticity with increased tendon reflexes, extensor plantar responses and loss of the abdominal reflexes. With the spread of the upper and lower motor neuron degeneration, the characteristic picture arises of exaggerated tendon reflexes in wasted muscles. Occasional patients are seen in whom the upper motor neuron features alone are present, and the picture being one of a progressive spastic paraparesis. The diagnosis in such cases is extremely difficult unless or until the lower motor neuron signs appear, though electromyography may help by revealing subclinical denervation of the muscles.

In progressive bulbar palsy there is early embarrassment of the airways with food and secretions tending to tip into the larynx. Patients become dysarthric or even anarthric. Weakness of the accessory muscles of respiration make the cough ineffective, and aspiration pneumonia frequently occurs. Often upper motor neuron pseudobulbar palsy is also present.

A characteristic feature of motor neuron disease is the absence of sensory involvement, though paraesthesiae or loss of vibration sensation at the ankles may rarely be noted. The average period from onset to death is about 3 years in most forms of the disease, and 2 years in progressive bulbar palsy. The clinical picture is a depressing one, the patient becoming more incapacitated, unable to feed himself and eventually to cough or swallow though with no impairment of higher mental function. However occasional cases have a more benign course with survival for 10 or 15 years.

Pathology

The diagnostic lesion at autopsy is degeneration and loss of the anterior horn cells of the spinal cord and skeletal motor nuclei of the medulla, together with degeneration of the corticospinal tracts. The α-motor neurons and probably γ-motor neurons accumulate lipofuscin, undergo degeneration with shrinkage and pyknosis, and eventual phagocytosis. An occasional cell may be seen showing the changes of central chromatolysis which usually indicate an axonal lesion. The anterior grey horns of the spinal cord are thus left with almost no large neurons and an increased number of astrocytes and residual macrophages (Hirano et al. 1969). Similar changes are seen in the pyramidal neurons, especially the Betz cells of the precentral gyrus. There is resultant degeneration with loss of fibres in the corticospinal tracts, usually worse in the lumbosacral and lower thoracic cord. The picture has certain features of a 'dying back' disease, except that the corticospinal tract in the upper thoracic cord is relatively spared while degeneration is again marked at the cervical level. The basis of this curious distribution is not clear.

In rare cases the pathological changes in the motoneurons differ from the classical. Alzheimer-like neurofibrillary tangles, hyaline cytoplasmic inclusions, and widespread central chromatolysis have been reported (Hirano et al. 1967, 1969, Schochet et al. 1969). Presumably the underlying disease process is different in each of these instances.

Aetiology

The aetiology of motor neuron disease is unknown, though there are a number of pointers which may be of significance. It is likely that several diseases with different aetiologies exist in this group, and certainly anterior horn cell degeneration can occur in a number of other diseases (see below). About 5–10 per cent of patients with motor neuron disease have a family history of similar disease, though the vast majority are sporadic (Thomson and Alvarez 1969, Amick et al. 1971). The incidence of previous acute anterior poliomyelitis in patients with motor neuron disease is about ten times that which might be expected and it is possible that the poliomyelitis virus may change its character from an 'acute' to a 'slow' virus (Poskanzer *et al.* 1969). Alternatively the increased metabolic load imposed on anterior horn cells innervating a greatly increased number of muscle fibres may perhaps be responsible for premature metabolic failure and degeneration. The disease has also been supposed to be due to an unrelated slow virus (Johnson 1969).

Lead intoxication causes a neuropathy which is often purely motor (see page 166 *et seq.*) and may be confused with progressive muscular atrophy. Lead intoxication has also been advanced as one of the causes of motor neuron disease. A history of exposure to lead may be elicited in up to 15 per cent of patients with motor neuron disease, and Campbell *et al.* (1970) found such patients survived longer than those without such a history. An increased incidence of gastric carcinoma and previous gastrectomy has been noted in patients with motor neuron disease, and a number of conflicting reports have dealt with endocrine and exocrine dysfunction in this disease (Quick and Greer 1967, Brown and Kater 1969).

A picture indistinguishable from motor neuron disease has been reported in patients with macroglobulinaemia (Peters and Clatanoff 1967), Hodgkin's disease (Walton *et al.* 1968), and a variety of carcinomata (Brain *et al.* 1965). The importance of this association is that the neurological disease may remit if the neoplasia is adequately treated. It is uncertain whether such a remission has ever been demonstrated in a case of motor neuron disease associated with carcinoma, and therefore this association may be purely fortuitous. Ischaemia particularly of the lower part of the spinal cord due to arteriosclerosis has been suggested as a cause of motor neuron disease in some patients (Skinhøj 1954, Fieschi *et al.* 1970).

Treatment

Different theories of the aetiology have led to suggestions of a variety of different therapies including vitamins, low fat diets, and antiviral, chelating and cytotoxic agents. So far none has proved successful. Current treatment is purely symptomatic, including spasmolytic agents such as baclofen and diazepam, and appliances for home and nursing care. Section of the cricopharyngeus muscle and injection of silicone implants lateral to the vocal cords may help patients with bulbar palsy. For the more advanced case laryngectomy is sometimes justified.

Anterior horn cell degeneration in other neurological diseases

The Chamorro people living in Guam and the other Mariana Islands in the Pacific Ocean have a remarkable incidence of a group of degenerative neurological diseases. Different patients have varying elements of Parkinsonism, dementia and amyotrophic lateral sclerosis. Neurofibrillary degeneration is a frequent pathological finding both in the anterior horn cells and brain (Hirano *et al.* 1966, 1969). A similar disease has less commonly been found in other races including Caucasians. Evidence is against the disease being inherited in the Chamorros. One suggestion concerning aetiology is that a cyanogen, cycasin, in the staple starch food derived from *Cycas circinalis* is responsible. This agent causes neurological disease in experimental animals (Hirono and Shibuya 1967).

Amyotrophy may also be striking in patients with spongiform encephalopathy of the Jakob-Creutzfeld type (Allen *et al.* 1971). A number of metabolic diseases affecting neurons, including the lipidoses, result in damage and degeneration of the anterior horn cells. Glycogen accumulation in the neurons in Pompe's disease (hereditary amylo-$1,4$-α-glucosidase deficiency) may lead to anterior horn cell death.

Hereditary spinal muscular atrophies

In addition to the occasional cases of inherited motor neuron disease, a number of inherited disease entities are recognized in which the patient suffers from progressive weakness and wasting of the skeletal muscles, and in which degeneration of the anterior horn cells in the spinal cord and to a lesser extent the brainstem is responsible. There is debate about exactly how many diseases can be separated from this group (Emery 1971), but for practical purposes three main groups based upon age of presentation will be described. In none is the aetiology of the condition known, and in all the treatment can therefore only be symptomatic.

Infantile spinal muscular atrophy (Werdnig-Hoffmann disease)

This disease usually presents in the first six months of life, the baby being noticed to have decreasing movements and increased floppiness (Byres and Banker 1961, Dubowitz 1966). In some the mother gives a history of decreased fetal movements suggesting prenatal onset. Muscle atrophy is not easy to detect at this stage, but hypotonicity and poverty of movements progress and involve all four limbs. The condition is purely motor. Progressive difficulty in feeding and respiration develops, and the child eventually dies, usually of pneumonia at about the age of 1 year. The age of onset and prognosis are however very variable, and occasional cases appear to arrest or show an unusually benign picture. The pattern of inheritance in most families is indicative of an autosomal recessive gene.

The pathological changes differ from adult spinal muscular atrophy in the striking frequency of central chromatolysis in the anterior horn cells. Chou and Fakadej (1971) have found these cells to be full of mitochondria unlike chromatolytic neurons due to axonal lesions. They found a striking abnormality of thick masses of glial fibrils in the anterior root of these cases which they suggested was responsible for the disease by causing compression of the motor nerve fibres. Occasional cases have shown differing pathological pictures including hyaline inclusions and peripheral vacuolation of the neurons (Kohn 1971).

Juvenile spinal muscular atrophy (Kugelberg-Welander disease)

The onset of this condition is from late infancy to adolescence, and the picture is often mistaken before further investigation for a muscular dystrophy (Gardner-Medwin *et al.* 1967). True or pseudohypertrophy of the calves and other muscles, and electrocardiographic abnormalities, which are occasionally seen, may be taken to confirm the diagnosis of a muscular dystrophy until electromyography and muscle biopsy reveal that the disease is due to progressive denervation. The term pseudomyopathic spinal muscular atrophy is often applied as a result. Proximal muscles are usually predominantly involved. In many the condition is slowly progressive, though the rate is slower than in infantile spinal muscular atrophy. Some patients die 5–15 years after the onset of the condition, but in a few patients the condition appears to arrest or even improve, particularly during the adolescent growth spurts.

Adult onset spinal muscular atrophy

This is a heterogeneous group of diseases. All have a more benign picture than motor neuron disease, the patients often surviving 20 or more years after the onset which usually is in the third or fourth decade. Five main subgroups may be recognized. The *limb-girdle syndrome* may be due to spinal muscular atrophy in about half the cases, the pattern of muscle involvement being similar to cases due to primary limb-girdle muscular dystrophy. The cases may be sporadic or recessively inherited. Similarly up to half the patients with the *facioscapulohumeral syndrome* may in fact have spinal muscular atrophy. The clinical picture again is similar to that of primary facioscapulohumeral muscular dystrophy. One form of *peroneal muscular atrophy* appears to be due to spinal muscular atrophy (see page 190). *Scapuloperoneal muscular atrophy*, sometimes inherited as an X-linked recessive disease, has also been recognized. *Other cases* do not fit into any typical picture unless it be the *atypical* pattern of muscle involvement. The atrophy often affects distal muscles as much as proximal, and may be asymmetric and involve muscles like the triceps and deltoid which are frequently spared in the muscular dystrophies. More work remains to be done in clarifying the nosology of the spinal muscular atrophies.

Anterior horn cell damage in myelopathies

The anterior horn cells, lying in the spinal cord, may be damaged by many conditions which are truly diseases of the central nervous system. Almost invariably such damage is associated with signs of lesions of the upper motor neuron or of the spinal cord sensory tracts which make diagnosis relatively easy (see page 79). Special investigations including myelography may however be required to confirm the diagnosis and localize the lesion. This group of diseases has recently been reviewed by the author (Bradley 1974).

Obstruction to the feeding arteries of the spinal cord may produce infarction with consequent damage to the anterior horn cells. This arterial occlusion may arise in one of the small spinal arteries such as the anterior spinal artery lying in the anterior sulcus and supplying the anterior half of the spinal cord, or it may be due to stenosis or occlusion of one of the major feeding vessels at their origin from the vertebral artery or aorta. Arteriosclerosis is the commonest cause, but other sources of emboli must be considered. The extent of anterior horn cell damage depends upon the site of infarction, and may be extensive in the lumbar and cervical enlargements where there is a large concentration of neurons. The clinical picture is usually of a sudden onset of an established lesion, but occasionally a gradually progressive syndrome results. The possible role of ischaemia in the aetiology of motor neuron disease has already been mentioned (page 240).

Ischaemia is probably the final common path for a number of other diseases damaging the spinal cord. Arachnoiditis, the chronic meningitides such as those due to syphilis, tuberculosis and fungus infections, and spinal cord compression may all be mentioned in this context. Excessive irradiation of the spinal cord causes both direct damage to the neural elements and endarteritis obliterans leading to infarction. A condition resembling intermittent claudication due to ischaemia of the calf muscles may arise from ischaemia of the spinal cord or nerve roots. Patients suffer pain and neurological symptoms of weakness, numbness and paraesthesiae in the affected region, brought on by exercise. A compressive lesion including a chronic disc prolapse, or lumbar canal stenosis is often surgically correctable.

Venous infarction of the spinal cord may also occur, though damage is mainly to the posterior half of the cord. Arteriovenous malformations of the spinal cord may produce damage in any part due either to direct expansion and compression, haemorrhage, thrombosis, or the 'stealing' of blood from the remainder of the cord. A rare condition is subacute necrotizing myelitis of Foix and Alajouanine in which there is a gradually ascending paraplegia which is at first spastic and later flaccid. It affects especially males with cor pulmonale, and there is debate whether it is due to an underlying angioma or to thrombophlebitis.

A tumour growing within the spinal cord, such as an astrocytoma or ependymoma, may damage the anterior horn cells. Similarly enlargement of the central canal (hydromyelia) or of a syrinx (syringomyelia) causes marked damage to the anterior horn cells, particularly in the cervical enlargement. A suspended dissociated sensory loss is the diagnostic feature.

Acute damage to the cord by a vertebral fracture or displacement, or a penetrating wound will damage the anterior horn cell. A haemorrhage within the central part of the cord (haematomyelia) may produce signs indistinguishable from syringomyelia. Occasionally there may arise several years after a traumatic paraplegia, an ascending picture indistinguishable from syringomyelia. This is due to an ascending syrinx, though its mode of formation is not certain. Anterior horn cell damage is extensive in these conditions where the lumbar and cervical enlargements are involved.

Cervical spondylotic myelopathy predominantly affects the C4 to C7 levels of the cord and may cause extensive lower motor neuron signs and symptoms which are partly due to root damage (see page 259), and partly due to anterior horn cell damage within the spinal cord.

Diseases of posterior root ganglia

Hereditary sensory radicular neuropathy

This condition is described on page 187. It is associated with primary degeneration and loss of the small neurons of the posterior root ganglia, producing dissociated loss of pain and temperature sensation with resultant neuropathic ulcers and arthropathy.

Friedreich's ataxia

In this disease, the major lesion is a progressive loss of large nerve fibres in the posterior columns (Greenfield 1954). Lesser degrees of degeneration occur in the corticospinal and posterior spinocerebellar tracts. The cause of the posterior column degeneration probably lies in the posterior root ganglia where particularly the larger neurons of the lumbosacral region show shrinkage and loss (Greenfield 1963a). This leads to loss of myelinated nerve fibres in both the posterior roots and posterior columns and consequent loss of joint position and vibration sense with sensory ataxia.

The disorder usually has an autosomal recessive inheritance, though occasional dominant and X-linked patterns have been recorded (Pratt 1966). It usually presents about the age of 10 years, though in occasional cases which have a similar progressive neurological degeneration, symptoms do not begin until the age of 20 or 30 years. The course is gradually downhill, patients becoming increasingly ataxic and spastic. Most patients have died within 15 years of the onset of the illness. The aetiology of the condition is at present unknown.

Similar though less extensive posterior root ganglion degeneration occurs in a number of the other hereditary spinocerebellar degenerations.

Herpes zoster (shingles)

Clinical

Shingles is a condition most commonly affecting the middle-aged and elderly, though no age is exempt. The usual picture is of a girdle-like pain on one side of the chest or neck and arm lasting for 3 or 4 days, followed by the vesicular eruption appearing in the same distribution. The latter patchily conforms to the distribution of one or sometimes more sensory roots. Unless secondary infection supervenes, the vesicles dry and scab in 5–10 days, and the pain gradually subsides. The area is now found to be hypaesthetic, but also painful to the touch. Healing of the skin occurs with permanent scar formation, and after some months there is gradual return of sensation by collateral reinnervation from the adjacent dermatomes.

Postherpetic neuralgia is a great problem occurring in about 20 per cent of patients, particularly in women, those with more severe vesiculation, and those more than 65 years of age (Molin 1969). In this condition the pain preceding the eruption usually remains permanently unabated, exacerbated by the painful sensation resulting from stimulation of the dysaesthetic skin. The severity of this pain may necessitate the strongest analgesics including opiates, and may lead to suicide. The treatment of postherpetic neuralgia is considered below.

Herpes zoster may involve other nerves of the body including the trigeminal nerve and the geniculate ganglion of the facial nerve. *Herpes ophthalmicus* is the commonest form of trigeminal nerve involvement. Corneal damage and scarring is an important hazard requiring treatment with antibiotic eye-drops and careful ocular hygiene. Geniculate herpes (Ramsay Hunt syndrome) is one of the causes of an acute facial palsy. It differs from the classic idiopathic Bell's palsy in that there is usually severe pain in the ear and pharynx preceding the paralysis, at the onset of which a few vesicles may be found in the external auditory canal and on the anterior pillars of the fauces. The prognosis for recovery of the facial paralysis tends to be somewhat worse than idiopathic Bell's palsy (Dalton 1960).

Though primarily a disease of the posterior root ganglia with consequent pain and sensory disturbances, the acute inflammation may spread to involve the underlying meninges and central nervous system. A meningeal inflammatory response is common and may at times produce an overt meningitis (Biggart and Fisher 1938). Inflammatory involvement of the cord may lead to anterior horn cell damage as described above (page 237), and is seen in up to 5 per cent of patients where the rash involves the limbs (Gupta *et al.* 1969). In the thoracolumbar region, lower motor neuron paralysis may be difficult to detect, though segmental abdominal paralysis may lead to a pseudohernia. The phrenic nerve may also be involved (*British Medical Journal* 1970). The long tracts of the spinal cord, particularly the corticospinal tract may be damaged in the process with an ipsilateral spastic paralysis of the leg. The inflammatory process in herpes ophthalmicus may spread to involve the II, III, IV and VI cranial nerves with consequent loss of vision and optic atrophy, or diplopia. Personally observed cases of herpes ophthalmicus have developed temporary dementia from frontal lobe involvement, and temporary contralateral choreoatheotosis from basal ganglia damage.

Aetiology

Shingles is due to the zoster-varicella virus, and non-immune subjects may develop chickenpox when in contact with a patient with shingles. In most cases, the patient with shingles has previously had varicella, and it is suggested that the virus remains dormant in the posterior root ganglia often for several decades until reactivation produces the shingles. Rarely, primary exposure to either condition may lead to an attack of shingles after an incubation period which is usually about 2 weeks. Reactivation of the virus may occur without cause, though it is commonest in the elderly and in those debilitated with various conditions including carcinomata, vertebral fractures, and the reticuloses such as Hodgkin's disease.

Pathology

The virus particles may be found in the vesicle fluid, and are presumed to reach there via the sensory nerve. The posterior root ganglia show marked damage with inflammatory cell infiltration, engorged blood vessels, haemorrhage and oedema (Greenfield 1963b). The neurons are severely damaged, and the sensory root and sensory fibres of the mixed spinal nerve consequently show changes of axonal degeneration. Often the inflammatory process spreads both into the peripheral nerve and underlying central nervous system. In the Ramsay Hunt syndrome, the lesion may lie either in the geniculate ganglion or perhaps in the brainstem.

Treatment

Patients with the acute syndrome require analgesics, sedatives and measures to prevent secondary infection. Postherpetic neuralgia and damage to the eye in herpes ophthalmicus are the most serious complications of shingles. Despite the theoretical risk of dissemination of the virus, treatment with corticosteroids (prednisone 60 mg/day for a week, tailing off over the next 2 weeks) if begun within 2 days of the appearance of the rash rapidly reduces pain and probably reduces both the incidence of postherpetic neuralgia and of ocular complications (Elliott 1964, Bergaust and

Westby 1967). Once postherpetic neuralgia has become established, treatment is not easy. Carbamazepine 200–400 mg four times daily helps relieve the pain in a small proportion of cases. Massage with a vibrator after spraying with a freezing spray three times a day will often slowly reduce the pain. Intravenous procaine infusions (three doses of 500 mg in 500 ml of dextrose solution in a half an hour at daily intervals) are sometimes helpful (Shanbrom 1961). Psychotropic drugs are often useful adjuvants, though occasionally therapy has to resort to unilateral spinothalamic tractotomy.

Carcinomatous ganglionitis

The neuropathies resulting from non-metastatic complications of carcinomata have been mentioned on page 191. The commonest form is a mixed sensorimotor neuropathy, and a pure sensory neuropathy is the next most common. The condition usually affects larger rather than smaller fibre function, though both may be equally involved. The picture is usually of a progressive distal symmetrical polyneuropathy. Carcinoma of the lung, particularly of the oat cell type, is by far the most frequent cause. Extensive degeneration of neurons and perivascular and diffuse infiltration with lymphocytes and inflammatory cells in the posterior root ganglia are seen in both conditions (Henson and Urich 1970). Attempts should be made to find and resect an underlying carcinoma in such patients, for in some the neuropathy is the earliest sign of a non-invasive carcinoma, and the clinical picture remits with total excision of the growth.

Diabetic ganglionopathy

The posterior root ganglia in diabetes often show various degenerative changes including swelling and degeneration of the neurons, and proliferation of the interstitial cells (Bruyn and Garland 1970). These changes may in part be responsible for the sensory neuropathy of diabetes mellitus, and in part the result of the peripheral damage to sensory axons. Diabetic neuropathy is considered on page 158.

Hereditary amyloidosis

In the Andrade type of amyloidosis, there is a preferential loss of the smallest nerve fibres. As discussed on page 182, this may well be due to amyloid infiltration of the posterior root ganglia. The neurons are reported to be replaced by amyloid, but the detailed structure of this process awaits clarification.

Idiopathic acquired posterior root ganglion degeneration

Occasional patients are encountered with an atypical sensory neuropathy. This may show an asymmetric radicular distribution, and different roots may be damaged in recurrent attacks. A number of such cases were reported by Dyck *et al.* (1968). The pathogenesis and the morphological changes in the ganglia have not been elucidated.

REFERENCES

ALLEN I. V., DERMOTT E., CONNOLLY J. H. and HURWITZ L. J. (1971) A study of a patient with the amyotrophic form of Creutzfeld-Jakob disease. *Brain* **94**, 715–724.

AMICK L. D., NELSON J. W. and ZELLWEGER H. (1971) Familial motor neuron disease, non-Chamorro type. *Acta neurol. Scand.* **47**, 341–349.

BERGAUST B. and WESTBY, R. K. (1967) Zoster ophthalmicus. Local treatment with cortisone. *Acta ophthalmol.* **45**, 787–793.

BIGGART J. H. and FISHER J. A. (1938) Meningo-encephalitis complicating herpes zoster. *Lancet* **2**, 944–946.

BODIAN D. (1948) *Trans. 1st. International Poliomyelitis Conference.* Lippincott, Philadelphia.

BODIAN D. (1959) In *Viral and Rickettsial Infections in Man*, 3rd edn., ed. Rivers T. and Horsfall F. L., pp. 479–498. Lippincott, Philadelphia.

BRADLEY W. G. (1974) Myelopathies affecting anterior horn cells. In *Peripheral Neuropathy*, ed. Dyck P. J., Thomas P. K. and Lambert E. H., part V. section C, ch. 1. Saunders, Philadelphia, in press.

BRAIN LORD, CROFT P. B. and WILKINSON M. (1965). Motor neurone disease as a manifestation of neoplasm (with a note on the course of classical motor neurone disease). *Brain* **88**, 479–500.

British Medical Journal (1970) Leading article: Paralysed hemidiaphragm and shingles. **1**, 382–383.

BROWN J. C. and KATER R. M. H. (1969) Pancreatic function in patients with amyotrophic lateral sclerosis. *Neurol. (Minneap.)* **19**, 185–189.

BRUYN G. W. and GARLAND H. (1970) Neuropathies of endocrine origin. In *Handbook of Clinical Neurology*, vol. 8, ed. Vinken P. J. and Bruyn G. W., pp. 29–71. North-Holland, Amsterdam.

BYERS R. K. and BANKER B. Q. (1961) Infantile muscular atrophy. *Arch. Neurol. (Chic.)* **5**, 140–164.

CAMPBELL A. G. M., WILLIAMS E. R. and BARLTROP D. (1970) Motor neurone disease and exposure to lead. *J. Neurol. Neurosurg. Psychiat.* **33**, 877–885.

CHOU S.M. and FAKADEJ A.V. (1971) Ultrastructure of chromatolytic motoneu-
rons and anterior spinal roots in a case of Werdnig-Hoffmann disease. *J. Neuropath. exp. Neurol.* **30**, 368–379.

DALTON G.A. (1960) Bell's palsy: some problems of prognosis and treatment. *Brit. med. J.* **1**, 1765–1770.

DUBOWITZ V. (1966) Hereditary proximal spinal muscular atrophy. *Brit. med. J.* **2**, 173–174.

DYCK P.J., GUTRECHT J.A., BASTRON J.A., KARNES W.E. and DALE A.J.D. (1968) Histologic and teased-fiber measurements of sural nerve in disorders of lower motor and primary sensory neurons. *Proc. Mayo Clin.* **43**, 81–123.

ELLIOTT F.A. (1964) Treatment of herpes zoster with high doses of prednisone. *Lancet* **2**, 610–611.

EMERY A.E.H. (1971) The nosology of the spinal muscular atrophies. *J. med. Gen.* **8**, 481–495.

FIESCHI C., GOTTLIEB A. and DE CAROLIS V. (1970) Ischemic lacunae in the spinal cord of arteriosclerotic subjects. *J. Neurol. Neurosurg. Psychiat.* **33**, 138–146.

GARDNER-MEDWIN D., HUDGSON P. and WALTON J.N. (1967) Benign spinal muscular atrophy arising in childhood and adolescence. *J. neurol. Sci.* **5**, 121–158.

GORDON I.R.S. and TUCKER J.F. (1945) Lesions of the central nervous system in herpes zoster. *J. Neurol. Neurosurg. Psychiat.* **8**, 40–46.

GREENFIELD J.G. (1954) *The Spinocerebellar Degenerations.* Blackwell, Oxford.

GREENFIELD J.G. (1963a) System degenerations of the cerebellum, brain stem and spinal cord. In *Greenfield's Neuropathology,* ed. Blackwood W., McMenemy W.H., Meyer A., Norman R.M. and Russell D.S., pp. 581–601. Arnold, London.

GREENFIELD J.G. (1963b) Infectious diseases of the central nervous system. In *Greenfield's Neuropathology,* ed. Blackwood W., McMenemy W.H., Meyer A., Norman R.M. and Russell D.S., pp. 138–234. Arnold, London.

GUPTA S.K., HELAL B.H. and KIELY P. (1969) The prognosis in zoster paralysis. *J. Bone Jt. Surg.* **51**B, 593–603.

HATTWICH M.A.W., WIES T.T., STECHSCHULTE C.J., BAER G.M. and GREGG M.B. (1972) Recovery from rabies. *Ann. int. Med.* **76**, 931–942.

HENSON R.A., and URICH H. (1970) Peripheral neuropathy associated with malig-
nant disease. In *Handbook of Clinical Neurology,* vol. 8, ed. Vinken P.J. and Bruyn G.W., pp. 131–148. North-Holland, Amsterdam.

HIRANO A., KURLAND L.T. and SAYER G.P. (1967) Familial amyotrophic lateral sclerosis. *Arch. Neurol. (Chic.)* **16**, 232–243.

HIRANO A., MALAMUD N., ELIZAN T.S. and KURLAND L.T. (1966) Amyotrophic lateral sclerosis and Parkinsonism-dementia complex on Guam. *Arch. Neurol. (Chic.)* **15**, 35–51.

HIRANO A., MALAMUD N., KURLAND L.T. and ZIMMERMAN H.M. (1969) A review of the pathological findings in amyotrophic lateral sclerosis. In *Motor Neuron Disease. Research in amyotrophic lateral sclerosis and related disorders,* ed. Norris F.H. and Kurland L.T., pp. 51–60. Grune and Stratton, New York.

HIRONO I. and SHIBUYA C. (1967) Induction of a neurological disorder by cycasin in mice. *Nature* **216**, 1311–1312.

HORSTMANN D.M., McCOLLUM R.W. and MASCOLA A.D. (1954) Viremia in human poliomyelitis. *J. exp. Med.* **99**, 355–369.

JOHNSON R.T. (1969) Virological studies and summary of Soviet experiments on the transmission of amyotrophic lateral sclerosis to monkeys. In *Motor Neuron Disease Research in amyotrophic lateral sclerosis and related disorders*, ed. Norris F.H. and Kurland L.T., pp. 280–283. Grune and Stratton, New York.

KOHN R. (1971) Clinical and pathological findings in an unusual infantile motor neuron disease. *J. Neurol. Neurosurg. Psychiat.* **34**, 427–431.

Lancet (1972) Newer rabies vaccines. **1**, 132.

MELNICK J.L. and LEDINKO N. (1953) Development of neutralizing antibodies against three types of poliomyelitis virus during an epidemic period. *Amer. J. Hyg.* **58**, 207.

MOLIN L. (1969) Aspects of the natural history of herpes zoster. *Acta derm.-venereol.* **49**, 569–583.

NORRIS F.H. and KURLAND L.T. ed. (1969) *Motor neuron disease. Research in amyotrophic lateral sclerosis and related disorders.* Grune and Stratton, New York.

PAUL J.R. (1971) *A History of Poliomyelitis.* Yale University Press, New York.

PAUL J.R., MELNICK J.L., BARNETT V.H. and GOLDBLOM N. (1952) A survey of neutralizing antibodies to poliomyelitis in Cairo, Egypt. *Amer. J. Hyg.* **55**, 402.

PETERS H.A. and CLATANOFF D.V. (1967) Spinal muscular atrophy secondary to macroglobulinaemia. *Neurol. (Minneap.)* **18**, 101–108.

POSKANZER D.C., CANTOR H.M. and KAPLAN G.S. (1969) The frequency of preceding poliomyelitis in amyotrophic lateral sclerosis. In *Motor Neuron Disease. Research in amyotrophic lateral sclerosis and related disorders*, ed. Norris F.H. and Kurland L.T., pp. 286–290. Grune and Stratton, New York.

PRATT R.T.C. (1967) *The Genetics of Neurological Disorders.* Oxford University Press, London.

QUICK D.T. and GREER M. (1967) Pancreatic dysfunction in patients with amyotrophic lateral sclerosis. *Neurol. (Minneap.)* **17**, 112–116.

RUSSELL W.R. (1956) *Poliomyelitis*, 2nd edn. Arnold, London.

SCHOCHET S.C., HARDMAN J.M., LADEWIG P.P. and EARLE K.M. (1969) Intraneuronal conglomerates in sporadic motor neuron disease. *Arch. Neurol. (Chic.)* **20**, 548–553.

SHANBROM E. (1961) Treatment of herpetic pain and postherpetic neuralgia with intravenous procaine. *J. Amer. med. Ass.* **176**, 1041–1043.

SKINHØJ E. (1954) Arteriosclerosis of the spinal cord. Three cases of pure 'syndrome of the anterior spinal artery'. *Acta Psych Neurol. (Scand.)* **29**, 139–144.

SÜKRÜ-AKSEL I. (1958) Pathologische Anatomie der Lyssa. In *Handbuch der Speziellen Pathologischen Anatomie und Histologie*, vol. XIII, 2A, ed. Scholz W. p. 417–435. Springer, Berlin.

TANGCHAI P. and VEJJAJIVA A. (1971) Pathology of the peripheral nervous system and human rabies. A study of nine autopsy cases. *Brain* **94**, 299–306.

THOMSON A.F. and ALVAREZ F.A.E. (1969) Hereditary amyotrophic lateral sclerosis. *J. neurol. Sci.* **8**, 101–110.

VAN BOGAERT L. (1958) Poliomyelite anterieure aiguë. (Maladi de Heine-Medin). In *Handbuch der Speziellen Pathologischen Anatomie und Histologie.* vol. XIII, 2A, ed. Scholz W. p. 244–297. Springer, Berlin.

VEJJAJIVA A., FOSTER J. B. and MILLER H. (1967) Motor neuron disease. A clinical study. *J. neurol. Sci.* **4**, 299–314.

WALTON J. N., TOMLINSON B. E. and PEARCE G. W. (1968) Subacute 'poliomyelitis' and Hodgkin's disease. *J. neurol. Sci.* **6**, 435–445.

9

Diseases of the Spinal Nerve Roots

The spinal nerve roots may be specifically damaged either because of their inherent susceptibility to certain diseases, or by processes specific to the spinal canal and subarachnoid space. Certain diseases show an especial predilection for the spinal roots, including idiopathic postinfectious polyneuropathy and diphtheria. Hereditary hypertrophic neuropathies are usually diffuse, but may occasionally centre upon the spinal roots and their enlargement may even cause spinal cord compression (Symonds and Blackwood 1962). These and other diseases which may involve the nerve roots as part of a diffuse polyneuropathy or perikaryal disease are considered in chapter 6 and chapter 8. It is interesting to speculate on why the roots are especially involved in some diseases. This may perhaps be due to the absence of the normal blood-nerve barrier in the nerve roots (Waksman 1961, Olsson 1966) allowing the easier access of toxins and antibodies to the roots.

This chapter will deal mainly with diseases of the nerve roots resulting from their anatomical site within the spinal canal. This topic has also been reviewed by the author elsewhere (Bradley 1974).

PATHOLOGICAL CONSIDERATIONS

The nerve root, like the peripheral nerve fibre in general, has a relatively limited repertoire of pathological reactions, though these can be evoked by a large number of stimuli. Minor forms of damage, whether compressive, ischaemic or toxic, may simply damage the Schwann cells producing segmental demyelination. This may block nerve conduction, with rapid recovery when the noxious agent is removed. More severe injury causes Wallerian degeneration and retrograde changes in the neuronal perikaryon.

Even if this does not lead to cell death, the distance for the axons to re-generate from the roots to the peripheral muscles is so long that permanent muscular denervation is common. Functional regeneration of the primary sensory neuron into the spinal cord does not occur. Thus if the damage to the nerve root is sufficiently severe to cause Wallerian degeneration, it is usually permanent.

DIAGNOSTIC FEATURES OF RADICULOPATHIES

As outlined on page 80, lesions of many different parts of the long cell which is the neuron may produce very similar symptoms and signs. Various clinical features may however help to indicate a lesion of the spinal nerve roots, while certain investigations may help to confirm this localization.

Clinical features

Lesions of the spinal nerve roots generally produce sensory loss and muscle weakness and wasting in a dermatomal and myotomal pattern. Compres-sion of a root will produce radicular or 'girdle' pain in the distribution of a dermatome. A unilateral lesion of the fifth and sixth cervical roots will pro-duce sensory loss on the outer aspect of the shoulder and upper arm, with weakness of the supraspinatus, infraspinatus, subscapularis, deltoid, biceps and brachioradialis muscles, as well as loss of the biceps and brachioradialis reflexes on that side. As can be seen from a study of tables 2.1 and 2.2 such a pattern can result only from a lesion of the nerve roots, and could not be due to damage to any one nerve or part of the brachial plexus.

However when the disease process is more diffuse as in arachnoiditis (see page 244), the radicular pattern may be much more difficult to discern. In these instances the clinical picture may imitate a diffuse polyneuropathy. A clue may be found in involvement of the trunk which is uncommon in the diffuse polyneuropathies described in chapter 6. Many of the diseases producing diffuse radiculopathies also damage the spinal cord. Therefore the finding of spinal cord and peripheral nerve abnormalities should sug-gest the possibility of a disease process within the spinal canal.

Investigations aiding in diagnosis of radiculopathies

Certain investigations may help to confirm the clinical suggestion of radi-cular damage. Lesions of the sensory roots do not usually affect the peripheral branch of the sensory axon. The sensory loss therefore occurs with preservation of the sensory nerve action potential (page 88) and axon flare in the insensitive area (see page 74). This preservation, however, simply indicates that the lesion causing sensory loss lies somewhere between the posterior root ganglion and the cerebral cortex, and is not diagnostic of a radicular lesion.

Electromyography of the spinalis muscles may be of help, for if they show signs of denervation this indicates a very proximal lesion. The damage may be in the anterior horn cell or the anterior root. Particularly where there are signs of spinal cord damage, neuroradiological investigations are required both to define the site of the lesion and sometimes to suggest its nature. Radiographs of the spine may show collapse, or the enlargement of the intervertebral foramen indicating a neuroma, and myelography may indicate the level and type of the disease in, for instance, arachnoiditis. Examination of the cerebrospinal fluid may aid in the diagnosis, for instance, by finding carcinoma cells or bacteria in chronic meningitides. Laminectomy may sometimes be required both for diagnosis and for treatment of the lesion.

DISEASES DAMAGING THE SPINAL NERVE ROOTS

Trauma

Acute intervertebral disc prolapse

The cervical and lumbar regions are the most prone to suffer intervertebral disc degeneration being the most mobile parts of the spine. The frequency of disc prolapse is highest in the lumbar region due to the greater forces there. All movements of the spine impose deformational changes on the intervertebral discs, and if excessive, or if degenerative changes are present in the disc, the annulus fibrosus may rupture allowing partial or total prolapse of the softer central nucleus pulposus into the spinal canal (Greenfield 1963a). This is more frequently lateral than central, and thus the spinal roots are more often compressed than the cord, and in the lumbar region sciatica is more usually unilateral.

Clinical

As a result of an excessive or sudden movement, the patient feels a sudden click and pain in the neck or lumbar region, and develops a sudden pain in a radicular distribution. The commonest disc prolapse in the cervical region is of the C5/6 interspace, and therefore pain is most frequently on the outside of the shoulder and arm. Movement exacerbates the pain. If the compression is mild, paraesthesiae and loss of tendon reflexes in the affected spinal segments may be the only result. If it is severe then sensory loss and muscle weakness in the appropriate segments occur. The commonest signs are of a C5–6 lesion (see page 254 above). There is often mild corticospinal tract damage at C5 with resultant hyper-reflexia below this level. This produces spread of activation to the C7/8 innervated finger flexors on percussion over the radial tubercle, the so-called 'inverted radial jerk'. Different clinical patterns appear when the prolapse is at different levels.

In the lumbar region the commonest prolapse is of the L5/S1 disc, producing low lumbar pain (lumbago) radiating down the back of one leg (sciatica). Major sensory and motor signs are relatively uncommon, but depression of the ankle jerk and a small area of impairment of pin-prick sensation under the lateral malleolus may often be found. Stretching the root over the disc prolapse during straight-leg raising causes pain. A high lumbar disc lesion (L2/3) causes pain radiating to the thigh and knee, and loss of the knee jerk. In this instance pain is elicited by lying the patient prone, and hyperextending the leg with the knee flexed (the femoral nerve stretch test). An L4/5 disc prolapse may produce pain in a sciatic distribution, and the only physical sign may be weakness of dorsiflexion of the big toe.

Investigations

The signs are often sufficient to define the level of the lesion, though plain radiography and myelography are occasionally required. The latter, however, is frequently normal despite a large lumbar disc prolapse. There may be signs of denervation on electromyography or loss of sensory nerve action potentials in the affected segments. Pain of a type indistinguishable from that due to a disc prolapse often occurs with no neurological signs. A lesion of the vertebral articular joints may perhaps be responsible in these cases.

Treatment

The pain may be so severe that opiates are required to control it. Various forms of deep heat therapy may bring symptomatic relief. Restriction of movements in a cervical collar or lumbar corset aids the resolution of the condition, probably by preventing continuing friction of the root over the disc prolapse, and perhaps by allowing gradual lengthening of the root to occur. Traction is useful for the severe case, probably providing effective immobilization. Where the pain and neurological signs are not relieved by conservative measures, surgical removal of the disc prolapse is required. If the motor and sensory roots are severely compressed, then the lesion is likely to be permanent, and recovery dependent upon sprouting from fibres of the adjacent motor and sensory segments.

Spinal nerve root avulsion

Injuries causing distraction of the head and shoulder may rupture the brachial plexus or avulse the spinal nerve roots from the cord, producing in both cases severe paralysis and sensory loss. Separation of these two conditions is important because the prognosis is different. As indicated above (pages 150–151) no recovery occurs with a severe radicular lesion such as avulsion, but some regeneration may occur with brachial plexus lesions, particularly if the anatomical disruption (neurotmesis, see page 150) is not extensive. Recovery is nevertheless delayed and often incomplete.

Separation of the two conditions may be achieved by the investigations described above (pages 254–255). However loss of the sensory nerve action potential and axon flare may not indicate the better prognosis of a brachial plexus lesion if there is also a root avulsion proximal to the brachial plexus lesion. The most direct indication of root avulsion is the myelographic demonstration of disrupted root sleeves through which the nerve roots have been torn (fig. 9.1.).

Compression

Intraspinal tumours

Any expanding lesion within the spinal canal will compress the nerve roots, and the spinal cord if present at that level. Due to condensation of the tracts within the spinal cord, compression of the latter usually produces a far more dramatic picture than the root compression.

Clinical

The pain of an intramedullary spinal cord tumour such as an astrocytoma or ependymoma may be due to root compression, but signs of damage to the

lower motor neuron and primary sensory neuron are probably due to intramedullary damage rather than to that of the roots. Intradural extramedul-
lary compression of the nerve roots may be due to a meningioma (Russell
and Rubinstein 1963) or a Schwannoma (neurofibroma) (see page 200). The

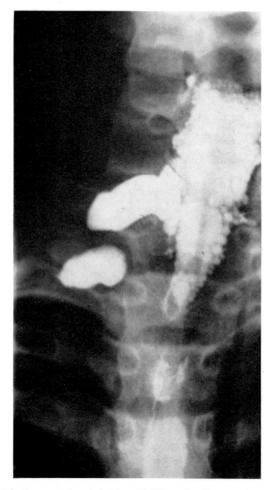

F IG. 9.1. Myelogram showing Myodil filling the disrupted root sleeves at
the C7 and C8 levels of a patient who suffered nerve root avulsion.

latter generally causes compression of only one nerve root. In von
Recklinghausen's disease (generalized neurofibromatosis), multiple neurofibromata may occur with consequently complex physical signs. Meningiomata are commonest in the thoracic region and in middle aged women, and

may compress more than one nerve root. Lipomata and dermoid cysts are associated with spina bifida occulta, and are considered below (page 262). Extradural compression due to carcinoma is usually focal, and radicular signs and symptoms are mild. The local pain is due to bone involvement. Extradural reticuloses produce more extensive damage to nerve roots and the mixed spinal nerves as they run through the extradural space.

The anatomical arrangements of the cauda equina make this a region for special consideration. In addition to pain and sensory and motor loss in the sacral segments, sphincter impairment is an early symptom. The loss of the anal and bulbocavernosus reflexes, as well as loss of knee and ankle jerks are useful diagnostic signs. The commonest intradural lesion responsible is an ependymoma of the filum terminale or conus medullaris. Intraspinal lipomata or dermoid cysts may be associated with dysraphism (see page 262). An implantation dermoid is a rare complication of a previous lumbar puncture carried out without a stylette. Extradural compression of the cauda equina may be due to intervertebral disc degeneration, carcinoma or chordoma in that order of frequency.

Treatment

Surgical decompression with the removal of the compressive lesion should be undertaken wherever possible, and is often required to make the exact diagnosis, and to suggest the use of radiotherapy.

Chronic intervertebral disc degeneration (spondylosis)

Continual bending and twisting of the intervertebral disc may produce gradual splaying of the fibrocartilaginous disc, which may bulge into the spinal canal and intervertebral foramina. Secondary calcification of the junction of this bulge with the vertebrae produces a bony osteophyte on each side of the disc. The consequent narrowing of the intervertebral disc space shortens the spinal canal, thereby tending to produce thickening of the spinal cord and roots and forward bulging of the ligamenta flava, at the same time as the canal and intervertebral foramen are being narrowed by osteophytes and chronic disc protrusion (Breig 1960, Breig and El-Nadi 1966, Hughes 1966, Waltz 1967). The effect of this on the spinal cord has already been mentioned (page 244). Individuals with a congenitally narrow spinal canal, including those with achondroplasia, are particularly liable to suffer neurological damage from disc degeneration (Pallis *et al* 1954, Duvoisin and Yahr 1962).

Clinical

The degenerative changes of cervical spondylosis compress the spinal roots and nerves predominantly in the intervertebral foramina rather than within the spinal canal. As in other radicular compressions, and many nerve entrapments elsewhere in the body, pain is one of the most prominent features (British Association of Physical Medicine 1966). This may occur spontaneously, or develop after a minor neck injury, often of whiplash type. The pain is radicular in distribution, and since disc degeneration is most commonly at C4/5 and C5/6, the shoulder and arm are the commonest sites for referral of pain.

Sensory symptoms may include a subjective numbness and paraesthesiae, though rarely does clinical testing reveal gross sensory loss. Motor weakness and wasting may occur in severely affected cases, and loss of tendon reflexes is frequent.

One clinical syndrome which most commonly results from lumbar spondylosis combined with a congenital narrowing of the lumbar canal is intermittent ischaemia of the cauda equina. There is usually disc degeneration with osteophyte formation, and marked sclerosis and hypertrophy of the lumbar laminae posteriorly (Verbiest 1955, Joffe *et al.* 1966). The symptoms are similar to intermittent claudication of the calves with pain in the legs on exertion, relieved by rest, but the peripheral pulses are normal. Two features aid in the recognition of this syndrome, first the development of neurological symptoms and signs at the time of the pain, often with loss of reflexes and power. Secondly the interval between cessation of exertion and relief of the pain is important. In intermittent claudication of the calves, relief occurs within a minute of cessation of exercise, but in intermittent ischaemia of the cauda equina up to 5 or 10 minutes may be required. This syndrome may arise from other causes of compression of the cauda equina, including tumours like ependymomatas, and also from ischaemia of the roots due to peripheral vascular disease.

Investigations

Plain spinal x-rays will reveal disc degeneration. On the lateral radiographs osteophytes can be seen encroaching posteriorly into the spinal canal, and on the oblique radiographs in the cervical region they can be seen in the

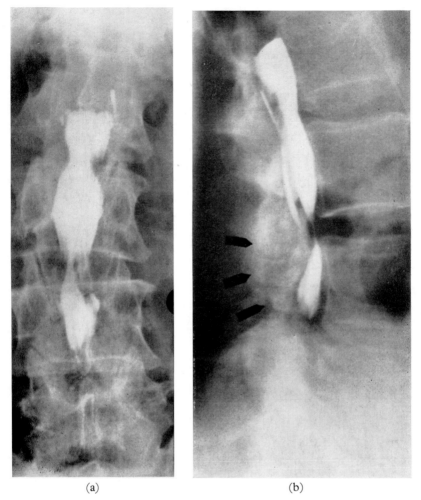

FIG. 9.2. Myelogram in a patient with lumbar canal stenosis showing the typical hour-glass deformity, and markedly sclerotic laminae compressing the theca from behind (*arrows*). *a* PA radiograph. *b* Lateral radiograph. (Kindly provided by Dr Arnold Appleby.)

intervertebral foramina. These changes are so frequently present over the age of fifty that it is important to remember that they may be coincidental, some other process being responsible for the syndrome. Myelography will aid by excluding a compression tumour, and showing typical disc degeneration. In lumbar canal stenosis the typical myelographic picture is of an hour-glass deformity (fig. 9.2).

Treatment

Clinical symptoms of both lumbar and cervical spondylotic radiculopathy quite frequently show a relapsing and remitting course making assessment of the efficacy of treatment difficult (Lees and Turner 1963). Restriction of movements by a collar or corset often helps, as does heat therapy (British Association of Physical Medicine 1966). Continuous traction for a week or ten days may sometimes be of use, probably by maintaining immobility. Occasionally surgical decompression is required for unremitting pain or neurological signs, particularly in the syndrome of intermittent ischaemia of the cauda equina.

Other causes of spinal root compression

Perineurial cysts may compress the first part of the mixed spinal nerve (Tarlov 1970). Occurring mainly in the sacral region, these cysts arise as focal outpouchings of the dural root sleeve (not of the perineurium), the nerve comprising part of the wall. Their lumen is in partial but not free communication with the subarachnoid space and thus they tend not to fill initially during myelography, but may do so after 24 hours. Patients usually present with symptoms and signs indistinguishable from the radiculopathy of a chronic disc protrusion. Excision of the dome of the cyst, perhaps with section of the root, is the recommended treatment.

A spinal extradural or subdural abscess, usually due to *Staphylococcus aureus*, presents with local spinal and radicular pain, exquisite local tenderness, toxaemia and fever (Hirson 1965). The spinal cord is frequently severely compressed, and surgical decompression and antibiotic therapy are urgently required. Chou and Fakadej (1971) noted a peculiar abnormality of the anterior roots in two patients with infantile spinal muscular atrophy (Werdnig-Hoffmann disease), consisting of large masses of glial processes full of glial fibrils (see page 242). This produced an appearance of hypertrophy of the nerve roots. They suggested that the aberrant glial tissue compressed the motor axons in the anterior roots, causing denervation and also retrograde neuronal death.

Dysraphism

Defects of closure of the neural tube during fetal development may result in a number of conditions damaging the cauda equina. In spina bifida occulta no major external abnormality is visible, there being simply a gap between the laminae (James and Lassman 1972). Occasionally a small dimple or tag of hair over the lumbosacral region may be a clue. Dermoid cysts, lipomata and meningeal diverticulae may be associated with spina bifida occulta, and by expansion compress the cauda equina. In the more gross spina bifida cystica seen in the newborn, total cauda equina damage or agenesis is not uncommon.

Toxic radiculopathies

The nerve roots are affected by many of the conditions which damage the peripheral nervous system in general. They are also specifically damaged by toxins injected into the subarachnoid space, either by accident or by design. The use of intrathecal alcohol to destroy the roots to relieve intractable pain due to carcinomatous infiltration of the pelvic plexus was introduced by Dogliotti (1931). Phenol was later used for the same purpose and for the relief of flexor spasms (Nathan 1959). Though it was originally suggested that the non-myelinated and small myelinated pain-carrying fibres were specifically damaged by phenol, it is now clear that fibres of all diameters are equally affected (Schaumberg et al. 1970). Phenol and alcohol damage both the axons and the Schwann cells of the nerve fibres with consequent Wallerian degeneration.

Other substances accidentally allowed to contaminate the cerebrospinal fluid may also damage the roots and spinal cord. Outbreaks of radiculopathy and arachnoiditis have resulted from contamination of spinal anaesthetics with detergents or preservatives (Winkleman et al. 1953, Hurst 1955). Occasionally disastrous reactions arise from the administration of the incorrect dose of antibiotics intrathecally. Contrast media used in the past for myelography may sometimes damage the nerve roots. Thorium dioxide was used for some time, but was taken up by macrophages and remained in the subarachnoid space indefinitely. The radioactive emissions of the thorium have been responsible for a number of cases of chronic radiculomyelopathy (Dale and Love 1967). Lipiodol which was introduced later also produced a number of acute irritative reactions, sometimes followed by permanent damage. Myodil, which is in current use, occasionally produces radicular pain for a few days, though serious long-term effects are extremely rare.

Chronic meningitis and arachnoiditis

The nerve roots are prey not only to toxic damage as described above, but also to any infective, inflammatory or neoplastic process affecting the cerebrospinal fluid.

Chronic infective meningitis

Any chronic meningitis such as that due to *Mycobacterium tuberculi* or to *Cryptococcus neoformans*, may damage the nerve roots by a process of inflammation, endarteritis and infarction. An inadequately treated or unusually indolent acute meningitis, particularly that due to the pneumococcus, may cause a similar process.

Syphilis

Syphilis may damage the nerve roots in three main ways. The commonest form, meningovascular syphilis, produces a chronic diffuse inflammatory meningitis with endarteritis and thrombosis of the small arteries. The spinal cord is particularly involved, the radiculopathy often being indicated only by areflexia. Tabes dorsalis (locomotor ataxia) is the clinical syndrome resulting from loss of joint position and deep pain sensation. Superficial pain and temperature sensation over most of the body is preserved, though classically there is either loss or profoundly delayed perception of superficial pain over the bridge of the nose, the front of the chest, the inside of the arms, the outside of the legs and the perianal area. Though posterior column degeneration in the spinal cord is most striking, and gave rise to the name of the syndrome, it is unlikely that this is primary, since degeneration of the posterior roots is often found. The site of the lesion affecting the large nerve fibres carrying joint position sense has given rise to much dispute (Greenfield 1963b, Hughes 1966). Obersteiner and Redlich (1894–95) believed the site of damage to be the root entry zone, whilst Nageotte (1903) believed that it lay in the posterior root itself. Both theories have difficulty in explaining why mainly the larger fibres are damaged, and a lesion of the larger posterior root ganglion neurons might be more attractive. However only minor changes are found in the ganglia, while significant inflammation and degeneration of the posterior root make this the most likely site of damage. Large gummata of the meninges, which are rare, compress the nerve roots as any other space occupying lesion, and also produce ischaemia due to endarteritis.

Uveomeningitic syndromes

Sarcoidosis

Sarcoidosis is the commonest disease in this category (Colover 1948, Matthews 1965). Uveitis, damage to the facial nerve in the parotid gland, a diffuse polyneuropathy and hypothalamic damage are the most frequent neurological complications of this disease. A few patients develop symptoms from granulomata in the meninges. A diffuse radiculopathy is difficult to separate from a polyneuropathy. Most such patients have one or more peripheral manifestations of sarcoidosis such as lung, skin or bone changes, lymphadenopathy or hypercalcaemia. Rarely a patient may be encountered with no systemic evidence of sarcoidosis, who pathologically has the typical sarcoid granulomata in the meninges. These should be accepted as cases of true sarcoidosis, until such time as they are shown to have a cause or a clinical course different from that of disseminated sarcoidosis.

Behçet's disease

Behçet's disease is another condition in this group (Wolf et al. 1964). The diagnostic features are recurrent attacks of uveitis with oral and genital ulceration and frequently thrombophlebitis. In a few cases viruses have been isolated from such patients. The nervous system may be involved, predominantly with a relapsing encephalomyelitis, though occasionally a radiculopathy or neuropathy are associated (O'Duffy et al. 1971, Lobo-Antunes 1972). The uveoencephalomeningitic syndromes (Vogt-Koyanagi-Harada) should also be considered (Riehl and Andrews 1966). These have uveitis, meningoencephalitis, and poliosis (tufts of white hair) as their features. The nerve roots may be damaged by the chronic meningitis.

Neoplastic radiculopathy

Primary tumours of the central nervous system such as medulloblastoma, and secondary carcinoma, particularly from the bronchus, breast and gastrointestinal tract, may become disseminated throughout the subarachnoid pathways, producing compression and damage of the nerve roots. Myelography may show multiple rounded filling defects on the roots or granular irregularities, neoplastic cells may be found in the cerebrospinal fluid, and the cerebrospinal fluid sugar may be low. However, often the carcinoma cells form a tight sheet around the affected roots, without free cells in the cerebrospinal fluid. Though most patients with this condition die fairly quickly, in a few the progress is slow and painful, and the diagnosis extremely difficult without surgical exploration and biopsy.

With a radiosensitive neoplasm like a medulloblastoma, neuraxis radiotherapy can be remarkably effective, but with carcinomatous meningitis this is much less effective. Systemic cytotoxic agents may also be effective in a few cases. Intrathecal cytotoxic agents may be tried, though many are hazardous by this route.

Radiculopathy due to endogenous toxins

A dermoid cyst may leak into the subarachnoid space either spontaneously or postoperatively, to produce a severe granulomatous, inflammatory reaction (Cantu and Wright 1968). Cholesterol crystals are probably the agent responsible. Corticosteroids may have a dramatic benefit in the acute phase (Cantu and Ojeman 1968). The clinical signs and symptoms are indistinguishable from an acute or chronic meningitis, though the diagnosis can be made by the recognition of cholesterol crystals and squames in the cerebrospinal fluid. Occasionally the picture is more indolent with progressive encephalopathy and deafness, cranial nerve signs and areflexia indicating radicular damage (Tomlinson and Walton 1967).

The leakage of blood into the cerebrospinal fluid produces a similar picture. Acute subarachnoid harmorrhage almost invariably produces signs of meningeal irritation. Chronic subarachnoid leakage of blood may produce the syndrome of superficial haemosiderosis of the central nervous system (Tomlinson and Walton 1964), where the deposition of iron pigment in the meninges and subjacent nervous tissue damages the brain, cranial nerves and nerve roots. This may occur with repeated small haemorrhages from an arteriovenous malformation, an aneurysm, or a vascular tumour such as an ependymoma or choroid plexus papilloma. Haemosiderin-laden macrophages in the cerebrospinal fluid will confirm the diagnosis.

Chronic idiopathic adhesive arachnoiditis

All of the conditions described above which damage the nerve roots lead to fibrosis and thickening of the adjacent arachnoid. Diffuse thickening of the arachnoid, forming adhesions within the subarachnoid space, occurs in a few patients in whom no cause for the condition can be found. The term chronic idiopathic adhesive arachnoiditis is given to this group. Full investigations, including biopsy are indicated since occasionally a treatable cause may be found (Davidson 1968). Spinal cord involvement often dominates the picture, but a radiculopathy may also occur.

Radiation radiculopathy

The peripheral nerves including the roots are more resistant to radiation damage than the central nervous system (Kristensson *et al.* 1967). Thus a radiation myelopathy is the usual result of excessive irradiation of the spinal canal. The cauda equina may be damaged by radiotherapy for pelvic lesions, or a cauda equina tumour like an ependymoma, the clinical and pathological picture being essentially the same as described on page 198. It may be difficult to decide whether deterioration in a patient who has had previous radiotherapy for a cauda equina tumour is due to extension of the tumour or to a radiation radiculopathy.

REFERENCES

BRADLEY W. G. (1974) Diseases of spinal roots. In *Peripheral Neuropathy*, ed. Dyck P. J., Thomas P. K. and Lambert E. H. Saunders, Philadelphia, in press.

BREIG A. (1960) *Biomechanics of the Central Nervous System. Some basic normal and pathologic phenomena.* Almquist and Wiksell, Stockholm.

BREIG A. and EL-NADI A. F. (1966) Biomechanics of the cervical spine cord. *Acta. Radiol. Scand. Diagnosis* **4**, 602–624.

BRITISH ASSOCIATION OF PHYSICAL MEDICINE (1966) Pain in the neck and arm: a multicentre trial of the effects of physiotherapy. *Brit. med. J.* **1**, 253–258.

CANTU R. C. and OJEMAN R. D. (1968) Glucosteroid treatment of keratin meningitis following the removal of a fourth ventricle epidermoid tumour. *J. Neurol. Neurosurg. Psychiat.* **31**, 73–75.

CANTU R. C. and WRIGHT R. L. (1968) Aseptic meningitis syndrome with cauda equina epidermoid tumour. *J. Ped.* **73**, 113–116.

CHOU S. M. and FAKADEJ A. V. (1971) Ultrastructure of chromatolytic motoneurons and anterior spinal roots in a case of Werdnig-Hoffmann disease. *J. Neuropath. exp. Neurol.* **30**, 368–379.

COLOVER J. (1948) Sarcoidosis with involvement of the nervous system. *Brain* **71**, 451–475.

DALE A. J. D. and LOVE J. C. (1967) Thorium dioxide myelopathy. *J. Amer. med. Ass.* **199**, 606–609.

DAVIDSON S. (1968) Cryptococcal spinal arachnoiditis. *J. Neurol. Neurosurg. Psychiat.* **31**, 76–80.

DOGLIOTTI A. M. (1931) Traitment des syndromes douloureux de la périphérie par l'alcoholisation sub-arachnoidienne des racines posterieres à leur emergence de la moelle épinière. *Press. méd.*, 1249–1252.

DUVOISIN R. C. and YAHR M. D. (1962) Compressive spinal cord and root syndromes in achondroplastic dwarfs. *Neurol. (Minneap.)* **12**, 202–207.

GREENFIELD J.G. (1963a) Lesions of the nervous system associated with diseases or malformations of the cranium and spinal column. In *Greenfield's Neuropathology*, ed. Blackwood W., McMenemey W.H., Meyer A., Norman R.M. and Russell D.S., pp. 650–665. Arnold, London.

GREENFIELD J.G. (1963b) Infectious diseases of the central nervous system. In *Greenfield's Neuropathology*, ed. Blackwood W., McMenemey W.H., Meyer A., Norman R.M. and Russell D.S., pp. 138–234. Arnold, London.

HIRSON C. (1965) Spinal subdural abscess. *Lancet* **2**, 1215–1217.

HUGHES J.T. (1966) *Pathology of the Spinal Cord*. Lloyd-Duke, London.

HURST E.W. (1955) Adhesive arachnoiditis and vascular blockage caused by detergents and other chemical irritants: experimental study. *J. Path. Bact.* **70**, 167–178.

JAMES C.C.M. and LASSMAN L.P. (1972) *Spina. Dysraphism: spina bifida occulta*. Butterworth, London.

JOFFE R., APPLEBY A. and ARJONA V. (1966) 'Intermittent ischaemia' of the cauda equina due to stenosis of the lumbar canal. *J. Neurol. Neurosurg. Psychiat.* **29**, 315–318.

KRISTENSSON K., MOLIN B. and SOURANDER P. (1967) Delayed radiation lesions of human spinal cord. Report of five cases. *Acta neuropath.* **9**, 34–44.

LEES F. and ALDREN TURNER J.W. (1963) Natural history and prognosis of cervical spondylosis. *Brit. med. J.* **4**, 1607–1610.

LOBO-ANTUNES J. (1972) Behçet's disease. *Ann. Int. Med.* **76**, 332–333.

MATTHEWS W.B. (1965) Sarcoidosis of the nervous system. *J. Neurol. Neurosurg. Psychiat.* **28**, 23–29.

NAGEOTTE J. (1903) *Pathogenie du Tabes Dorsal*. Naud, Paris.

NATHAN P.W. (1959) Intrathecal phenol to relieve spasticity in paraplegia. *Lancet* **2**, 1099–1012.

OBERSTEINER H. and REDLICH E. (1894–1895) Quoted by Greenfield J.G. (1963b).

O'DUFFY J.D., CARNEY J.A. and DEODHAR S. (1971) Behçet's disease. Report of ten cases, three with new manifestations. *Ann. Int. Med.* **75**, 561–570.

OLSSON Y. (1966) Studies on vascular permeability in peripheral nerves. I: Distribution of circulating fluorescent serum albumin in normal, crushed and sectioned peripheral nerve. *Acta neuropath. (Berl.)* **7**, 1–15.

PALLIS C., JONES A.M. and SPILLANE J.D. (1954) Cervical spondylosis. Incidence and implications. *Brain* **77**, 274–289.

RIEHL J.-L. and ANDREWS J.M. (1966) The uveomeningoencephalitic syndrome. *Neurol. (Minneap.)* **16**, 603–609.

RUSSELL D.S. and RUBINSTEIN L.J. (1963) *Pathology of Tumours of the Nervous System*. 2nd edn. Arnold, London.

SCHAUMBERG H.H., BYCK R. and WELLER R.O. (1970) The effect of phenol on peripheral nerve. A histological and electrophysiological study. *J. Neuropath. exp. Neurol.* **29**, 615–630.

SYMONDS C.P. and BLACKWOOD W. (1962) Spinal cord compression in hypertrophic neuritis. *Brain* **85**, 251–260.

TARLOV I.M. (1970) Spinal perineurial and meningeal cysts. *J. Neurol. Neurosurg. Psychiat.* **33**, 833–843.

TOMLINSON B. E. and WALTON J. N. (1964) Superficial haemosiderosis of the central nervous system. *J. Neurol. Neurosurg. Psychiat.* **27**, 332–339.

TOMLINSON B. E. and WALTON J. N. (1967) Granulomatous meningitis and diffuse parenchymatous degeneration of the nervous system due to an intracranial epidermoid cyst. *J. Neurol. Neurosurg. Psychiat.* **30**, 341–348.

VERIBIEST H. (1955) Further experience on the pathological influence of developmental narrowness of the bony lumbar vertebral canal. *J. Bone Jt. Surg.* **37**B, 576–583.

WAKSMAN B. H. (1961) Experimental study of diphtheritic polyneuritis in the rabbit and guinea pig. III. The blood-nerve barrier in the rabbit. *J. Neuropath. exp. Neurol.* **20**, 35–77.

WALTZ T. A. (1967) Physical factors in the production of the myelopathy of cervical spondylosis. *Brain* **90**, 395–404.

WINKELMAN N. W., GOTTEN N. and SCHEIBERT D. (1953) Localized adhesive spinal arachnoiditis. A study of 25 cases with reference of aetiology. *Trans. Amer. Neurol. Ass.* (78th), 15–17.

WOLF S. M., SCHOTLAND D. L. and PHILLIPS L. L. (1965) Involvement of the nervous system in Behçet's syndrome. *Arch. Neurol.* (Chic.) **12**, 315–325.

10

Disorders of Neuromuscular Transmission and Skeletal Muscle

A patient with a pure motor weakness may suffer from corticospinal tract or anterior horn cell disease, from a pure motor neuropathy, from a defect of neuromuscular transmission, or from a primary muscle disease. The separation of upper motor neuron weakness from the remainder is discussed in chapter 3. Diseases of the anterior horn cell are considered in chapter 8. Pure motor neuropathies have been mentioned elsewhere (page 81 and chapters 6 and 8), and will also be considered below. Disorders of the neuromuscular junction and skeletal muscle are grouped together in this chapter for convenience. An outline of each condition is given in the following sections to provide a basis for the separation of these conditions from those mainly considered in this book, namely diseases of the peripheral nerve. This separation, which depends both on the clinical picture and results of investigations, is of great importance because each condition potentially has its own special treatment. For a more detailed consideration reviews by Cambier (1968) and Walton (1974) should be consulted.

DISORDERS OF NEUROMUSCULAR TRANSMISSION

Myasthenia gravis

This condition affects females twice as frequently as males, and the peak incidence of both sexes is about 20 years. The condition usually begins insidiously with weakness predominantly affecting the extraocular muscles, muscles of the face, neck and mastication, and proximal muscles of the upper and lower limbs. These muscles are involved in about 90 per cent of patients at some time in the course of the disease. The patient therefore complains of drooping of the eyelids and double vision, difficulty in chewing and holding the mouth shut, and of weakness of the neck. She also has difficulty in lifting her arms and climbing stairs. The characteristic feature is the marked fatiguability. She may be relatively strong first thing in the morning but becomes increasingly weak as the day wears on. Repetitive actions may also be used to demonstrate this fatiguability. The patient is asked to look up or bite repeatedly, and will become increasingly weak in the performance of this task, which a few minutes earlier was performed without difficulty.

Apart from the weakness and fatiguability, clinical examination is rarely abnormal. Mild muscular atrophy may occur, but sensation and the tendon reflexes are normal. If the diagnosis is suspected, electrophysiological and pharmacological tests described on page 98 *et seq.* should be undertaken. The finding of electrophysiological evidence of a marked decremental response to repetitive nerve stimulation at 5–20 stimuli per second, and correction of the weakness of the fatigued muscle and the electrical decrement by edrophonium are the most widely used tests to diagnose myasthenia gravis. Pathological studies of muscle are seldom helpful. A few collections of lymphocytes ('lymphorrhages') and a variety of changes in the morphology of the terminal ramifications of the nerves in the motor end plates may be seen, but are not diagnostic (Santa *et al.* 1972).

The aetiology of the disease is still not fully understood ('*Myasthenia gravis*', 1966). Abnormalities of the thymus are found in about 80 per cent of patients with myasthenia gravis. In most this is thymic hyperplasia with numerous germinal centres indicating active lymphoid proliferation. In about 15 per cent, particularly in males, there is a thymoma which may be malignant. The relationship of the thymic abnormalities to myasthenia gravis is undoubted, and in particular in young women and those in whom the condition has been present for less than 5 years, thymectomy often produces a dramatic relief of symptoms (Simpson 1958). Removal of a thymoma is usually indicated on the grounds of potential malignancy alone, though improvement in the myasthenia is less common after thymectomy in those with thymomata.

The serum of a high proportion of myasthenics contains 7S γ-globulin antibodies to the A bands of skeletal muscle (Strauss *et al.* 1960) as well as γ-globulin antibodies binding to neuronal nuclei (Kornguth *et al.* 1970). Myasthenia gravis is frequently associated with a whole group of autoimmune diseases and in particular with systemic lupus erythematosus, thyroid disease particularly thyrotoxicosis, and rheumatoid arthritis. It seems likely that the thymus produces lymphocytes which are responsible for the abnormal antibodies and the production of the electrophysiological defect in myasthenia gravis. The role of the myoid cells which are present in the thymus, and have a structure very similar to striated muscle, is uncertain.

The physiological studies of myasthenia gravis have been interpreted as suggesting the presence of a circulating agent which competes with acetylcholine at the motor end plates (Simpson 1969). The occurrence of myasthenia gravis lasting for the first 1–12 weeks of life in about 12 per cent of babies born to myasthenic mothers supports this suggestion. Electrophysiological studies of human intercostal muscle biopsies suggest a deficiency of the amount of acetylcholine in each quantum or a decreased responsiveness of the post-synaptic membrane (Elmqvist et al. 1964). Desmedt (1966) has argued strongly for the hypothesis that the disease process is a preterminal failure of acetylcholine synthesis similar to that induced by hemicholinium. The antineuronal antibodies may perhaps be the mechanism of damage to the neuron.

The treatment of myasthenia gravis rests firstly upon anticholinesterase drugs such as neostigmine and pyridostigmine, which increase the concentration and effect of released acetylcholine by inhibiting the acetylcholinesterase of motor end plates. Atropine is usually required to block the muscarinic effects upon the viscera. The control of anticholinesterase therapy is difficult, and excess may cause cholinergic block. Moreover different muscles require different amounts of acetylclolinesterase for maximum potentiation. Ephedrine, potassium and spironolactone may sometimes act as adjuvants. If this treatment fails to produce an almost complete control of symptoms, particularly in women in the early years of their disease, thymectomy is indicated. In many patients, despite thymectomy, the disease produces a parlous state requiring artificial respiration and tracheostomy. Treatment with intermittent courses of adrenocorticotrophin (Namba et al. 1971), or prednisone in high dosage (Jenkins 1972) in an intensive therapy unit may produce deterioration for a short period, followed by a relative or absolute remission for a further period. Long-term immunosuppression has been advocated by some (Mertens et al. 1969).

This is a disease with a fickle natural history, occasional patients being on an artificial respirator for years and then spontaneously remitting, only later to return to the respirator. It leads to a very great deal of morbidity because of unrelieved muscle weakness, and the death rate is considerable from weakness of the muscles of respiration and swallowing.

The myasthenic syndrome

This is a rare condition first described by Eaton and Lambert (1957). The patient complains of progressive weakness, mainly of the proximal muscles of the upper and lower limbs, and may complain of increasing fatiguability which is why the term 'the myasthenic syndrome' was applied. However, some patients notice the diagnostic feature, which may be brought out on clinical examination, namely that repeated maximum efforts induce a marked *facilitation* in the strength of contraction. The tendon reflexes in these patients are usually very depressed, but there are rarely other signs of abnormality of the neuromuscular system. Unlike myasthenia gravis, the extraocular, facial and masticatory muscles are rarely involved. Electrophysiological tests of weak muscles show a very reduced amplitude of the evoked motor action potential on nerve stimulation with single shocks, and this may show a myasthenic type of decrement with slow repetitive stimulation at 1–5/s. A rapidly *incremental* response to tetanic rates of stimulation of about 30/s is the diagnostic feature, however (see pages 98–99). In strong muscles with a normal amplitude of evoked motor action potential, a decrement may be seen with slow rates of stimulation. The patients report, and the electrophysiological tests confirm, little effect of anticholinesterase drugs upon neuromuscular transmission. However calcium or guanidine, both of which increase the number of quanta of acetylcholine released by each nerve impulse, abolish the electrophysiological changes and relieve the patient's symptoms (McQuillen and Johns 1967). The defect in the myasthenic syndrome is thus believed to be a deficiency in the release of acetylcholine quanta at the motor end plates.

Most patients have this syndrome in relation to an underlying carcinoma. This is often detected at the time of presentation, or may appear within 2 years. Carcinoma of the bronchus is the most common type responsible. Instances have been reported of patients without an underlying carcinoma, but are so uncommon that a full search for a neoplasm is indicated in any patient with this syndrome. Removal of the cancer may cure the syndrome.

Other causes of neuromuscular blockade

Aside from the drugs which cause neuromuscular blockade and are used in anaesthesia, a few other agents may also cause deficient neuromuscular conduction. Very high plasma levels of antibiotics of the streptomycin-kanamycin-colistin group may block neuromuscular function (McQuillen *et al.* 1968). Botulism probably prevents the release of acetylcholine from the nerve terminals; recovery requires the growth of new nerve terminals (Duchen 1971). Hypercalcaemia may impair the release of acetylcholine.

DISEASES OF SKELETAL MUSCLE

Like the list of causes of peripheral neuropathy, the list of diseases of skeletal muscle is extremely long. This section is intended only to point out the major diagnostic features of the most important of the muscle diseases. For a fuller consideration, reference should be made to Walton (1974).

Primary muscular dystrophies

The muscular dystrophies are a group of inherited diseases of skeletal muscle. The grouping has a historic basis, and is thus somewhat arbitrary. A number of other diseases of muscle, which are also inherited, have been recognized since the grouping was defined, and are not usually included in this classification. The classification, however, has certain advantages. Early in the diseases there is often specific involvement of certain muscle groups, sparing others until later; the diseases are progressive, and to a greater or lesser extent the muscle is damaged by a process of focal fibre necrosis, phagocytosis and regeneration. It is becoming recognized that specific muscle involvement can occur in cases of spinal muscular atrophy, whose clinical appearance may be indistinguishable from one of the primary muscular dystrophies. Also acute fibre necrosis is not specific for these diseases. Nevertheless this is still the best form of classification for clinical purposes at present.

X-linked muscular dystrophies

The most frequent type of muscular dystrophy encountered is the *pseudo-hypertrophic progressive muscular dystrophy of Duchenne*, manifesting in boys and carried by asymptomatic mothers. From the first weeks of life there is a very high serum creatine kinase activity, and muscle degeneration and regeneration is prominent from the age of a year. At about the age of 2–3 years, it leads to progressive weakness and wasting of the proximal muscles, particularly of the lower limbs with lumbar hyperlordosis, a waddling gait, and atrophy of the quadriceps and hamstring muscles. The biceps, brachioradialis, serrati and pectoral muscles are also involved early in the disease. The calf muscles are often abnormally large, but of normal power (pseudohypertrophy). The condition progresses until the child becomes unable to walk at around the age of 9–12 years, and death often occurs from a cardiomyopathy or respiratory complications at the age of 15 or 20 years. A more benign X-linked form (the *Becker type*) produces a similar pattern of muscle involvement but symptoms begin in the teens and the progression is much slower.

Autosomal recessive limb-girdle muscular dystrophy

Patients with muscular weakness and wasting of specific muscles of the shoulder and pelvic girdles and proximal parts of the limbs, beginning in early adult life and progressing to confinement in a wheelchair in 10–15 years, are often grouped together as suffering from *limb-girdle muscular dystrophy*. In some, the family history is suggestive of an autosomal recessive mode of inheritance. Supraspinati, serrati, pectorals, flexors, extensors and abductors of the hips, and the quadriceps muscles are especially involved. It is now recognized that this is not a homogeneous group. Many suffer from a form of spinal muscular atrophy, and other primary muscle diseases may also be found in this group. Many, however, have a primary progressive myopathy, and still can be called limb-girdle muscular dystrophy.

Facioscapulohumeral muscular dystrophy

The third most common form of muscular dystrophy is that involving especially the muscles of the face, those around the scapulae, particularly the serrati, supra- and infra-spinati, trapezii and rhomboids, and the biceps, brachioradialis and triceps muscles. Early involvement of the anterior tibial group of muscles is usually seen. The onset of symptoms is frequently in early middle life, though it can be most variable. Most patients have a family history indicating a dominant inheritance. This clinical group of patients is again mixed, with some cases of spinal muscular atrophy, and also other primary muscle diseases contained within it. Many however are still considered to have a muscular dystrophy.

Oculopharyngeal muscular dystrophy

This is a rare type of muscular dystrophy involving the extraocular muscles, spreading progressively to the facial and bulbar musculature. Often there is a dominant form of inheritance, and muscle fibres usually show the changes of an accumulation of abnormal mitochondria (*mitochondrial myopathy*). The onset is usually in the third or fourth decade, and the condition progresses very slowly. It may be difficult in the early stages of the disease to separate oculopharyngeal muscular dystrophy from ocular myopathy, some cases of which are probably due to neuronal atrophy. The latter, however, usually begin earlier in life, and does not produce dysphagia.

Distal muscular dystrophy

Rare cases have been reported of patients with mainly distal progressive muscle weakness and wasting, where electrophysiological and pathological studies of the muscle indicate a primary myopathy. This clinical pattern is of course very like that of a chronic peripheral neuropathy or spinal muscular atrophy. In view of the well-known development of secondary myopathic changes in chronically denervated muscle, the existence of this disease can only be accepted after a full autopsy study.

Disorders associated with myotonia

The commonest of this group, *dystrophia myotonica*, would perhaps better be classified with the muscular dystrophies since muscle degeneration is an important part of the disease. However myotonia is a feature, and the condition is generally included with the non-progressive conditions, *myotonia congenita* and *paramyotonia congenita*. Myotonia is seen clinically as difficulty in relaxing a muscle immediately after maximum contraction, and may be demonstrated by prolonged contraction after percussion (percussion myotonia). Microelectrode studies demonstrate a progressive decrement of the resting membrane potential of muscle fibres producing an action potential, recovery from which restores the resting membrane potential to normal, but is followed by a further decrement to produce a further action potential. Myotonia is recognized in electromyography by sustained trains of muscle fibre action potentials of high frequency, usually waxing and waning and heard as a 'dive-bomber' sound on the loud-speaker.

Dystrophia myotonica

This disease is inherited as an autosomal dominant with variable degrees of expressivity. Patients carrying the gene may never have symptoms, or may have only the peculiar characteristic cataracts in the senium. On the other hand, they may have symptoms of muscle weakness and myotonia beginning in adult life, or may present as floppy babies. No cause of these differences has yet been identified. The signs of the condition are ptosis, and weakness and wasting of the facial, masseter, temporalis and sternomastoid muscles. These signs are often present long before the patient presents with symptoms which are usually related to the onset of proximal muscle weakness. The disease affects many systems, producing progressive dementia, cardiomyopathy, gonadal atrophy and frontal baldness. Electromyography shows both myotonic high-frequency discharges and myopathic changes. Muscle biopsy shows both focal necrotizing change, and bizarre sarcolemmal masses and circumferentially orientated myofibrils (*ringbinden*).

Myotonia congenita

Inherited by an autosomal dominant mode, this condition (Thomsen's disease) has pure and often severe myotonia of all the skeletal muscles of the body, but no progressive muscle weakness. Patients often have bulky muscles, and are bothered by difficulty in relaxing these muscles after forced effort. A recessively inherited form of myotonia congenita (Becker) is also recognized, in which the onset is often delayed until after the first decade, and a progressive mild myopathy may develop.

Paramyotonia congenita

This condition is a bridge between myotonia congenita and hyperkalaemic periodic paralysis, though it is a disease *sui generis*. Myotonia, particularly exacerbated by cold, is characteristic, together with occasional attacks of weakness of the muscles particularly induced by cold. The administration of potassium may also induce attacks of weakness. Again, this disease is not generally associated with progressive muscular weakness.

Periodic paralysis

Patients having periodic paralysis suffer, as the name indicates, recurrent attacks of weakness usually affecting the legs more than the arms, and often sufficiently severe to render them unable to lift their arms or legs from the bed. Two major types of periodic paralysis are recognized, and both are usually inherited in an autosomal dominant mode.

Hypokalaemic familial periodic paralysis

In this condition, attacks often occur a half to two hours after a heavy carbohydrate meal, and on resting after exertion. The attacks may occur as infrequently as once every few months and last a few hours or more with spontaneous remission. In the attack, the plasma potassium falls dramatically, often as low as 2·0 mEq/1. There may be vacuolation of the muscle fibres, perhaps due to dilatation of the sarcoplasmic reticulum. The condition is probably due to an as yet unidentified abnormality of the sarcolemmal membrane and the process of excitation-contraction coupling. Between the attacks the patients are usually entirely normal, though in later life some develop a progressive vacuolar myopathy. Myotonia may at times be present, both clinically in the eyelids and on electromyography of other muscles. This form of periodic paralysis may occur in thyrotoxicosis, an association which is particularly frequent in Orientals.

Hyperkalaemic periodic paralysis (adynamia episodica hereditaria)

This condition is generally less common than hypokalaemic familial periodic paralysis, though it arises particularly in those with Scandinavian blood. The attacks are often precipitated by rest after exertion, or occur spontaneously on waking in the morning. They are usually described as shorter, less severe and more frequent than in hypokalaemic periodic paralysis, though this generalization is not always true. The attacks are associated with a rise of serum potassium, particularly in the venous blood draining paralysed muscles. The basic abnormality is probably a periodic increase in sarcolemmal membrane permeability to sodium, leading to a lowering of the resting membrane potential and a loss of intracellular potassium. Myotonia is more common than in hypokalaemic familial periodic paralysis, and a fixed myopathy rarely develops.

Normokalaemic periodic paralysis

This third form has many of the characteristics of hyperkalaemic periodic paralysis, and may be a variant of it.

Polymyositis

The skeletal muscle may be damaged by an autoimmune inflammatory necrotizing process producing the histological picture of inflammation of many muscles. Inflammatory cells, particularly lymphocytes and occasional plasmocytes with macrophages, occur both in the perivascular area and predominantly in the connective tissue septa surrounding fasciculi. The process is patchy, and the absence of inflammatory change in any one biopsy is not proof against the diagnosis. Patients often are aware of pain and tenderness of the muscles, as well as of progressive weakness and wasting. The proximal muscles including those of the neck are mainly involved, and dysphagia due to bulbar muscle involvement is not infrequent. The tendon reflexes are generally preserved until there is severe muscle weakness and wasting, and may even be exaggerated in the early stages. Paraesthesiae may occur perhaps due to some peripheral sensory nerve damage, and may make the diagnosis difficult. An inflammatory cardiomyopathy may also develop.

The damage is usually extensive with a rise of serum creatine kinase activity to high levels. Electromyography shows increased insertional activity, pseudomyotonic discharges (ill-sustained high frequency discharges), and fibrillation potentials, perhaps indicating the presence either of intramuscular nerve damage or of many intact segments of muscle separated from motor end plates by necrotic segments.

Polymyositis may be divided into four groups by reference to associated phenomena (Rose and Walton 1966):

Type I Acute polymyositis with myoglobinuria; sub-acute pure polymyositis

Type II Polymyositis with dominant muscle weakness, associated with minor evidence of collagen-vascular disease, such as raised ESR or positive antinuclear factor

Type III Polymyositis complicating severe collagen-vascular disease, for instance rheumatoid arthritis, scleroderma or systemic lupus erythematosus

Type IV Polymyositis complicating malignant disease.

This division has practical importance, because the prognosis is different in the different groups. A division based on age is also important, since the form and prognosis differs in the young and old patient. In children, polymyositis is often of type II or III, but the prognosis with sustained high dose corticosteroid therapy is universally good. In adults with type III polymyositis, the prognosis is generally poorer despite this treatment, and is better in type I. In patients over the age of 50 years, type IV polymyositis is much commoner, and it is important to search for an underlying carcinoma. The polymyositis may present several years before the carcinoma reveals itself by local or metastatic effects. Total removal of the carcinoma may result in a cure of the polymyositis in some patients, but failing this the prognosis is usually poor.

The reason why the body reacts against its own skeletal muscle, activating lymphocytes and antibodies inducing muscle fibre death, is not known. A similar process seems to occur in all autoimmune diseases. It has been suggested that certain viruses may enter the muscle fibre, reproduce there and become the source of antigen against which the body reacts. The findings under the electron microscope of virus-like particles adds to this suggestion, but as yet there is no confirmation. The treatment of all forms of polymyositis, aside from removal of an underlying carcinoma, is immunosuppression with high doses of corticosteroids with or without cytotoxic agents such as azathioprine or cyclophosphamide.

Polymyalgia rheumatica should be mentioned in this section for it presents with severe muscle pains and resultant weakness. The erythrocyte sedimentation rate is high, and patients are older than 55 years. The muscle often shows no pathological change, though giant cell arteritis is often found in the cranial arteries. Corticosteroid therapy for 6 months to 2 years is curative.

Metabolic myopathies

Under this heading may be grouped diseases where a clue exists to the underlying metabolic cause of the myopathy. The division is arbitrary and it must be hoped that eventually all diseases including the muscular dystrophies will come into this category. The periodic paralyses with abnormalities of potassium and sodium metabolism might also have been included here. The often painful proximal myopathies of renal failure and metabolic bone disease, which may be due to abnormalities of calcium metabolism, should also be mentioned.

Glycogen storage disease

Myophosphorylase deficiency (McArdle's disease; type V glycogenosis) is associated with a block in the energy metabolism of the muscle and the accumulation of glycogen as a result. The deficiency of myophosphorylase prevents the splitting of glucose-1-phosphate from glycogen, and the energy metabolism must rest wholly upon aerobic pathways. On severe muscle exertion, particularly during ischaemia, the muscle becomes very anoxic. There are pain and cramps, and the normal rise of venous lactate in these circumstances does not develop. Glycogen accumulates in the sarcoplasm up to a level of 5 per cent.

α-1,4, glucosidase deficiency also results in glycogen accumulation and impaired carbohydrate oxidation. The enzyme which hydrolyses the α-1,4, glucoside link of glycogen to release glucose from glycogen is deficient. Two forms of the condition are recognized, the more common infantile *Pompe's disease* in which glycogen accumulates in most of the cells of the body including the heart, neurons and skeletal muscle; and an adult form in which the deficit is mainly in the skeletal muscle. The enzyme is a lysosomal enzyme, but glycogen accumulates both in lysosomes and in the cytoplasm.

Mitochondrial myopathies

In a number of different disease entities, there has been shown to be an accumulation of normal and abnormal mitochondria in the skeletal muscle fibres. The disease pictures range from muscle weakness in childhood to familial facioscapulohumeral muscular dystrophy. Two instances of hypermetabolism due to uncontrolled oxidation of substrates by abnormal mitochondria have been described. Non-specific mitochondrial abnormalities may occur in many diseases, and only where the mitochondrial change is extensive should cases be accepted into this group.

Lipid storage myopathy

Rare instances of myopathy associated with accumulation of lipid in muscle have been reported.

Endocrine myopathies

Associated with thyroid disease

Muscle involvement in hyperthyroidism is very frequent. About a quarter of patients complain of muscle weakness, a half have signs of muscle weakness on clinical examination, and 90 per cent have electromyographic evidence of a proximal myopathy affecting especially the shoulder girdle muscles. Muscular weakness with hypertrophy, slow contraction and sometimes painful cramps may be seen in hypothyroidism.

Associated with adrenal disease

Hypercorticism, whether from an adrenal tumour or adrenal cortical hyperplasia, or from corticosteroid therapy, may produce a severe proximal myopathy. Addison's disease is associated with some weakness, as may be hypopituitarism.

Associated with abnormalities of calcium metabolism

The disorders of neuromuscular transmission associated with hypercalcaemia have been mentioned above (page 274). Hypoparathyroidism may also produce proximal muscle weakness and cramps. A proximal myopathy can develop in many conditions causing osteomalacia, and responds specifically to vitamin D therapy.

Vitamin deficiency myopathies

In animals deficiency of vitamin E produces a profound necrotizing myopathy, but so far this deficiency has not been recognized as a cause of muscle disease in man.

Toxic myopathies

A large number of toxic agents may damage muscle. Haff disease results from eating contaminated fish, and several snake venoms produce acute destruction of muscle fibres (*rhabdomyolysis*). Certain drugs, including corticosteroids (especially 9α-fluoro derivatives), chloroquine, emetine and vincristine can damage muscle fibres.

Idiopathic rhabdomyolysis

Rare individuals suffer from acute attacks of necrosis of muscle with profound paralysis and myoglobinuria. If death does not occur from profound paralysis. the patient recovers with virtually complete regeneration of the damaged skeletal muscle. Exertion and mild illnesses may precipitate attacks.

Obscure congenital myopathies

These rare conditions may be found particularly in patients presenting with the floppy baby syndrome, or with childhood myopathies. They include *nemaline myopathy*, where all the fibres have many abnormal paracrystalline rods; *central core disease* where the centre of the fibres shows an absence of sarcoplasmic organelles, the abnormal myofibrils being tightly collected together into a 'core'; and *centronuclear myopathy* where many of the muscle fibres are abnormally small with nuclei lined up in the central region as in a myotube. The biochemical basis of none of these diseases is understood.

DIFFERENTIAL DIAGNOSIS OF PURE MOTOR WEAKNESS

A large group of patients present with pure weakness involving several muscle groups. Patients with no more suggestion of sensory involvement than occasional paraesthesiae or areflexia must also be considered in this context. These patients present a problem of differential diagnosis. However the separation of the various conditions is usually possible on clinical grounds with recourse to confirmation by the various methods of investigation outlined in chapter 4.

The separation of cases with psychogenic or upper motor neuron causes of muscle weakness is usually relatively easy as discussed in page 78 *et seq.* Clinically obvious fasciculation and electromyographic evidence of fibrillation potentials with motor units which are giant both in amplitude and spread are characteristic of anterior horn cell diseases or chronic motor neuropathies. The reflexes are generally preserved until the muscle is severely atrophied, and in motor neuron disease the associated upper motor neuron degeneration causes exaggerated reflexes.

A pure motor neuropathy is difficult to diagnose, and two pointers are helpful. Widespread areflexia at an early stage points to the involvement of the peripheral nerves. A raised cerebrospinal fluid protein level may also suggest a neuropathy or radiculopathy. Electrophysiological studies may show a decreased nerve conduction velocity or nerve action potential amplitude. The causes of a pure motor neuropathy include lead intoxication, acute porphyric neuropathy, acute idiopathic polyneuritis of the Guillain-Barré-Strohl syndrome, and chronic and recurrent idiopathic polyneuritis. One personally observed patient had recurrent attacks of proximal pure muscle weakness associated with areflexia and an increased cerebrospinal fluid concentration. These developed both spontaneously, and after mild infections, as well as on reduction of corticosteroid therapy. Only in the fourth attack did distal sensory changes confirm the previous electrophysiological evidence that the site of damage was in the peripheral nerves.

Disorders of neuromuscular transmission should always be considered where fatigue rather than constant weakness is a feature. The clinical pattern of myasthenia gravis and the myasthenic syndrome allow easy separation. Only ocular myopathy, oculopharyngeal muscular dystrophy and polyneuritis cranialis can be confused with myasthenia gravis, and the demonstration of marked fatiguability cured by anticholinesterase therapy is diagnostic of the latter. In general, diseases of the neuromuscular junction and muscle do not affect the muscle spindle until late in the disease, and thus the tendon reflexes are generally preserved until the muscle is very weak. In many muscular dystrophies, the pattern of involvement of the muscles is relatively specific, while in most other myopathies involvement is non-selective though often proximal. Muscle pains, cramps and pain on exertion are useful diagnostic hints to polymyositis or disorders of energy metabolism.

REFERENCES

CAMBIER J. (1968) *La Myasthenie.* Baillière et Fils, Paris.

DESMEDT J.E. (1966) Presynaptic mechanisms in myasthenia gravis. *Ann. N.Y. Acad. Sci.* **135**, 209–246.

DUCHEN L.W. (1971) An electron microscopic study of the changes induced by botulinum toxin in the motor end-plates of slow and fast skeletal muscle fibres of the mouse. *J. neurol. Sci.* **14**, 47–60.

EATON L.M. and LAMBERT E.H. (1957) Electromyography and electrical stimulation of nerves in diseases of motor unit: observations on myasthenic malignant tumours. *J. Amer. med. Ass.* **163**, 1117–1124.

ELMQVIST D., HOFMANN W.W., KUGELBERG J. and QUASTEL D.M.J. (1964) An electrophysiological investigation of neuromuscular transmission in myasthenia gravis. *J. Physiol. (Lond.)* **174**, 417–434.

JENKINS R.B. (1972) The treatment of myasthenia gravis with prednisone. *Lancet* **1**, 765–767.

KORNGUTH S.E., HANSON J.C. and CHUN R.W.M. (1970) Antineuronal antibodies in patients with myasthenia gravis. *Neurol. (Minneap.)* **20**, 749–755.

McQUILLEN M.P. and JOHNS R.J. (1967) The nature of the defect in the Eaton-Lambert syndrome. *Neurol. (Minneap.)* **17**, 527–536.

McQUILLEN M.P., CANTOR H.E. and O'ROURKE J.R. (1968) Myasthenic syndrome associated with antibiotics. *Arch. Neurol. (Chic.)* **18**, 402–415.

MERTENS H.G., BALZEREIT F. and LEIPERT M. (1969) The treatment of severe myasthenia gravis with immunosuppressive agents. *Europ. Neurol.* **2**, 321–339.

MYASTHENIA GRAVIS (1966) *Ann. N.Y. Acad. Sci.* **135**, 1–680.

NAMBA T., BRUNNER N.G., SHAPIRO M.S. and GROB D. (1971) Corticotropin therapy in myasthenia gravis: effects, indications and limitations. *Neurol. (Minneap.)* **21**, 1008–1018.

ROSE A.L. and WALTON J.N. (1966) Polymyositis: survey of 89 cases with particular reference to treatment and prognosis. *Brain* **89**, 747–768.

SANTA T., ENGEL A.G. and LAMBERT E.H. (1972) Histometric studies of neuromuscular junction ultrastructure. I. Myasthenia gravis. *Neurol. (Minneap.)* **22**, 71–82.

SIMPSON J.A. (1958) An evaluation of thymectomy in myasthenia gravis. *Brain* **81**, 112–144.

SIMPSON J.A. (1969) Myasthenia gravis and myasthenic syndromes. In *Diseases of Voluntary Muscle*, ed. Walton J.N. pp. 541–578. Churchill, London.

STRAUSS A.J.L., SEEGAL B.C., HSU K.C., BURKHOLDER P.M., NASTUK W.L. and OSSERMAN K.E. (1960) Immunofluorescent demonstration of a muscle-binding, complement-fixing serum globulin fraction in myasthenia gravis. *Proc. Soc., exp. Biol. Med.* **105**, 184–191.

WALTON J.N. ed. (1974) *Disorders of Voluntary Muscle*. Churchill Livingstone, Edinburgh.

II

Synopsis: A Diagnostic Approach to Peripheral Nerve Disease

Diagnostic staircase

To achieve the pinnacle of the diagnosis in a patient with peripheral nerve disease, the doctor must ascend the same diagnostic staircase as in any other disease. The steps of this staircase must be carefully followed.

History

The history must be carefully taken, clearly to document the first and subsequent symptoms, their distribution and rate of development, and the current position, both concerning the patient's symptoms and his functional capabilities. The cause of the neuropathy is often difficult to discover, and its identification frequently rests upon a searching series of direct questions. Peripheral nerve disease is so often associated with systemic diseases like renal or hepatic failure or diabetes mellitus that symptoms in all systems must be diligently sought. Exposure to toxins frequently goes unnoticed, and a careful history of all medications and of the occupation and hobbies of the patient is required. Nerves may be injured in various repetitive manoeuvres, and a demonstration of the activities of work and play may be of value. A history of past illness and operations can sometimes point to the cause of the neuropathy. A few neuropathies are familial, and the recognition of this aids in their diagnosis. It may be helpful to examine other members of the family, even though they deny symptoms. A family history of diabetes mellitus, pernicious anaemia or other autoimmune disease may suggest valuable lines of investigation.

Examination

Chapter 3 details the points of importance in the examination of the peripheral nervous system. The key to a quick and accurate examination is to have a technique which provides a rapid survey of the whole of the peripheral nervous system. Upon this is grafted a careful search for the deficits indicated by the patient's history. Efforts must be made to decide upon the distribution of the deficits, and the sensory boundaries, muscle and reflex involvement must clearly be defined to allow the next step to be taken on the diagnostic staircase.

Anatomical localization

During the examination, every deficit will have been probed to define as well as possible the anatomical site of the lesion. At the end of the examination a summary must be made of the overall picture of the lesions. Are the deficits of psychological origin, or is the lesion in the central or peripheral nervous systems? If the latter, what degree of involvement is there of the sensory, motor and autonomic parts? Do the lesions lie in the perikarya, nerve roots, or proximal or distal parts of the nerves? Is the condition a mononeuropathy, a mononeuritis multiplex, or a polyneuropathy? Might the disease lie in the neuromuscular junction or muscle?

Upon this anatomical summary rests the next step, the formulation of a differential diagnosis.

Differential diagnosis

The construction of a list of conditions affecting the peripheral nervous system which might give rise to the pattern of symptoms, the findings on examination, and the deduced distribution of the anatomical lesions, is the next step. This requires the full understanding of all the diseases which may affect the peripheral nervous system, and which are detailed in chapters 6–10. If the disease pattern is an acute mononeuritis multiplex, then ischaemic and collagen vascular diseases are very likely to be responsible. A list of such diseases is easy to construct. If the pattern is a chronic distal sensorimotor polyneuropathy, then another, much larger list of conditions, which may be responsible, can be constructed.

From such a list, it is possible to undertake various tests seeking to confirm or rule out each of the conditions on the list.

Investigations

In diseases of the peripheral nervous system, it is sometimes necessary to enlist the help of special investigations before it is possible clearly to formulate the anatomical localization or differential diagnosis. Electrophysiological and pathological studies (see chapter 4) are often required to point to the site of the lesion, and define whether the pathology is predominantly segmental demyelination or axonal degeneration. With this information, it is possible more accurately to formulate a differential diagnosis, and undertake a series of diagnostic tests for each of the conditions on the list. These investigations are detailed in chapters 4 and 6–10.

Final diagnosis

If the clinician has correctly ascended the diagnostic staircase, then one test will confirm the presence of one of the diseases on the list of the differential diagnosis, and all the other tests will be negative. If every test is negative, the condition falls into the idiopathic group, for which as yet no causes have been found.

Methods of classification of peripheral nerve disease

Numerous methods have been advanced for the classification of peripheral nerve disease. Some have been based upon the medical student's 'life-belt', the check list of aetiological categories. This spans inherited, toxic, metabolic, endocrine, deficiency, traumatic, infective, autoimmune, vascular, neoplastic and other categories eventually finishing with idiopathic. Upon this check list may be strung all the diseases of the peripheral nervous system, but unfortunately such a list is of no great help in expediting arrival at the diagnosis.

Many other classifications of peripheral nerve disease have been produced, including those of Krücke (1959) and Simpson (1971). Some have been based on the pathological picture, some on the distribution of the lesions, and some on the rate of onset. The scheme below incorporates most of these features, with the object of leading quickly and logically to the diagnosis.

Practical classification of peripheral nerve diseases

Once the disease has been recognized as affecting the peripheral nerves, the difficulty of deciding the aetiology arises. This section attempts to provide a simplified practical and logical approach to this task. The diagnostic synopsis is based on the clinical features of the disease. Firstly, is the neuro-

TABLE 11.1. Diagnostic synopsis of peripheral nerve disease

Rate	Distribution	Pattern	Predominant pathological change	Predominant type of fibre involved	Disease
ACUTE		Mononeuritis/m. multiplex	Axonal degeneration		Trauma Vascular. Diabetes
	Distal/diffuse	Polyneuropathy	Axonal degeneration		Toxic. Metabolic
			Segmental demyelination		Diphtheria
	Proximal	Mononeuritis/radiculopathy		[Painful]	Diphtheria
	Proximal/diffuse	Polyneuropathy	Axonal degeneration		Porphyria
ACUTE/SUBACUTE	Proximal/diffuse	Polyneuropathy/radiculopathy	Segmental demyelination		Guillain-Barré-Strohl syndrome
SUBACUTE/CHRONIC		Mononeuritis/m. multiplex			Entrapment
CHRONIC		Mononeuritis/m. multiplex			Entrapment. Tumour. Leprosy
		Radiculopathy			Radiculopathies
	Distal	Polyneuropathy		Sensory-large	Hereditary neuropathy. Carcinoma
				Sensory-small	Familial amyloidosis
				Sensory-general	Diabetes
			Axonal degeneration	Motor	Toxic. Hereditary peroneal muscular atrophy Hereditary neuropathies. Vitamin deficiencies. Toxic. Carcinoma. Metabolic. Old age. Leprosy Vascular. Diabetes
	Proximal	Mononeuritis			Vascular
RECURRENT	Distal/diffuse	Polyneuropathy	Axonal degeneration		Vascular
HYPERTROPHIC/RECURRENT	Distal/diffuse	Polyneuropathy	Segmental demyelination		Hereditary peroneal muscular atrophy. Dejerine-Sottas disease. Steroid-sensitive recurrent neuropathy

pathy acute, subacute, chronic, recurrent or associated with nerve hyper-trophy? Secondly, what is the distribution of the disease; is it proximal, distal or diffuse? Is it a mononeuropathy, mononeuritis multiplex, radicul-opathy or polyneuropathy? Within this clinical framework it is possible to separate certain groups of disorders by whether the major type of fibre involved is sensory or motor, or large or small, and whether the pre-dominant pathological change is segmental demyelination or axonal de-generation. The latter may be differentiated either by electrophysiological or pathological studies.

Such a simplified diagnostic synopsis is shown in table 11.1. It is by no means comprehensive. Many other diseases could be added after a careful study of chapter 6. Moreover some diseases may present clinically in several different ways. The synopsis given here is based upon an original personal suggestion by A. K. Asbury (1967), and has the advantage of offer-ing an outline of the clinical principles upon which the diagnosis of peri-pheral nerve disease is based.

REFERENCES

KRÜCKE W. (1959) Histopathologie der Polyneuritis und Polyneuropathie. *Dtsch. Z. Nervenheilk* **180**, 1–39.
SIMPSON J. A. (1971) Peripheral neuropathy. Ætiological and clinical aspects. *Proc. roy. Soc. Med.* **64**, 291–293.

12

Treatment of Peripheral Nerve Disease

It is a common misconception that there is no treatment for most neurological diseases including those of the peripheral nervous system. This short chapter is included to show that such a belief is erroneous. Specific and curative therapy is available for the treatment of a small number of diseases of the peripheral nerves, and for the remainder effective, if not curative, symptomatic therapy is possible.

Specific treatment

The specific treatment which is available for each individual disease is discussed in the consideration of each disease in chapter 6. Such treatments include the administration of vitamins like cyanocobalamin, and of hormones like insulin and triiodothyronine in specific deficiency states; the withdrawal of toxins damaging nerves, such as lead; the withdrawal of green plant products in Refsum's disease; the control of underlying metabolic and neoplastic diseases such as uraemia and leukaemia; the surgical relief of nerve compression or entrapment, and the restoration of transected nerves; and the prevention and treatment of specific infections affecting nerves like diphtheria and leprosy.

Symptomatic therapy

Symptomatic therapy covers the whole field of neurological and rehabilitative medicine and much besides. Only brief reference can be made here to the principles of treatment. For consideration in depth, reviews by Nichols (1971) and Brown and Opitz (1971) are recommended.

Symptomatic treatment may be divided into measures to overcome the motor, sensory and autonomic problems, and surgical, medical and psychological symptomatic therapy.

Treatment of muscle weakness

The whole specialty of physiotherapy plays a large part in overcoming and preventing the problems of muscle weakness from peripheral nerve disease. By a programme of passive and active movement, it is possible to increase the effectiveness of unaffected muscles, to strengthen weak muscles, and to prevent contractures and disuse atrophy. If physiotherapy is started early in the course of the disease, the muscles and joints will be kept in an optimal condition for the time when nerve regeneration occurs. The facilities of a complete physiotherapy department should include a gymnasium, swimming pool and methods of electrical stimulation of nerve and muscle. However often as much can be achieved with the enthusiastic application of simple apparatus.

Physical methods of aiding weak muscles include splints and braces, such as cock-up wrist splints, leg calipers of the light Rizolli back-spring type, or the full form with toe spring. 'Lively splints', in which springs aid action of the weak muscles, and the stronger muscles pull against the springs, may be used especially for arm nerve palsies. 'Artificial muscles', either powered by electricity or gas, may be used to replace the action of a totally paralysed muscle.

Patients with severe peripheral nerve disease may require extensive help from occupational therapists, including numerous aids, appliances and adaptations. These range from the simple adaptation of utensils, including larger diameter handles and the combined spoon and fork, to 'lazy-tongs', to wheelchairs, bath and toilet rails, hoists and specially adapted cars. Re-housing on a single level, or the adaptation of the patient's existing house with ramps for wheelchairs, stair lifts, and rails may be required. Nursing assistance in the home is frequently necessary.

Severely paralysed patients may require to be nursed in hospital, where treatment may extend even to artificial respiration in diseases such as acute idiopathic polyneuritis of the Guillain-Barré-Strohl syndrome or acute porphyric neuropathy. The provision of one of a number of currently available patient-operated, remotely controlled electronic appliances such as the POSSUM (POSSUM Controls Ltd, 63 Mandeville Road, Aylesbury, Bucks) or the System 7 (System 7, 3 Avon Way, Shoeburyness, Essex), offers a new dimension to home care for such chronically disabled patients into whose groups sufferers of peripheral nerve disease fortunately rarely come.

Treatment of sensory denervation

Of the positive sensory disturbances of peripheral nerve disease, causalgia is the most severe. As described on page 152, sympathectomy is often curative. Postherpetic neuralgia and many other positive sensory disturbances may be suppressed by carbamazepine, phenytoin or procaine infusions as described on page 247.

Skin which is denervated is readily burned or otherwise injured, leading to various infections including abscesses and osteomyelitis. Joints which are denervated are similarly readily injured leading eventually to painless disorganized neuropathic (Charcot) joints. The prevention of such injuries by careful advice, protection and frequent examination is far better than attempted treatment when the complication has occurred.

Treatment of autonomic dysfunction

As described in chapter 7, autonomic neuropathies may lead to disturbances of bowel and bladder control, and to cardiovascular disturbances. The bladder may need to be stimulated to empty by carbachol, bethanecol or distigmine, or the sphincters may need to be stimulated by propantheline in cases of incontinence. Autonomic diarrhoea may be treated with tetracycline, codeine phosphate etc. Constipation may require bulk laxatives, lubricatory suppositories and stimulators like bisacodyl or Senokot (Westminster). Catheterization and enemata may eventually be required. Postural hypotension may require fludrocortisone or rarely pressure suits for the lower limbs and abdomen.

Surgical treatment

Symptomatic surgical therapy is relatively limited to the grafting of nerves which have had an irreversible complete focal lesion, in patients where the other nerves are normal. Cured leprosy is such an instance as described on page 157. Tendon transplantation may occasionally help by restoring some degree of active movement which was otherwise lost.

Medical treatment

Vitamins of the B group are often given either as multivitamin tablets or as vitamin B_{12} injections, where no specific medical treatment is available. The tenuous rationale is that some of this group of vitamins are required for peripheral nerve function, and that certain disorders of peripheral nerve have abnormal pyruvate tolerance tests indicating dysfunction in carbohydrate metabolic pathways involving thiamine. Few if any patients benefit other than by the psychological effect mentioned below.

Corticosteroid therapy is sometimes given to patients, particularly those with idiopathic chronic recurrent or hypertrophic neuropathy without a family history. In some, a definite improvement occurs, but occasionally an equally and even more dramatic deterioration occurs upon withdrawal of the therapy. Thus it is important to recognize that patients may have a severe relapse precipitated by attempted withdrawal of corticosteroid therapy, and to assess whether the severity of the neuropathy is sufficient to warrant this risk. The state may eventually be reached of increasing corticosteroid dependency in rare patients (Matthews *et al.* 1970). It might be considered wise to avoid corticosteroid therapy in all but severe neuropathies. However, the chances of encountering such an unfortunate patient are relatively slight, and most clinicians accept this risk for the benefit of a larger number of patients. If a profound relapse develops on reducing the dose of corticosteroids, then the dose must be returned to the previous level or above, maintained there for perhaps a further month, and then gradually reduced by about 5 per cent per month with extreme caution. The place of immunosuppressants in these patients responding to corticosteroids has yet to be determined.

Psychological treatment

As in all diseases, it is important that the patient understands the nature and effects of his condition within the limits of his comprehension and psychological ability to cope with this information. The relatives must certainly know the full picture. In chronic diseases of the peripheral nerves, the physician must have frequent and regular discussions with the patient and relatives about the personal, psychological, social and economic effects of the disorder. The cooperation of the patient and relatives in various aids and adaptations, and in changes of the way of life imposed by the disease is essential if the patient is to be treated in the best way. The prompt recognition of reactive anxiety and depression, and their treatment by frank discussion and appropriate psychotropic drugs is of great importance. An approach based upon the sympathetic care of the patient and his family is just as important as the dispassionate scientific approach to the investigation, diagnosis and treatment of the disease.

REFERENCES

BROWN J.R. and OPITZ J.L. (1971) Treatment of neuropathies. In *Handbook of Clinical Neurology*, vol. 8, ed. Vinken P.J. and Bruyn G.W. pp. 373–411. North-Holland, Amsterdam.

MATHEWS W.B., HOWELL D.A. and HUGHES R.C. (1970) Relapsing corticosteroid-dependent polyneuritis. *J. Neurol. Neurosurg. Psychiat.* **33**, 330–337.

NICHOLS P.J.R. (1971) *Rehabilitation of the Severely Disabled.* Vol. 2: Management. Butterworth, London.

13

Perspective

A considerable body of knowledge now exists about the peripheral nervous system in health and in disease. However an even greater body of knowledge awaits to be discovered, particularly in the biochemical field. Now is the time to pause and to outline our areas of knowledge, our areas of ignorance, and, with a certain amount of guessing, to forecast the likely growing points in the next decade.

In the field of the basic sciences, a great deal is already known about the anatomy and physiology of the normal peripheral nervous system. Uncertainty still exists about the relationship between axonal diameter, internodal length and conduction velocity in myelinated nerve fibres. Our understanding of the biochemistry of normal perikarya, axons, Schwann cells and myelin is however much more limited, though an outline of most processes has been recognized. We have little knowledge about the turnover of Schwann cells, myelin or axoplasm. The metabolic relationship between the perikaryon and its satellite cells and the axons and Schwann cells requires to be clarified. We have the glimmerings of understanding about axoplasmic flow, and the interrelationship of the perikaryon, axon and nerve terminals. A very great deal more information is required before these glimmerings are bright enough to read the whole story.

Turning to disease states, a large number of individual diseases have now been characterized, and to a greater or lesser extent the physiological and pathological changes occurring in the axons, perikarya, Schwann cells and myelin sheaths have been determined. However in few diseases is the biochemical basis known, or a specific treatment available. The various hereditary neuropathies might seem to be the diseases most capable of elucidation, being presumably due to a single abnormality in one of the metabolic pathways. As yet they have generally resisted efforts to determine these abnormalities. We have only suggestions about the mechanism by which metabolic diseases like uraemia, diabetes and liver disease damage nerves. The cause of the neuropathies of carcinoma and old age await discovery. The action of most toxins damaging the peripheral nervous system is unknown. The hypothesis of the dying-back of nerves in many distal neuropathies may well be correct, but the physiological and biochemical basis of the pattern of disease remains to be clarified. While awaiting understanding of the biochemical basis and specific treatment of many diseases, it would be helpful to have available therapeutic agents which would stimulate nerve regeneration.

Forecasts of areas in which we can expect to see a significant breakthrough in the next decade must obviously be speculative, though nonetheless interesting. The current growing points which look most likely to yield worthwhile results are in the fields of the mechanism of action of neurotoxins, the metabolic basis of the hereditary neuropathies, and the basis of the 'dying-back' neuropathies. Axoplasmic flow will probably be increasingly understood both in health and disease, and knowledge of the interrelationship of the neuron and its satellite cells can be expected to enlarge greatly in the next decade. It is to be hoped that the large body of chronic idiopathic polyneuropathies may be split into aetiological groups, and that the cure of some of these may appear.

Appendix:
Histological Techniques in the
Study of Peripheral Nerve

MARGARET JENKISON FIMLT
& W. G. BRADLEY

FIXATIVES

Susa fixative

mercuric chloride	4·5 g
sodium chloride	0·5 g
trichloracetic acid	2·0 g
acetic acid	4·0 ml
formalin	20·0 ml
distilled water	80·0 ml

Block size 3–8 mm diameter. Fixation time 3–24 h. Transfer directly to 95 per cent alcohol. Remove mercury pigment before staining by taking sections to water and treating with 0·5 per cent iodine in 70 per cent alcohol for 3–5 min. Rinse briefly in tap water. Treat with 2·5 per cent sodium thiosulphate for $\frac{1}{2}$–2 min until bleached. Wash in running tap water, 5 min. Proceed with staining.

Formol-calcium solution

formalin (40 per cent w/v)	10 ml
calcium chloride	1 g
distilled water	100 ml

Block size 3–10 mm diameter. Fixation time 24 h.

Flemming's solution

1 per cent chromic acid solution	15 ml
2 per cent osmium tetroxide solution	4 ml
acetic acid	1 ml

Block size 2 mm diameter. Fixation time 12–24 h. Wash in running water 24 h.

EMBEDDING

Modified Pertefi double embedding technique for automatic tissue processor

1	70 per cent alcohol	$1\frac{1}{2}$ h
2	95 per cent alcohol	2 h
3	Absolute alcohol	$1\frac{1}{2}$ h
4	Absolute alcohol	2 h
5	Equal parts absolute alcohol and methyl benzoate	2 h
6	1 per cent celloidin in equal parts parts absolute alcohol and methyl benzoate	3 h
7	1 per cent celloidin in equal parts of absolute alcohol and methyl benzoate	4 h
8	Toluene I	1 h
9	Toluene II	2 h
10	Wax I	$2\frac{1}{2}$ h
11	Wax II	$1\frac{1}{2}$ h
12	Transfer to wax II in vacuum embedding oven	$1\frac{1}{2}$ h
13	Embed in paraffin wax	

Methacrylate embedding

Solution A

glycol methacrylate	80 ml
2-butoxyethanol	16 ml
benzoyl peroxide	270 mg

Solution B

polyethylene glycol 400	15 vol
N,N-dimethylaniline	1 vol

Following fixation, take tissue through ascending concentrations of alcohol as follows:

1 70 per cent alcohol—two changes each of 30 min.
2 90 per cent alcohol—two changes each of 30 min.
3 Absolute alcohol—two changes each of 30 min.
4 Place in solution A for 1 h followed by fresh solution A and leave in this overnight.
5 Embed in a mixture of 42 parts solution A to 1 part solution B. Leave for 2–3 h to harden.

STAINS

Haematoxylin and eosin

Mayer's haemalum

haematoxylin	1 g
sodium iodate	0·2 g
potassium alum or ammonium alum	50 g
citric acid	1 g
chloral hydrate	50 g
distilled water	1000 ml

Dissolve haematoxylin, alum and sodium iodate overnight. Add chloral hydrate and citric acid and boil for 5 min.

Eosin solution

eosin Y	9 g
erythrosin	4 g
phloxine	2 g
methylated spirits	200 ml
distilled water	800 ml

Fixative Susa

Embedding Paraffin or methacrylate

Section 5 μm thickness

1 Remove mercury pigment.
2 Take sections to water.
3 Mayer's haemalum 5–10 min.
4 Wash.
5 Differentiate in 1 per cent acid-alcohol.
6 Wash.
7 Blue in running tap water 5 min.
8 Stain in eosin 2 min.

Palmgren axon stain

Acid-formalin

formalin (40 per cent w/v)	25 ml
distilled water	75 ml
1 per cent nitric acid	6 drops

Silver solution

silver nitrate	15 g
potassium nitrate	10 g
distilled water	100 ml
1 per cent glycerine	5 ml

Reducer

pyrogallol	10 g
distilled water	450 ml
absolute alcohol	550 ml
1 per cent nitric acid	2 ml

Fixative Susa or formol-calcium

Embedding Paraffin or methacrylate

Section 5 μm thickness

1   Sections to water.
2   Remove mercury pigment (page 298).
3   Sections through ascending grades of alcohol to absolute alcohol.
4   Place slides in 1 per cent celloidin in equal parts ether and absolute alcohol for 1 min.
5   Drain and harden in 70 per cent alcohol for 2 min.
6   Rinse well in distilled water.
7   Place in acid-formalin for 5 min.
8   Wash well in distilled water; 8 changes in 5 min.
9   Place in silver solution for 15 min.
10 Drain and reduce in reducer preheated to 56°C for 1 min agitating vigorously. Any precipitate should be washed off with fresh reducer.
11 Wash in distilled water.
12 Fix in 5 per cent sodium thiosulphate for 5 min.
13 Rinse in tap water.
14 Dehydrate, clear and mount.

Results Axons—brown-black on golden background.

Myelin stains

Solochrome cyanin

Staining solution Place 0·2 g solochrome cyanin RS in a flask. Add 0·5 ml concentrated sulphuric acid. Mix well and incorporate all the dye in the sludge. Add 90 ml distilled water and 10 ml of 4 per cent iron alum. Mix and filter.

Fixative Susa

Embedding Paraffin or methacrylate

Section 5 μm thickness

1   Sections to water. Remove mercury pigment (page 298).
2   Stain in solochrome cyanin for 10 min at room temperature.
3   Wash well in running water.
4   Differentiate in 10 per cent iron alum until nuclei are scarcely visible.
5   Wash well in running water.
6   Counterstain with eosin if desired.

Results Myelin neurokeratin—bright blue. Erythrocytes—blue. Nuclei—pale blue.

Alternative method

Solochrome stock staining solution

distilled water	60 ml
concentrated sulphuric acid	1 drop

Solochrome working solution

solochrome stock solution	16 drops
distilled water	60 ml
concentrated sulphuric acid	1 drop

1 Sections to water. Remove mercury pigment (page 298).
2 Place in solochrome working solution overnight.
3 Wash well in running water.
4 Dehydrate, clear and mount.

Weigert-Pal method

Weigert's lithium carbonate-haematoxylin

haematoxylin	1 g
distilled water	100 ml
absolute alcohol	5 ml
saturated lithium carbonate (about	
1·3 per cent)	1 ml

Dissolve haematoxylin in the water by heating gently. Allow to cool, then add the alcohol and lithium carbonate. The solution should be freshly prepared just before use.

Pal's solution

Equal parts of 1 per cent oxalic acid and 1 per cent sodium sulphate.

Fixative Flemming's solution

Embedding Paraffin

Sections 2–5 μm thickness

1   Sections to water. Celloidinise (see above page 302).
2   Wash in distilled water.
3   Place in Weigert's solution overnight at room temperature.
4   Wash in water.
5   Treat with 0·25 per cent potassium permanganate for 30 s.
6   Wash in water.
7   Treat with Pal's differentiator until the background is almost colourless (about 30 s), steps 5–7 being repeated until desired differentiation is reached.
8   Wash thoroughly in tap water.
9   Dehydrate, clear and mount.

Results Myelin sheath—brown-black.

Lipid stains

Sudan black B

Sudan black B staining solution

Sudan black B	1 g
triethyl phosphate	60 ml
distilled water	40 ml

The distilled water is added to the triethyl phosphate; the Sudan black B is added to this solution. Heat the mixture to 100°C for 5 min, stirring constantly. Filter hot. The solution keeps well but must be refiltered immediately before use.

Mayer's carmalum

Dissolve 2 g of carmine in 100 ml of 5 per cent ammonium alum solution by boiling for 1 h. Make up to original volume and add a few crystals of thymol to prevent growth of moulds.

Fixative 10 per cent formol-calcium solution

Sections Frozen, 15–20 μm thickness

1   Wash sections well in distilled water.
2   Rinse in 60 per cent triethyl phosphate.

3   Stain in Sudan black B solution for 10 min.
4   Rinse in 60 per cent triethyl phosphate for 30 s.
5   Wash in distilled water.
6   Stain in Mayer's carmalum for 3 min.
7   Wash in distilled water.
8   Mount in glycerine jelly.

Results Lipids—black. Nuclei—red.

Oil red O

Staining solution

Oil red O	1 g
triethyl phosphate	60 ml
distilled water	40 ml

Add the distilled water to the triethyl phosphate; followed by the Oil red O.
Heat to 100°C for 5 min, stirring constantly. Filter hot. The stock solution
keeps well but must be refiltered before use.

Fixative 10 per cent formol-calcium solution

Sections Frozen, 15–20 μm

1   Wash in distilled water.
2   Rinse in 60 per cent triethyl phosphate.
3   Stain in oil red O solution for 15 min.
4   Wash in 60 per cent triethyl phosphate for 30 s.
5   Wash in distilled water.
6   Stain in haematoxylin for 1 min.
7   Wash in tap water for 5 min.

Results Neutral lipid—red. Nuclei—blue.

Metachromatic stains

Acid cresyl violet stain

Acid cresyl violet solution

cresyl violet	0·02 g
1 per cent acetic acid	100 ml

Fixative Formol-calcium solution

Sections Frozen, 15–20 μm

1   Wash in distilled water.
2   Stain in acid cresyl violet solution at 60°C for 10 min.
3   Cool to room temperature.
4   Wash in distilled water.
5   Mount in glycerine jelly.

Results Metachromatic material—red. Other tissue—purple.

Toluidine blue stain

1   Section to distilled water.
2   Stain in 0·25 per cent toluidine blue in veronal buffer pH 4·5 for 10 s.
3   Rinse in distilled water.
4   Mount in glycerine jelly.

Results Metachromatic material—red. Other tissue—blue.

Amyloid stains

Congo red stain

Stock solution

80 per cent alcohol saturated with Congo red and sodium chloride.

Working solution

Stock solution   50 ml
1 per cent aqueous sodium hydroxide   0·5 ml

Filter and use within 15 min.

Fixative Preferably in alcoholic fixative but adequate results are obtained after formalin or Susa

Sections Paraffin embedding or frozen. 5–20 μm thickness
1   Sections to water.
2   Stain nuclei with Mayer's haemalum for 5 min.
3   Wash well in water.
4   Treat with alkaline solution for 20 min.
5   Stain in Congo red solution for 20 min.
6   Dehydrate with three brief rinses in absolute alcohol.
7   Clear and mount.

Results Nuclei—blue. Amyloid—deep pink to red.

Thioflavine T stain

Fixative and *Sections* as above

1 Sections to water.
2 Stain in Mayer's haemalum for 2 min to quench nuclear fluorescence.
3 Wash in water for a few minutes.
4 Stain in 1 per cent aqueous thioflavine T for 3 min.
5 Rinse in water.
6 Differentiate in 1 per cent acetic acid for 20 min.
7 Wash in water.
8 Mount in Apathy's medium.

Results Amyloid—bright yellow fluorescence. Mast cell granules—yellow.

PREPARATION OF NERVES FOR TEASING FOR LIGHT MICROSCOPY

1 Fix in 10 per cent formalin for 24 h.
2 Wash in distilled water.
3 Place in 1 per cent osmic acid solution for 24 h.
4 Wash in distilled water.
5 Place successively in 15, 45 and 60 per cent glycerol in water over a period of 2 days.
6 Leave in 66 per cent glycerol for teasing.

PREPARATION FOR ELECTRON MICROSCOPY

Phosphate buffer pH 7·4

Solution A 0·2 M sodium dihydrogen phosphate

Solution B 0·2 M disodium hydrogen phosphate

To make 100 ml 0·1 M phosphate buffer pH 7·4

solution A	9·5 ml
solution B	40·5 ml
distilled water	50 ml

Check pH and correct as necessary.

3·6 per cent phosphate-buffered glutaraldehyde

glutaraldehyde (25 per cent stock solution)	14·4 ml
phosphate buffer pH 7·4	86·6 ml

2 per cent phosphate-buffered osmium tetroxide

osmium tetroxide	2 g
phosphate buffer pH 7·4	100 ml

Araldite mixture (Durcupan)

resin A/M	50 ml
hardener 964 B	50 ml
plasticizer dibutyl phthalate	2 ml
accelerator 964	1 ml

1 Place stretched nerve into 3·6 per cent glutaraldehyde in phosphate buffer pH 7·4 at 4°C for 1 h. After 1 h make several small longitudinal incisions in the nerve leaving it still stretched and then fixed for a further 1 h at 4°C.
2 Rinse in 0·1 M phosphate buffer at pH 7·4.
3 Chop the nerve into small pieces discarding 3 mm at either end of nerve.
4 Rinse three times in 0·1 M phosphate buffer at pH 7·4 10 min each.
5 Place in 2 per cent osmium tetroxide in phosphate buffer for 2 h at 4°C.
6 Rinse three times in 0·1 M phosphate buffer 10 min each.
7 Dehydrate in 50, 70, 80, 90, 95 per cent alcohol 10–15 min each.
8 Three changes of absolute alcohol 20 min each.
9 Three changes of propylene oxide 20 min each.
10 Equal parts of propylene oxide–Araldite 2 h.
11 Three changes Araldite mixture over 24 h.
12 Embed and place in 60°C oven to harden 24 h.

Preparation of nerves for teasing for electron microscopy

1 Fix 0·5–1 cm lengths of nerve in 3·6 per cent glutaraldehyde in 0·1 M phosphate buffer at pH 7·4 for 2 h.

2   Wash well in 0·1 M phosphate buffer.
3   Fix in 1 per cent osmium tetroxide in 0·1 M phosphate buffer at pH 7·4.
4   Wash well in distilled water.
5   Dehydrate in 50, 70, 80, 90, 95 per cent alcohol 15–30 min each.
6   Three changes absolute alcohol 1 h each.
7   Clear in toluene 1 h.
8   Equal parts of Araldite–toluene 1 h.
9   Three parts Araldite–1 part toluene overnight.
10 Place in fresh Araldite mixture for at least 1 h.
11 Store in freezer compartment of domestic refrigerator until the speci-
    men is required for teasing. If it is necessary to store for a long period
    it is safer to omit the accelerator.
12 A single fibre can be teased, mounted in Araldite which is allowed to
    solidify to produce a permanent preparation. The teased fibre can be
    examined and internodal lengths measured. This fibre is then blocked
    out in moulds prior to sectioning for electron microscopy.

Toluidine blue staining of Araldite sections

Staining solution 1 per cent toluidine blue in 1 per cent sodium borate solution

Sections 1–2 μm in Araldite

1   Sections are dried on to slides on a hot plate at 85°C for 1 min.
2   1 drop of 1 per cent toluidine blue is placed on section at 85°C for 1 min.
3   Rinse in distilled water.
4   *Either* Dehydrate in absolute alcohol.
    or   Dry on hot plate.
5   Clear in xylene and mount.

Vital staining of motor end-plates using methylene blue solution

1   Trim the muscle biopsy to 3–5 mm in diameter.
2   Inject with 0·015 per cent methylene blue in 0·9 per cent sodium
    chloride solution. Multiple injections using a fine needle are adminis-
    tered along the whole length of the biopsy using a minimum of 10 ml of
    the dye solution. Injections should be continued until the solution runs
    freely from the punctured surfaces.
3   Split specimen longitudinally into strips.

4   Place strips on a saline-soaked gauze in a stream of oxygen delivered at 4 l/min for a minimum of 1 h.

5   Immerse in freshly filtered saturated aqueous ammonium molybdate solution at 4°C overnight.

6   Wash in several changes of distilled water for a minimum of 30 min.

7   Hand-cut longitudinal sections as thinly as possible. Place between thin glass slides.

8   Crush first with fingers and then by means of a heavy weight for 30 min.

9   Dehydrate, clear and mount.

Index

Individual diseases affecting nerve will be found under the heading of Neuropathy.